Contents

World directory of medical schools

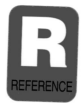

World directory of medical schools

•••

Seventh edition

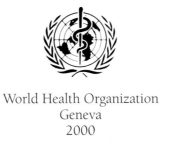

World Health Organization
Geneva
2000

WHO Library Cataloguing-in-Publication Data

World directory of medical schools.—7th ed.

  1. Schools, Medical—directories

  ISBN 92 4 150010 7   (NLM classification: W 19)

The World Health Organization welcomes requests for permission to reproduce or translate its publications, in part or in full. Applications and enquiries should be addressed to the Office of Publications, World Health Organization, Geneva, Switzerland, which will be glad to provide the latest information on any changes made to the text, plans for new editions, and reprints and translations already available.

The designations employed and the presentation of the material in this publication do not imply the expression of any opinion whatsoever on the part of the Secretariat of the World Health Organization concerning the legal status of any country, territory, city or area or of its authorities, or concerning the delimitation of its frontiers or boundaries.

The mention of specific companies or of certain manufacturers' products does not imply that they are endorsed or recommended by the World Health Organization in preference to others of a similar nature that are not mentioned. Errors and omissions excepted, the names of proprietary products are distinguished by initial capital letters.

Designed in New Zealand
Typeset in Hong Kong
Printed in Spain
98/12327—minimum graphics/Best-set/Policrom—5000

Preface

The seventh edition of the *World directory of medical schools* is the result of a wide and coordinated effort encompassing the design, field-testing and translation of questionnaires, the development of an electronic database, and editing, printing and dissemination. The resulting directory provides information on 1642 schools worldwide and is a continuation of the work carried out in previous editions.

The electronic database on which the directory is based provides additional information relevant to medical curricula, educational approaches, the assessment of students, the availability and use of facilities and equipment, staff activities, continuing education, the mutual recognition of qualifications, and the evaluation or accreditation of medical school programmes. For those concerned with and committed to improving the quality of medical education and its relevance to the health needs of society, this database will provide information on the status and trends of medical education worldwide.

While medical education must be adapted to respond to the specific needs of individuals and the populations they intend to serve in a given environment, certain capacities of a physician are universal. In a world where borders are becoming increasingly illusory, there are growing opportunities and expectations for international collaboration to enhance quality assurance in medical education through research and development.[1,2] Interest in the contribution of medical schools to respond to people's health needs and to participate in shaping the future health system through their education, research and service-delivery missions is also growing worldwide.[3–6] Benchmarks and

[1] *Towards the assessment of quality in medical education.* Geneva, World Health Organization, 1992 (unpublished document WHO/HRH/92.7; available on request from Department of Organization of Health Services Delivery, World Health Organization, 1211 Geneva 27, Switzerland).

[2] Towards a global consensus on quality medical education: serving the needs of populations and individuals. Proceedings of the 1994 World Health Organization/Educational Commission for Foreign Medical Graduates Invitational Consultation, Geneva, 3–6 October 1994. *Academic Medicine*, 1995, 70 (7, Suppl.):S1–S90.

[3] *Defining and measuring the social accountability of medical schools.* Geneva, World Health Organization, 1995 (unpublished document WHO/HRH/95.7; available on request from Department of Organization of Health Services Delivery, World Health Organization, 1211 Geneva 27, Switzerland).

[4] Improving the social responsiveness of medical schools. Proceedings of the 1998 Educational Commission for Foreign Medical Graduates/World Health Organization Invitational Conference. *Academic Medicine*, 1999, 74 (8, Suppl.):Svii–Sviii, S1–S94.

evaluation mechanisms are required to assess and promote the role of medical schools in educating future generations of doctors and in influencing the features of their future practice environment for an optimal response to the health needs of society. In particular, action is needed at the institutional, national and global level to design and promote the most appropriate approaches to allow medical schools to be the principal contributors to people's health.

Dr C. Boelen
Department of Organization of Health Services Delivery

---

[5] Reorientation of medical education and medical practice for health for all. In: *Forty-eighth World Health Assembly, Geneva, 1–12 May 1995. Volume 1. Resolutions and decisions, and list of participants*. Geneva, World Health Organization, 1995 (unpublished document WHA48/1995/REC/1):8–10.

[6] *Doctors for health. A WHO global strategy for changing medical education and medical practice for health for all*. Geneva, World Health Organization, 1996 (unpublished document WHO/HRH/96.1; available on request from Department of Organization of Health Services Delivery, World Health Organization, 1211 Geneva 27, Switzerland).

Introduction

The seventh edition of the *World directory of medical schools* lists institutions of basic medical education in 157 countries or areas. It also provides information on the conditions for obtaining the licence to practise medicine in 14 countries or areas that do not have medical schools. The information presented in general reflects the situation during the academic year 1995–96, and is based primarily on answers to two questionnaires designed by the World Health Organization and sent: (i) to ministerial authorities requesting information of a general nature on medical education and conditions for practice in the country; and (ii) to all medical schools of whose existence the World Health Organization has been informed by the national government, either by confirming existing lists or by providing specific information. The questionnaires were field-tested in several parts of the world, but it sometimes proved difficult to accommodate data provided from ministerial authorities or medical schools within the suggested layout.

At the time of going to press, and in spite of follow-up, a number of governments and medical schools had not replied to the questionnaires. In these cases only those schools that were previously recognized by the government concerned have been listed. It is therefore not possible to guarantee in all cases the complete accuracy of the information presented, particularly in regard to up-to-date addresses. In addition, compatible information was not always provided by the authorities of the countries cited, particularly concerning agreements between countries. Schools that have been established but where instruction has not yet started have not been listed.

The World Health Organization would appreciate notification of any errors and omissions. These should be addressed to the Department of Organization of Health Services Delivery, World Health Organization, 1211 Geneva 27, Switzerland.

The population figures were made available to WHO by the United Nations Population Division following their 1996 revision of *World population prospects*. The number of physicians per 100 000 population (1993) was taken from *The world health report 1997* (WHO, Geneva, 1997). The medical schools in each country are listed alphabetically by city, except in the case of Brazil, Canada, China, Colombia, India, Mexico and the USA, where they are listed under the state or province; Japan, where they are listed by prefecture; and the United Kingdom, which is subdivided into England, Northern

Ireland, Scotland and Wales. The data were either submitted by the governments or obtained directly from the institutions. Where no information was available, this is indicated by a dash (—). As the information included in the Directory must of necessity be restricted in scope, the name and address, where available, of the national registration body or licensing authority from which further information can be obtained has been given for each country or area.

Scope of the directory

The following information is provided for most of the medical schools listed: the name and address, the year instruction started, the language of instruction, the length of the degree course, and whether the applicant is required to pass an entrance examination and foreign students are eligible for admission.

Name and address

The names and addresses of the medical schools are in the language of the country concerned, unless the language does not use the Roman alphabet. In that case an English or French version is given, depending on which of the two languages was used to answer the questionnaires. Capital letters have been used for all names and addresses; diacritical marks and accented characters have been omitted as these posed problems for the computerized database.

Year instruction started

This is the year in which medical education began at the institution; it does not necessarily correspond to the date when the institution was founded.

Language

This refers to the language(s) used in teaching. Where more than one language is used, they are listed in decreasing order of importance.

Duration of basic medical degree course, including practical training

The degree course is often followed by an internship of 1 or 2 years.

Database

A database is being constructed, based on the replies to the two question-naires. It covers the following areas:

Ministerial questionnaire

● Current number of medical schools within the country.
● Duration of the programme of medical education.
● Title of degree awarded.
● Medical registration/licence to practise.
● Mutual recognition of qualifications.
● Accreditation/recognition or equivalent system.

Medical school questionnaire

● General information.
● Curriculum.
● Assessment of students.
● Facilities/equipment.
● Staff activities.
● Continuing education.
● Interaction with other entities.
● Evaluation and accreditation.

Copies of the two questionnaires are available on request from the Department of Organization of Health Services Delivery, World Health Organization, 1211 Geneva 27, Switzerland.

Acknowledgements

The World Health Organization gratefully acknowledges the contribution of the Educational Commission for Foreign Medical Graduates (ECFMG) and in particular its late former President, Dr M. Wilson, ECFMG, Washington, DC, USA, and Professor A. Rothman, University of Toronto, Toronto, Canada, who assisted in designing the questionnaires on which the directory is based. The contribution of the deans and faculties from the medical schools that participated in the field-testing of the questionnaires is also gratefully acknowledged.

Description of medical education programmes
and lists of training institutions,
by country or area

AFGHANISTAN

Total population in 1995: **20 833 000**
Number of physicians per 100 000 population (1993): —
Number of medical schools: **4**
Duration of basic medical degree course, including practical training: **7 years**
Title of degree awarded: **Doctor of Medicine (MD)**
Medical registration/licence to practise: **Registration is obligatory with the Ministry of Public Health, Kabul. The licence to practise medicine is granted by the Department of Licentiate and Medical Registration, Ministry of Public Health, PO Box 33, Kabul, on successful completion of the 7-year course and receipt of an MD degree. Graduates of foreign medical schools must have their degree validated by an internationally recognized agency. Foreigners require official permission to practise.**
Work in government service after graduation: **Obligatory**
Agreements with other countries: **Agreements exist with France, Germany, the Islamic Republic of Iran, the Russian Federation, Tajikistan and Uzbekistan.**

HERAT MEDICAL SCHOOL
HERAT

FACULTY OF MEDICINE
STATE MEDICAL INSTITUTE OF NANGARHAR
JALALABAD
Year instruction started: **1964**

FACULTY OF MEDICINE
AVICENNA STATE MEDICAL INSTITUTE OF KABUL
KABUL
Year instruction started: **1932**

IBNE-SINA BALKH MEDICAL SCHOOL
MAZAR I SHARIF

ALBANIA

Total population in 1995: **3 401 000**
Number of physicians per 100 000 population (1993): **141**
Number of medical schools: **1**
Duration of basic medical degree course, including practical training: **6 years (a further year of supervised clinical practice is required before the degree is awarded)**
Title of degree awarded: ***Mjek i Përgjithshëm* (General Physician)**

Medical registration/licence to practise: **Registration is obligatory with the Order of Albanian Physicians. The licence to practise medicine is granted by the Ministry of Health, Tirana, on receipt of a copy of the final diploma and the marks achieved during the course.**
Work in government service after graduation: **Not obligatory**
Agreements with other countries: **None**

FAKULTETI I MJEKESISE
UNIVERSITETI I TIRANES
TIRANA
Year instruction started: **1952**

ALGERIA

Total population in 1995: **28 784 000**
Number of physicians per 100 000 population (1993): **83**
Number of medical schools: **11**
Duration of basic medical degree course, including practical training: **6 or 7 years**
Title of degree awarded: *Docteur en Médecine* (Doctor of Medicine)
Medical registration/licence to practise: **The licence to practise medicine is granted by the *Ministère de la Santé et de la Population, 128 chemin Mohamed Gacem, El-Madania, Alger.***
Work in government service after graduation: —
Agreements with other countries: —

INSTITUT NATIONAL D'ENSEIGNEMENT SUPERIEUR EN SCIENCES
      MEDICALES
UNIVERSITE D'ALGER
AVENUE AHMED GHERMOUL
BP 30
ALGER

INSTITUT NATIONAL D'ENSEIGNEMENT SUPERIEUR EN SCIENCES
      MEDICALES
ANNABA

INSTITUT DE SCIENCES MEDICALES[1]
UNIVERSITE DE BATNA
CHAHID BOUKHLOUF MOHAMMED EL-HADI
BATNA 05000

---

[1] Degree granted by the Institut national d'Enseignement supérieur en Sciences médicales, Constantine.

Tel.: +213 (4) 850 392/854 962
Fax: +213 (4) 850 392
Telex: 82805 iessm dz
Year instruction started: **1977**
Language of instruction: **French**
Duration of basic medical degree course, including practical training: **7 years**
Entrance examination: **No**
Foreign students eligible: **Yes**

INSTITUT DE SCIENCES MEDICALES[1]
UNIVERSITE DE BLIDA
ROUTE DE SOUMAA
BP 270
BLIDA 09000
Tel.: +213 (3) 415 853
Fax: +213 (3) 417 813/417 726
Year instruction started: **1982**
Language of instruction: **French**
Duration of basic medical degree course, including practical training: **7 years**
Entrance examination: **No**
Foreign students eligible: **Yes**

INSTITUT NATIONAL D'ENSEIGNEMENT SUPERIEUR EN SCIENCES
    MEDICALES
CONSTANTINE

INSTITUT NATIONAL D'ENSEIGNEMENT SUPERIEUR EN SCIENCES
    MEDICALES
MOSTAGANEM

INSTITUT NATIONAL D'ENSEIGNEMENT SUPERIEUR EN SCIENCES
    MEDICALES
CHEMIN VICINAL, ROUTE ES-SENIA
ELMENAOUER 1510
ORAN
Tel.: +213 (6) 340 602
Fax: +213 (6) 340 604
Year instruction started: **1958**
Language of instruction: **French**
Duration of basic medical degree course, including practical training: **7 years**
Entrance examination: **No**
Foreign students eligible: **Yes**

---

[1] Degree granted by the Institut national d'Enseignement supérieur en Sciences médicales, Algiers.

INSTITUT DE SCIENCES MEDICALES[1]
UNIVERSITE DE SETIF
SETIF

INSTITUT DE SCIENCES MEDICALES[2]
UNIVERSITE DE SIDI-BEL-ABBES
SIDI-BEL-ABBES

INSTITUT DE SCIENCES MEDICALES[3]
UNIVERSITE DE TIZI-OUZOU
ROUTE DE HASNAOUA
TIZI-OUZOU 15000
Tel.: +213 (3) 217 381
Fax: +213 (3) 211 960
Telex: 76970 cbmsm dz
Year instruction started: **1981**
Language of instruction: **French**
Duration of basic medical degree course, including practical training: **7 years**
Entrance examination: **No**
Foreign students eligible: **Yes**

INSTITUT DE SCIENCES MEDICALES[2]
UNIVERSITE DE TLEMCEN
TLEMCEN

ANGOLA

Total population in 1995: **11 185 000**
Number of physicians per 100 000 population (1993): —
Number of medical schools: **1**
Duration of basic medical degree course, including practical training: **6 years**
Title of degree awarded: ***Doctor em Medicina*** (**Doctor of Medicine**)
Medical registration/licence to practise: —
Work in government service after graduation: —
Agreements with other countries: —

---

[1] Degree granted by the Institut national d'Enseignement supérieur en Sciences médicales, Constantine.
[2] Degree granted by the Institut national d'Enseignement supérieur en Sciences médicales, Oran.
[3] Degree granted by the Institut national d'Enseignement supérieur en Sciences médicales, Algiers.

FACULDADE DE MEDECINA
CP 116
LUANDA
Tel.: +244 (2) 383 872/383 866
Year instruction started: **1975**
Language of instruction: **Portuguese**
Duration of basic medical degree course, including practical training: **6 years**
Entrance examination: **Yes**
Foreign students eligible: **Yes**

ANTIGUA AND BARBUDA

Total population in 1995: —
Number of physicians per 100 000 population (1993): **76**
Number of medical schools: **1**
Duration of basic medical degree course, including practical training: **4 years**
Title of degree awarded: **Doctor of Medicine (MD)**
Medical registration/licence to practise: **Registration is obligatory with the Ministry of Health. The licence to practise medicine is granted by the Medical Board of Antigua and Barbuda. Applications should be approved by the Medical Officer and submitted through the Ministry of Health, St John's Street, Antigua. Graduates of foreign medical schools must have their degree validated.**
Work in government service after graduation: **Not obligatory**
Agreements with other countries: **None**

SCHOOL OF MEDICINE
UNIVERSITY OF HEALTH SCIENCES ANTIGUA
DOWNHILL CAMPUS
PICCADILLY
PO BOX 510
ST JOHN'S
Tel.: +268 (1) 460 1391
Fax: +268 (1) 460 1477
E-mail: med-prog@uhsa.edu.ag
Year instruction started: **1983**
Language of instruction: **English**
Duration of basic medical degree course, including practical training: **4 years**
Entrance examination: **No**
Foreign students eligible: **Yes**

ARGENTINA

Total population in 1995: **35 219 000**
Number of physicians per 100 000 population (1993): **268**
Number of medical schools: **14**
Duration of basic medical degree course, including practical training: **6 or 7 years**
   (a further year of practice is required before the degree is awarded)
Title of degree awarded: *Médico* **(Physician)**
Medical registration/licence to practise: **Registration is obligatory with the**
   Dirección Nacional de Fiscalización Sanitaria, Ministerio de Salud y Acción
   ***Social, Avenida 9 de Julio 1925, Piso 7, 1395 Buenos Aires*, and with the**
   secretariat of one of the provincial health authorities. Graduates of foreign
   medical schools must have their degree validated.
Work in government service after graduation: **Not obligatory**
Agreements with other countries: **Agreements exist with Bolivia, Colombia and**
   Ecuador.

ESCUELA DE MEDICINA
INSTITUTO UNIVERSITARIO DE CIENCIAS BIOMEDICAS (IUCB)
SOLIS 453
1078 BUENOS AIRES-CF
Tel.: +54 (1) 384 8457
Fax: +54 (1) 384 8457
Year instruction started: **1993**
Language of instruction: **Spanish, English**
Duration of basic medical degree course, including practical training: **6 years**
Entrance examination: **Yes**
Foreign students eligible: **Yes**

FACULTAD DE CIENCIAS MEDICAS
UNIVERSIDAD AUSTRAL
AVENIDA JUAN DE GARAY 125
1063 BUENOS AIRES-CF

FACULTAD DE MEDICINA
UNIVERSIDAD DE BUENOS AIRES
PARAGUAY 2155
1121 BUENOS AIRES-CF
Tel.: +54 (1) 961 8961
Fax: +54 (1) 961 8961
E-mail: decanato@fmed.uba.ar

Year instruction started: **1852**
Language of instruction: **Spanish**
Duration of basic medical degree course, including practical training: **6 years**
Entrance examination: **Yes**
Foreign students eligible: **Yes**

FACULTAD DE MEDICINA
UNIVERSIDAD DEL SALVADOR
TUCUMAN 1845
1050 BUENOS AIRES-CF
Tel.: +54 (1) 811 8519/813 2935
Fax: +54 (1) 812 9846
Year instruction started: **1956**
Language of instruction: **Spanish**
Duration of basic medical degree course, including practical training: **6 years**
Entrance examination: **Yes**
Foreign students eligible: **Yes**

FACULTAD DE CIENCIAS BIOLOGICAS
UNIVERSIDAD HEBREA ARGENTINA BAR ILAN
CARRERA DE MEDICINA
TENIENTE GENERAL JUAN D. PERON 2933
1198 BUENOS AIRES-CF
Year instruction started: **1956**

FACULTAD DE MEDICINA
UNIVERSIDAD MAIMONIDES
FELIPE VALLESE 326
1405 BUENOS AIRES-CF
Tel.: +54 (1) 982 8488/982 3425
Fax: +54 (1) 982 7840
Year instruction started: **1991**
Language of instruction: **Spanish**
Duration of basic medical degree course, including practical training: **6 years**
Entrance examination: **Yes**
Foreign students eligible: **Yes**

FACULTAD DE MEDICINA
UNIVERSIDAD CATOLICA DE CORDOBA
JACINTO RIOS 571
5000 CORDOBA-CBA
Year instruction started: **1956**

FACULTAD DE CIENCIAS MEDICAS
UNIVERSIDAD NACIONAL DE CORDOBA
CIUDAD UNIVERSITARIA PABELLON PERU
APDO 32
5000 CORDOBA-CBA
Tel.: +54 (51) 334 040
Fax: +54 (51) 334 036/334 041
Year instruction started: **1877**
Language of instruction: **Spanish**
Duration of basic medical degree course, including practical training: **6 years**
Entrance examination: **No**
Foreign students eligible: **Yes**

FACULTAD DE MEDICINA
UNIVERSIDAD NACIONAL DEL NORDESTE
MORENO 1240
CASILLA DE CORREO 368
3400 CORRIENTES-CTS
Tel.: +54 (783) 360 85/214 74
Fax: +54 (783) 222 90
E-mail: informedi@fmunne.sld.ar
Year instruction started: **1953**
Language of instruction: **Spanish**
Duration of basic medical degree course, including practical training: **7 years**
Entrance examination: **No**
Foreign students eligible: **Yes**

FACULTAD DE CIENCIAS MEDICAS
UNIVERSIDAD NACIONAL DE LA PLATA
CALLE 60 Y 120
1900 LA PLATA-BA
Tel.: +54 (21) 258 989
Fax: +54 (21) 258 989
Year instruction started: **1934**
Language of instruction: **Spanish**
Duration of basic medical degree course, including practical training: **7 years**
Entrance examination: **No**
Foreign students eligible: **Yes**

FACULTAD DE CIENCIAS DE LA SALUD
UNIVERSIDAD ADVENTISTA DEL PLATA
25 DE MAYO 99
3101 LIBERTADOR S. MARTIN-ER
Year instruction started: **1956**

FACULTAD DE CIENCIAS MEDICAS
UNIVERSIDAD NACIONAL DE CUYO
AVENIDA LIBERTADOR 40 PARQUE GENERAL SAN MARTIN
CASILLA DE CORREO 33
5500 MENDOZA-MZA
Tel.: +54 (61) 494 046
Fax: +54 (61) 494 047
E-mail: post.master@fmed2.uncu.edu.ar
Year instruction started: **1951**
Language of instruction: **Spanish**
Duration of basic medical degree course, including practical training: **6 years**
Entrance examination: **Yes**
Foreign students eligible: **Yes**

FACULTAD DE MEDICINA
UNIVERSIDAD NACIONAL DE ROSARIO
SANTA FE 3100
2000 ROSARIO-SF
Tel.: +54 (41) 250 693/250 121
Fax: +54 (41) 251 533
Year instruction started: **1920**
Language of instruction: **Spanish**
Duration of basic medical degree course, including practical training: **6 years**
Entrance examination: **No**
Foreign students eligible: **Yes**

FACULTAD DE MEDICINA
UNIVERSIDAD NACIONAL DE TUCUMAN
LAMADRID 875
CASILLA DE CORREO 159
4000 SAN MIGUEL DE TUCUMAN-T
Year instruction started: **1950**
Language of instruction: **Spanish**
Entrance examination: **No**
Foreign students eligible: **Yes**

ARMENIA

Total population in 1995: **3 638 000**
Number of physicians per 100 000 population (1993): **312**
Number of medical schools: **1**
Duration of basic medical degree course, including practical training: **6 years (a further year of supervised clinical practice is required before the degree is awarded)**

Title of degree awarded: **Doctor of Medicine (MD)**
Medical registration/licence to practise: **Registration is obligatory with the Yerevan State Medical University, 2 Koryune Street, 375025 Yerevan. The licence to practise medicine is granted by the Ministry of Health following a 1-year internship.**
Work in government service after graduation: **Obligatory**
Agreements with other countries: **Agreements exist with the Catholic University of Louvain, Belgium, the Mediterranean University, Marseilles, France and the Aristotle University, Thessalonika, Greece (Tempus Compact Pre-Pec agreement) and with McGill University, Montreal, Canada, and Aleppo University, Syrian Arab Republic.**

YEREVAN STATE MEDICAL UNIVERSITY
2 KORYUNE STREET
YEREVAN 375025
Tel.: +374 (2) 560 594/581 812
Fax: +374 (2) 565 481/151 812
Year instruction started: **1922**
Language of instruction: **Armenian, Russian**
Duration of basic medical degree course, including practical training: **6 years**
Entrance examination: **Yes**
Foreign students eligible: **Yes**

AUSTRALIA

Total population in 1995: **18 957 000**
Number of physicians per 100 000 population (1993): **—**
Number of medical schools: **10**
Duration of basic medical degree course, including practical training: **4–6 years (a further year of clinical practice in a teaching hospital is required before the degree is awarded)**
Title of degree awarded: **Bachelor of Medicine and Bachelor of Surgery (MB, BS)**
Medical registration/licence to practise: **Registration is obligatory with the medical registration authority in any of the eight States and Territories comprising the Federation of Australia. The licence to practise medicine is granted to holders of an MB/BS degree from a medical school accredited by the Australian Medical Council (AMC) following a satisfactory 1-year internship in an approved teaching hospital. A certificate of good standing is required. Graduates who have qualified abroad are required to pass a two-part AMC examination.**
Work in government service after graduation: **Not obligatory**
Agreements with other countries: **Graduates of New Zealand medical schools accredited by the AMC are entitled to unconditional registration.**

SCHOOL OF MEDICINE
THE FLINDERS UNIVERSITY OF SOUTH AUSTRALIA
FLINDERS DRIVE
PO BOX 2100
ADELAIDE 5001
SA
Tel.: +61 (8) 820 441 60
Fax: +61 (8) 820 458 45
E-mail: deansom@flinders.edu.au
Year instruction started: **1975**
Language of instruction: **English**
Duration of basic medical degree course, including practical training: **4 years**
Entrance examination: **Yes**
Foreign students eligible: **Yes**

FACULTY OF MEDICINE
UNIVERSITY OF ADELAIDE
FROME ROAD
ADELAIDE 5005
SA
Tel.: +61 (8) 830 352 52
Fax: +61 (8) 823 237 41
E-mail: international.programs@registry.adelaide.edu.au
Year instruction started: **1885**
Language of instruction: **English**
Duration of basic medical degree course, including practical training: **6 years**
Entrance examination: **Yes**
Foreign students eligible: **Yes**

FACULTY OF MEDICINE
MONASH UNIVERSITY
WELLINGTON ROAD
CLAYTON 3168
VIC
Tel.: +61 (3) 990 543 01
Fax: +61 (3) 990 543 02
Year instruction started: **1961**
Language of instruction: **English**
Duration of basic medical degree course, including practical training: **6 years**
Entrance examination: **No**
Foreign students eligible: **Yes**

THE UNIVERSITY OF QUEENSLAND MEDICAL SCHOOL
HERSTON ROAD
HERSTON 4006
QLD
Tel.: +61 (7) 336 552 78
Fax: +61 (7) 336 554 33
E-mail: s.leuthner@mailbox.uq.oz.au
Year instruction started: **1936**
Language of instruction: **English**
Duration of basic medical degree course, including practical training: **4 years**
Entrance examination: **Yes**
Foreign students eligible: **Yes**

FACULTY OF MEDICINE
UNIVERSITY OF TASMANIA
43 COLLINS STREET
HOBART 7000
TAS
Year instruction started: **1965**

FACULTY OF MEDICINE AND HEALTH SCIENCES
UNIVERSITY OF NEWCASTLE
UNIVERSITY DRIVE
CALLAGHAN
NEWCASTLE 2308
NSW
Tel.: +61 (49) 215 676
Fax: +61 (49) 215 669
E-mail: ue.jmp@medicine.newcastle.edu.au
Year instruction started: **1978**
Language of instruction: **English**
Duration of basic medical degree course, including practical training: **5 years**
Entrance examination: **Yes**
Foreign students eligible: **Yes**

FACULTY OF MEDICINE
UNIVERSITY OF MELBOURNE
GRATTAN STREET
PARKVILLE 3050
VIC
Tel.: +61 (3) 934 458 90
Fax: +61 (3) 934 770 84

Year instruction started: **1862**
Language of instruction: **English**
Duration of basic medical degree course, including practical training: **6 years**
Entrance examination: **No**
Foreign students eligible: **Yes**

FACULTY OF MEDICINE AND DENTISTRY
UNIVERSITY OF WESTERN AUSTRALIA
MOUNTS BAY ROAD, NEDLANDS
PERTH 6907
WA
Tel.: +61 (8) 934 623 16
Fax: +61 (8) 934 623 69
E-mail: medinfo@cyllene.uwa.edu.au
Year instruction started: **1957**
Language of instruction: **English**
Duration of basic medical degree course, including practical training: **6 years**
Entrance examination: **Yes**
Foreign students eligible: **Yes**

FACULTY OF MEDICINE
UNIVERSITY OF NEW SOUTH WALES
ANZAC PARADE
SYDNEY 2052
NSW
Tel.: +61 (2) 938 524 54
Fax: +61 (2) 938 512 89
E-mail: enquiries@med.unsw.edu.au
Year instruction started: **1961**
Language of instruction: **English**
Duration of basic medical degree course, including practical training: **6 years**
Entrance examination: **No**
Foreign students eligible: **Yes**

FACULTY OF MEDICINE
UNIVERSITY OF SYDNEY
SYDNEY 2006
NSW
Tel.: +61 (2) 935 131 32
Fax: +61 (2) 935 131 96
Year instruction started: **1883**
Language of instruction: **English**
Duration of basic medical degree course, including practical training: **4 years**
Entrance examination: **Yes**
Foreign students eligible: **Yes**

AUSTRIA

Total population in 1995: **8 106 000**
Number of physicians per 100 000 population (1993): **327**
Number of medical schools: **3**
Duration of basic medical degree course, including practical training: **6–8 years (including 16 weeks' compulsory internship)**
Title of degree awarded: ***Medicinae Universalis Doctor* (*Dr med.univ.*, Doctor of Medicine)**
Medical registration/licence to practise: **Registration is obligatory with the *Oesterreichische Aerztekammer* (Austrian General Medical Council), *Weihburggasse 10–12, 1010 Wien.* The licence to practise medicine is granted to medical graduates with Austrian or European Union citizenship who have postgraduate training as a general practitioner or as a specialist. Graduates of foreign medical schools must also have their degree validated.**
Work in government service after graduation: **Not obligatory**
Agreements with other countries: **An agreement exists with other countries of the European Union (Directive 93/16/EEC governing the employment of doctors; the Italian *Laurea in Medicina* has automatic equal status with *Dr med.univ.*).**

MEDIZINISCHE FAKULTAET
KARL FRANZENS UNIVERSITAET GRAZ
UNIVERSITAETSPLATZ 3
A-8010 GRAZ
Tel.: +43 (316) 380 4100
Fax: +43 (316) 381 328
E-mail: meddekan@kfunigraz.ac.at
Year instruction started: **1863**
Language of instruction: **German**
Duration of basic medical degree course, including practical training: **6 years**
Entrance examination: **No**
Foreign students eligible: **Yes**

MEDIZINISCHE FAKULTAET
LEOPOLD-FRANZEN-UNIVERSITAET INNSBRUCK
CHRISTOPH PROBST PLATZ
A-6020 INNSBRUCK
Tel.: +43 (512) 507 3001
Fax: +43 (512) 507 2995

Year instruction started: **1670**
Language of instruction: **German**
Duration of basic medical degree course, including practical training: **6–8 years**
Entrance examination: **No**
Foreign students eligible: **No**

MEDIZINISCHE FAKULTAET
UNIVERSITAET WIEN
DR KARL LUEGER RING 1-3
A-1010 WIEN
Year instruction started: **1365**
Language of instruction: **German**
Entrance examination: **No**
Foreign students eligible: **Yes**

AZERBAIJAN

Total population in 1995: **7 594 000**
Number of physicians per 100 000 population (1993): **390**
Number of medical schools: **1**
Duration of basic medical degree course, including practical training: —
Title of degree awarded: —
Medical registration/licence to practise: —
Work in government service after graduation: —
Agreements with other countries: —

AZERBAIJAN STATE MEDICAL INSTITUTE N. NARIMANOV
ULICA BAKIHANOVA 23
BAKU 370008
Year instruction started: **1919**

BAHAMAS

Total population in 1995: **284 000**
Number of physicians per 100 000 population (1993): **141**
Number of medical schools: **None**
Medical registration/licence to practise: **Physicians wishing to practise must register with the Bahamas Medical Council, PO Box N-9802, Nassau. The licence to practise medicine is granted annually to graduates of a**

recognized medical school who have completed an approved internship. Foreigners must hold a work permit issued by the Department of Immigration.

Work in government service after graduation: **Not obligatory**

Agreements with other countries: **No formal agreements exist, but informal agreements exist with the Caribbean Region Medical Boards and the University of the West Indies.**

BAHRAIN

Total population in 1995: **570 000**

Number of physicians per 100 000 population (1993): **11**

Number of medical schools: **1**

Duration of basic medical degree course, including practical training: **6 years (a further year of supervised clinical practice is required before the degree is awarded)**

Title of degree awarded: **Doctor of Medicine (MD)**

Medical registration/licence to practise: **Medical registration and licensure are obligatory with the Licensure Office, Ministry of Health, PO Box 12, Manama, to graduates of a recognized medical school who have successfully completed an internship year and passed the licensure examination.**

Work in government service after graduation: **Not obligatory**

Agreements with other countries: **Agreements exist with all Gulf States and with the Arab Board of Medical Specialities.**

COLLEGE OF MEDICINE AND MEDICAL SCIENCES
ARABIAN GULF UNIVERSITY
PO BOX 22979
MANAMA
Tel.: +973 279 411/277 209
Fax: +973 270 370
Telex: 9494 agucm bn
Year instruction started: **1985**
Language of instruction: **English**
Duration of basic medical degree course, including practical training: **6 years**
Entrance examination: **Yes**
Foreign students eligible: **Yes**

BANGLADESH

Total population in 1995: **120 073 000**

Number of physicians per 100 000 population (1993): **18**

Number of medical schools: **11**

Duration of basic medical degree course, including practical training: **—**

Title of degree awarded: —
Medical registration/licence to practise: —
Work in government service after graduation: —
Agreements with other countries: —

SHER-E-BANGLA MEDICAL COLLEGE
BARISAL 8200
Tel.: +880 (43) 152 151
Year instruction started: **1968**
Language of instruction: **English**
Duration of basic medical degree course, including practical training: **5 years**
Entrance examination: **Yes**
Foreign students eligible: **Yes**

CHITTAGONG MEDICAL COLLEGE
K.B. FAZLUL KADER ROAD
CHITTAGONG 4203
Tel.: +880 (31) 226 762/212 157/618 894
Year instruction started: **1957**
Language of instruction: **English**
Duration of basic medical degree course, including practical training: **5 years**
Entrance examination: **Yes**
Foreign students eligible: **Yes**

INSTITUTE OF APPLIED HEALTH SCIENCES
UNIVERSITY OF SCIENCE AND TECHNOLOGY, CHITTAGONG
JANASHEBA COMPLEX, FOY'S LANE
PO BOX 1079
CHITTAGONG 1079
Tel.: +880 (31) 624 023/227 678/(2) 864 959
Fax: +880 (2) 868 300
Year instruction started: **1989**
Language of instruction: **English**
Duration of basic medical degree course, including practical training: **5 years**
Entrance examination: **Yes**

BANGLADESH MEDICAL COLLEGE (BMSRI)
DHAKA UNIVERSITY
HOUSE NO. 35
ROAD NO. 14/A
DHANMONDI RESIDENTIAL AREA
DHAKA 1209
Tel.: +880 (2) 816 699/815 843/318 202
Fax: +880 (2) 912 5655

E-mail: bmch@bangla.net
Year instruction started: **1984**
Language of instruction: **English**
Duration of basic medical degree course, including practical training: **5 years**
Entrance examination: **Yes**
Foreign students eligible: **Yes**

DHAKA MEDICAL COLLEGE
DHAKA 2
Year instruction started: **1946**

SIR SALIMULLAH MEDICAL COLLEGE
MITFORD
DHAKA
Year instruction started: **1972**

JAHURUL ISLAM MEDICAL COLLEGE AND HOSPITAL
UNIVERSITY OF DHAKA
BHAGALPUR
BAJITPUR
KISHOREGANJ
Year instruction started: **1992**

MYMENSINGH MEDICAL COLLEGE
MYMENSINGH
Year instruction started: **1962**

RAJSHAHI MEDICAL COLLEGE
RAJSHAHI
Year instruction started: **1958**

RANGPUR MEDICAL COLLEGE
RANGPUR 5400
Tel.: +880 (10) 521 2288
Year instruction started: **1970**
Language of instruction: **English**
Duration of basic medical degree course, including practical training: **5 years**
Entrance examination: **Yes**
Foreign students eligible: **Yes**

SYLHET MAG OSMANI MEDICAL COLLEGE
SYLHET 3100
Tel.: +880 (821) 714 368
Year instruction started: **1962**

Language of instruction: **English**
Duration of basic medical degree course, including practical training: **6 years**
Entrance examination: **Yes**
Foreign students eligible: **Yes**

BARBADOS

Total population in 1995: **261 000**
Number of physicians per 100 000 population (1993): **113**
Number of medical schools: **1**
Duration of basic medical degree course, including practical training: **5 years**
Title of degree awarded: **Bachelor of Medicine and Surgery (MB, BS)**
Medical registration/licence to practise: **Registration is obligatory with the Medical Council, Ministry of Health, Bridgetown, Barbados and is granted to graduates who have completed an 18-month internship. Graduates of foreign medical schools must complete a 15-month internship in specific disciplines.**
Work in government service after graduation: **Obligatory**
Agreements with other countries: **None**

SCHOOL OF CLINICAL MEDICINE AND RESEARCH
UNIVERSITY OF THE WEST INDIES
QUEEN ELIZABETH HOSPITAL
MARTINDALE'S ROAD
BRIDGETOWN
Tel.: +1246 429 5112/436 4650
Fax: +1246 429 6738
Year instruction started: **1967**
Language of instruction: **English**
Duration of basic medical degree course, including practical training: **5 years**
Entrance examination: **No**
Foreign students eligible: **Yes**

BELARUS

Total population in 1995: **10 348 000**
Number of physicians per 100 000 population (1993): **379**
Number of medical schools: **4**
Duration of basic medical degree course, including practical training: **5 or 6 years (a further 1 or 2 years of supervised clinical practice is required before the degree is awarded)**
Title of degree awarded: *Kvalifikacija* **(Physician)**
Medical registration/licence to practise: **Registration is obligatory with the**

Executive Committees on Health of the 7 oblasts following an examination on successful completion of a 1- or 2-year internship in government service. Graduates who have qualified abroad must have their degree certified by the Republic's Examination Board.

Work in government service after graduation: **Obligatory (1 or 2 years)**

Agreements with other countries: **Recognition of degrees received in countries of the Commonwealth of Independent States.**

GOMEL STATE MEDICAL INSTITUTE
LANGE STREET 5
GOMEL 246000
Tel.: +375 (232) 534 121/532 062
Fax: +375 (232) 539 831
E-mail: librex@intsect.gomel.by
Year instruction started: **1991**
Language of instruction: **Russian**
Duration of basic medical degree course, including practical training: **6 years**
Entrance examination: **Yes**

GRODNO MEDICAL INSTITUTE
ULICA GORKOGO 80
GRODNO 230015
Tel.: +375 (152) 335 561
Fax: +375 (152) 335 341
E-mail: indek@ggmi.belpak.grodno.by
Year instruction started: **1958**
Language of instruction: **Russian**
Duration of basic medical degree course, including practical training: **6 years**
Entrance examination: **Yes**
Foreign students eligible: **Yes**

MINSK MEDICAL INSTITUTE
PROSPEKT DZERZINSKOGO 83
MINSK 220798
Tel.: +375 (17) 271 9424
Fax: +375 (17) 272 6197
Year instruction started: **1921**
Language of instruction: **Belorussian, Russian**
Duration of basic medical degree course, including practical training: **6 years**
Entrance examination: **Yes**
Foreign students eligible: **Yes**

VITEBSK MEDICAL INSTITUTE
PROSPEKT FRUNZE 27
VITEBSK 210023
Year instruction started: **1934**

BELGIUM

Total population in 1995: **10 159 000**
Number of physicians per 100 000 population (1993): **365**
Number of medical schools: **11**
Duration of basic medical degree course, including practical training: **7 years**
Title of degree awarded: *Docteur en Médecine, Chirurgie et Accouchement*
  (**Doctor of Medicine, Surgery and Midwifery**) in the French-speaking
  community; *Aerts* (**Physician**) in the Flemish community
Medical registration/licence to practise: **Registration is obligatory with the
  provincial councils of the** *Ordre des Médecins*. **The provincial medical
  boards grant the licence to practise medicine after having examined the
  validity of the graduate's diploma. Every year each board issues a list of
  physicians authorized to practise in the province. Foreigners and holders
  of foreign medical qualifications must receive the authorization of the
  provincial authorities.**
Work in government service after graduation: **Not obligatory**
Agreements with other countries: **Agreements exist with other countries of the
  European Union (Directive 93/16/EEC governing the employment of
  doctors), as well as with Iceland, Liechtenstein, Norway and South Africa.**

FACULTEIT VOOR GENEESKUNDE[1]
UNIVERSITAIR CENTRUM VAN ANTWERPEN
GROENENBORGERLAAN 171
B-2020 ANTWERPEN
Tel.: +32 (3) 218 0305
Fax: +32 (3) 218 0304
E-mail: sdelaet@maze.ruca.ua.ac.be
Year instruction started: **1965**
Language of instruction: **Dutch**
Duration of basic medical degree course, including practical training: **7 years**
Entrance examination: **Yes**
Foreign students eligible: **Yes**

---

[1] Students study for the first part of their degree course (years 1–3) at the Universitair Centrum van
  Antwerpen and for the second part at the Universitair Instelling Antwerpen.

FACULTEIT VOOR GENEEESKUNDE[1]
UNIVERSITAIR INSTELLING ANTWERPEN
UNIVERSITEITSPLEIN 1
B-2610 ANTWERPEN
Tel.: +32 (3) 820 2540
Fax: +32 (3) 820 2501
E-mail: vliempt@uia.ua.ac.be
Year instruction started: **1972**
Language of instruction: **Dutch**
Duration of basic medical degree course, including practical training: **7 years**
Entrance examination: **Yes**
Foreign students eligible: **Yes**

FACULTE DE MEDECINE
UNIVERSITE CATHOLIQUE DE LOUVAIN
AVENUE EMMANUEL MOUNIER 50
UCL 5020
B-1200 BRUXELLES
Tel.: +32 (2) 764 5020/764 5028
Fax: +32 (2) 764 5035
Year instruction started: **1426**
Language of instruction: **French**
Duration of basic medical degree course, including practical training: **7 years**
Entrance examination: **No**
Foreign students eligible: **Yes**

FACULTE DE MEDECINE
UNIVERSITE LIBRE DE BRUXELLES
CAMPUS ERASME, ROUTE DE LENNIK 808
CP 610
B-1070 BRUXELLES
Tel.: +32 (2) 555 6024
Fax: +32 (2) 555 6798
Year instruction started: **1848**
Language of instruction: **French**
Duration of basic medical degree course, including practical training: **7 years**
Entrance examination: **No**
Foreign students eligible: **Yes**

---

[1] Students study for the first part of their degree course (years 1–3) at the Universitair Centrum van Antwerpen and for the second part at the Universitair Instelling Antwerpen.

FACULTEIT VAN DE GENEESKUNDE EN DE FARMACIE
VRIJE UNIVERSITEIT BRUSSEL
LAARBEEKLAAN 103
B-1090 BRUSSEL
Year instruction started: **1961**

FACULTEIT VOOR GENEESKUNDE
LIMBURGS UNIVERSITAIR CENTRUM
UNIVERSITAIR CAMPUS
B-3590 DIEPENBEEK
Tel.: +32 (11) 268 111
Fax: +32 (11) 268 199
Year instruction started: **1973**
Language of instruction: **Dutch**
Duration of basic medical degree course, including practical training: **7 years**
Entrance examination: **Yes**
Foreign students eligible: **Yes**

FACULTEIT DER GENEESKUNDE
RIJKSUNIVERSITEIT GENT
DE PINTELAAN 185
B-9000 GENT
Tel.: +32 (9) 240 4193
Fax: +32 (9) 240 4990
E-mail: jan.pollet@rug.ac.be
Year instruction started: **1817**
Language of instruction: **Dutch**
Duration of basic medical degree course, including practical training: **7 years**
Entrance examination: **Yes**
Foreign students eligible: **Yes**

FACULTEIT DER GENEESKUNDE
KATHOLIEKE UNIVERSITEIT LEUVEN
MINDERBROEDERSSTRAAT 17
B-3000 LEUVEN
Tel.: +32 (16) 337 462
Fax: +32 (16) 337 487
Year instruction started: **1425**
Language of instruction: **Dutch**
Duration of basic medical degree course, including practical training: **7 years**
Entrance examination: **Yes**
Foreign students eligible: **Yes**

FACULTE DE MEDECINE
UNIVERSITE DE L'ETAT A LIEGE
PLACE DU 20 AOUT 7
B-4000 LIEGE
Year instruction started: **1817**

FACULTE DE MEDECINE ET DE PHARMACIE
UNIVERSITE DE MONS HAINAUT
AVENUE DU CHAMP DE MARS 24
B-7000 MONS
Tel.: +32 (65) 373 501/373 502/373 503
Fax: +32 (65) 373 633
E-mail: secretariat.fmp@umh.ac.be
Year instruction started: **1975**
Language of instruction: **French**
Duration of basic medical degree course, including practical training: **7 years**
Entrance examination: **No**
Foreign students eligible: **Yes**

FACULTE DE MEDECINE
FACULTES UNIVERSITAIRES NOTRE-DAME DE LA PAIX
RUE DE BRUXELLES 61
B-5000 NAMUR
Tel.: +32 (81) 724 347
Fax: +32 (81) 724 272
Year instruction started: **1962**
Language of instruction: **French**
Duration of basic medical degree course, including practical training: **7 years**
Entrance examination: **No**
Foreign students eligible: **Yes**

BELIZE

Total population in 1995: **219 000**
Number of physicians per 100 000 population (1993): **47**
Number of medical schools: **2**
Duration of basic medical degree course, including practical training: 4 or 4.5 years
Title of degree awarded: —
Medical registration/licence to practise: —
Work in government service after graduation: —
Agreements with other countries: —

ST MATTHEWS UNIVERSITY SCHOOL OF MEDICINE
PO BOX 91
SAN PEDRO
AMBERGRIS CAYE
Tel.: +501 (2) 632 63
Fax: +501 (2) 632 60
E-mail: stmatthews@btl.net
Year instruction started: **1997**
Language of instruction: **English**
Duration of basic medical degree course, including practical training: **4 years**
Entrance examination: **No**
Foreign students eligible: **Yes**

SCHOOL OF MEDICINE
CENTRAL AMERICA HEALTH SCIENCES UNIVERSITY
PO BOX 989
BELIZE CITY
Tel.: +501 (2) 355 60
Fax: +501 (2) 356 51
E-mail: belizemed@btl.net
Year instruction started: **1996**
Language of instruction: **English**
Duration of basic medical degree course, including practical training: **4.5 years**
Entrance examination: **No**
Foreign students eligible: **Yes**

BENIN

Total population in 1995: **5 563 000**
Number of physicians per 100 000 population (1993): **6**
Number of medical schools: **1**
Duration of basic medical degree course, including practical training: **7 years**
Title of degree awarded: ***Docteur en Médecine* (Doctor of Medicine)**
Medical registration/licence to practise: —
Work in government service after graduation: —
Agreements with other countries: —

FACULTE DES SCIENCES DE LA SANTE
UNIVERSITE NATIONALE DU BENIN
BP 188
COTONOU
Year instruction started: **1970**

BOLIVIA

Total population in 1995: **7 593 000**
Number of physicians per 100 000 population (1993): **51**
Number of medical schools: **10**
Duration of basic medical degree course, including practical training: **6 years (a further year of supervised practice is required before the degree is awarded)**
Title of degree awarded: *Médico y Cirujano* (Physician and Surgeon)
Medical registration/licence to practise: **Registration is obligatory with the *Colegio Médico de Bolivia, C. Ballivian No. 1266, Casilla 2801, La Paz*. The licence to practise medicine is granted to graduates of a recognized medical school who have completed 1 year of service in a rural area. Graduates of foreign medical schools must have their degree certified by the university of origin.**
Work in government service after graduation: **Obligatory (1 year in a rural area)**
Agreements with other countries: —

FACULTAD DE MEDICINA
UNIVERSIDAD DEL VALLE
CAMPUS TIQUIPAYA
CASILLA 4742
COCHABAMBA
Tel.: +591 (42) 873 73/873 74
Fax: +591 (42) 885 50
Year instruction started: **1989**
Language of instruction: **Spanish**
Duration of basic medical degree course, including practical training: **6 years**
Foreign students eligible: **Yes**

FACULTAD DE MEDICINA
UNIVERSIDAD MAYOR DE SAN SIMON
AVENIDA ANICETO ARCE 0371
CASILLA 3119
COCHABAMBA
Tel.: +591 (42) 315 08/322 06
Fax: +591 (42) 316 90
E-mail: postmaster@umss.edu.bo
Year instruction started: **1932**
Language of instruction: **Spanish**
Duration of basic medical degree course, including practical training: **6 years**
Entrance examination: **Yes**
Foreign students eligible: **Yes**

FACULTAD DE MEDICINA
UNIVERSIDAD DEL VALLE
CASILLA 13602
LA PAZ
Tel.: +591 (2) 431 112/432 133
Fax: +591 (2) 433 261
Year instruction started: **1994**

FACULTAD DE MEDICINA
UNIVERSIDAD IBEROAMERICANA
AVENIDA 14 DE SEPTIEMBRE 5809
CASILLA 3498
LA PAZ
Tel.: +591 (2) 783 177/784 704
Fax: +591 (2) 782 431
Year instruction started: **1994**

FACULTAD DE MEDICINA
UNIVERSIDAD MAYOR DE SAN ANDRES
AVENIDA SAAVEDRA 2246
CASILLA 10367
LA PAZ
Tel.: +591 (2) 229 290/229 291
Fax: +591 (2) 229 589
Year instruction started: **1834**

FACULTAD DE MEDICINA
UNIVERSIDAD NUESTRA SENORA DE LA PAZ
CALLE PRESBITERO MEDINA 2412
CASILLA 5995
LA PAZ
Tel.: +591 (2) 418 167/418 290
Fax: +591 (2) 410 255
E-mail: unslp@caoba.entelnet.bo
Year instruction started: **1992**
Language of instruction: **Spanish, English**
Duration of basic medical degree course, including practical training: **6 years**
Entrance examination: **No**
Foreign students eligible: **Yes**

FACULTAD DE MEDICINA
UNIVERSIDAD DEL ALTIPLANO
CALLE LA PLATA ESQUINA MURGIA
ORURO
Tel.: +591 (52) 549 46
Year instruction started: **1994**

FACULTAD DE MEDICINA
UNIVERSIDAD CATOLICA BOLIVIANA
CALLE ESPANA 368
CASILLA 3201
SANTA CRUZ
Tel.: +591 (3) 351 549/337 815
Fax: +591 (3) 332 389
Year instruction started: **1995**

FACULTAD DE MEDICINA
UNIVERSIDAD CRISTIANA BOLIVIANA
CAMPUS UNIVERSITARIO KM 5
CALLE NORTE AVENIDA BANZER
CASILLA 4780
SANTA CRUZ
Tel.: +591 (3) 410 472
Fax: +591 (3) 426 311
Year instruction started: **1994**

FACULTAD DE MEDICINA
UNIVERSIDAD MAYOR, REAL Y PONTIFICIA SAN FRANCISCO XAVIER
CALLE JUNIN ESQUINA ESTUDIANTES
CASILLA 233
SUCRE
Tel.: +591 (64) 224 02/232 45
Year instruction started: **1846**

BOSNIA AND HERZEGOVINA

Total population in 1995: **3 628 000**
Number of physicians per 100 000 population (1993): —
Number of medical schools: **3**
Duration of basic medical degree course, including practical training: —
Title of degree awarded: —
Medical registration/licence to practise: —
Work in government service after graduation: —
Agreements with other countries: —

MEDICINSKI FAKULTET
UNIVERZITETA "DJURO PUCAR STARI" U BANJA LUCI
MUSTAFA SABINOVIC 10
BANJA LUKA 78000
Year instruction started: **1978**

MEDICINSKI FAKULTET
UNIVERZITETA U SARAJEVU
CEKALUSA 90
SARAJEVO 71000
Tel.: +387 (71) 203 670
Fax: +387 (71) 203 670
Year instruction started: **1946**
Language of instruction: **Bosnian**
Duration of basic medical degree course, including practical training: **6 years**
Entrance examination: **Yes**
Foreign students eligible: **Yes**

MEDICINSKI FAKULTET
UNIVERZITETA U TUZLI
BRATSTVA I JEDINSTVA 19
TUZLA 75000

BOTSWANA

Total population in 1995: **1 484 000**
Number of physicians per 100 000 population (1993): **26**
Number of medical schools: **None**
Medical registration/licence to practise: **Registration is obligatory with the Botswana Medical Council, Private Bag 0038, Gaborone. Foreigners must hold a work permit.**
Work in government service after graduation: **Not obligatory**
Agreements with other countries: **An agreement exists with Norway.**

BRAZIL

Total population in 1995: **161 087 000**
Number of physicians per 100 000 population (1993): **134**
Number of medical schools: **82**
Duration of basic medical degree course, including practical training: **6–9 years**
Title of degree awarded: *Médico* **(Doctor of Medicine)**
Medical registration/licence to practise: **Registration is obligatory with the university that awarded the degree or is empowered to register degrees**

awarded by independent medical schools. The licence to practise medicine is granted by the regional medical council. Graduates of foreign medical schools must have their degree accredited by a Brazilian university. Foreigners must hold a residence permit.

Work in government service after graduation: **Not obligatory**
Agreements with other countries: **None**

■ ALAGOAS

ESCOLA DE CIENCIAS MEDICAS DE ALAGOAS
FUNDACAO GOVERNADOR LAMENHA FIL'HO
AVENIDA SIQUEIRA CAMPOS 2095
TRAPICHE DA BARRA
MACEIO 57010
Fax: +55 (82) 326 5627
Year instruction started: **1970**

CENTRO DE CIENCIAS DA SAUDE
UNIVERSIDADE FEDERAL DE ALAGOAS
CAMPUS SIMOES KM 13
TABOLEIRO DOS
CP 2018
MACEIO 57000
Fax: +55 (82) 322 2345
Year instruction started: **1970**

■ AMAZONAS

FACULDADE DE CIENCIAS DA SAUDE
FUNDACAO UNIVERSIDADE DO AMAZONAS
RUA AFONSO PENA 1053
MANAUS 69000
Tel.: +55 (92) 232 3607
Fax: +55 (92) 232 3607
Year instruction started: **1967**
Language of instruction: **Portuguese**
Duration of basic medical degree course, including practical training: **6 years**
Entrance examination: **Yes**
Foreign students eligible: **Yes**

■ BAHIA
ESCOLA DE MEDICINA E SAUDE PUBLICA
FUNDACAO BAHIANA PARA O DESENVOLVIMENTO DA MEDICINA
RUA FREI HENRIQUE 8
NAZARE
SALVADOR 40050
Fax: +55 (71) 243 4928
Year instruction started: **1953**

FACULDADE DE MEDICINA
UNIVERSIDADE FEDERAL DA BAHIA
AVENIDA REITOR MIGUEL CALMON S/N
CANELA
SALVADOR 40000
Fax: +55 (71) 245 9002
Year instruction started: **1808**

■ CEARA
CENTRO DE CIENCIAS DA SAUDE
UNIVERSIDADE FEDERAL DO CEARA
RUA CAPITAO FRANCISCO PEDRO 1210
RODOLFO TEOFILO
FORTALEZA 60000
Fax: +55 (85) 243 4776
Year instruction started: **1948**

■ DISTRITO FEDERAL
FACULDADE DE CIENCIAS DA SAUDE
UNIVERSIDADE DE BRASILIA
CAMPUS UNIVERSITARIO
CP 15-3031
BRASILIA 70910-900
Tel.: +55 (61) 348 2574/348 2270
Fax: +55 (61) 273 0105
Year instruction started: **1966**
Language of instruction: **Portuguese**
Duration of basic medical degree course, including practical training: **6 years**
Entrance examination: **Yes**
Foreign students eligible: **Yes**

■ **ESPIRITO SANTO**
ESCOLA DE MEDICINA DA SANTA CASA DE MISERICORDIA DE VITORIA
  (EMES-CAM)
AVENIDA NOSSA SENHORA DA PENHA S/N
CP 5135
VITORIA 29045
Fax: +55 (27) 227 2150
Year instruction started: **1968**

CENTRO BIOMEDICO
UNIVERSIDADE FEDERAL DO ESPIRITO SANTO
AVENIDA MARECHAL CAMPOS S/N
CP 780
VITORIA 29000
Fax: +55 (27) 335 2243
Year instruction started: **1961**

■ **GOIAS**
FACULDADE DE MEDICINA
UNIVERSIDADE FEDERAL DE GOIAS
PRIMEIRA AVENIDA S/N
SETOR UNIVERSITARIO
GOIANIA 74605
Tel.: +55 (62) 202 2565
Fax: +55 (62) 202 2565
Year instruction started: **1960**
Language of instruction: **Portuguese**
Duration of basic medical degree course, including practical training: **6 years**
Entrance examination: **Yes**
Foreign students eligible: **Yes**

■ **MARANHAO**
CENTRO DE CIENCIAS DA SAUDE
UNIVERSIDADE FEDERAL DO MARANHAO
RUA BARAO DE ITAPARY 66
SAO LUIS 65000
Fax: +55 (98) 221 5285
Year instruction started: **1958**

■ **MATO GROSSO**
FACULDADE DE CIENCIAS MEDICAS
FUNDACAO UNIVERSIDADE FEDERAL DE MATO GROSSO
AVENIDA FERNANDO CORREA DA COSTA S/N
CUIABA 78000

Tel.: +55 (65) 315 8850
Fax: +55 (65) 315 8852
Year instruction started: **1980**
Language of instruction: **Portuguese**
Duration of basic medical degree course, including practical training: **6 years**
Entrance examination: **Yes**
Foreign students eligible: **No**

■ MATO GROSSO DO SUL
CENTRO DE CIENCIAS BIOLOGICAS E DA SAUDE
FUNDACAO UNIVERSIDADE FEDERAL DE MATO GROSSO DO SUL
CIDADE UNIVERSITARIA
CP 649
CAMPO GRANDE 79070
Fax: +55 (67) 787 1081
Year instruction started: **1968**

■ MINAS GERAIS
UNIVERSIDADE DE ALFENAS/UNIFENAS
CAMPUS UNIVERSITARIO
TREVO
CP 23
ALFENAS 37130
Fax: +55 (35) 921 4403

FACULDADE DE MEDICINA DE BARBACENA
FUNDACAO PRES. ANTONIO CARLOS
PRACA ANTONIO CARLOS S/N
CP 45
BARBACENA 36200
Fax: +55 (32) 332 2789

FACULDADE DE CIENCIAS MEDICAS DE MINAS GERAIS
FUNDACAO UNIVERSITARIA MINEIRA
ALAMEDA EZEQUIEL DIAS 275
CP 1756
BELO HORIZONTE 30130-100
Fax: +55 (31) 222 1324
Year instruction started: **1951**

FACULDADE DE MEDICINA
UNIVERSIDADE FEDERAL DE MINAS GERAIS
AVENIDA ALFREDO BALENA 190
SANTA EFIGENIA
CP 340
BELO HORIZONTE 30130-100
Tel.: +55 (31) 226 7600
Fax: +55 (31) 273 4985
Year instruction started: **1911**
Language of instruction: **Portuguese**
Duration of basic medical degree course, including practical training: **6 years**
Entrance examination: **Yes**
Foreign students eligible: **Yes**

FACULDADE DE MEDICINA DE ITAJUBA
AVENIDA RENO JUNIOR 368
CP 25
ITAJUBA 37500
Tel.: +55 (35) 621 4545
Fax: +55 (35) 621 4555
Year instruction started: **1968**
Language of instruction: **Portuguese**
Duration of basic medical degree course, including practical training: **6 years**
Entrance examination: **Yes**
Foreign students eligible: **Yes**

FACULDADE DE MEDICINA
UNIVERSIDADE FEDERAL DE JUIZ DE FORA (UFJF)
RUA CATULO BREVIGLIERI S/N
JUIZ DE FORA 36100
Fax: +55 (32) 215 6382
Year instruction started: **1953**

FACULDADE DE MEDICINA DO NORTE DE MINAS
FUNDACAO UNIVERSIDADE NORTE MINEIRA DE ENSINA SUPERIOR
AVENIDA UNIVERSITARIA S/N
VILA MAURICEIA
CP 126
MONTES CLAROS 39400
Fax: +55 (38) 222 1234
Year instruction started: **1969**

FACULDADE DE CIENCIAS MEDICAS "DR JOAO ANTONIO GARCIA
   COUTINHO"
FUNDACAO DE ENSINO SUPERIOR
AVENIDA ALFREDO CUSTODIO DE PAULA 320
CP 229
POUSO ALEGRE 37550
Tel.: +55 (35) 421 3504
Fax: +55 (35) 421 3501
Year instruction started: **1969**
Language of instruction: **Portuguese**
Duration of basic medical degree course, including practical training: **6 years**
Entrance examination: **Yes**
Foreign students eligible: **Yes**

FACULDADE DE MEDICINA DO TRIANGULO MINEIRO
FREI PAULINO 30
UBERABA 38025 180
Tel.: +55 (34) 312 7722
Fax: +55 (34) 312 6640
Year instruction started: **1953**
Language of instruction: **Portuguese**
Duration of basic medical degree course, including practical training: **6 years**
Entrance examination: **Yes**
Foreign students eligible: **Yes**

CENTRO DE CIENCIAS BIOMEDICAS
FUNDACAO UNIVERSIDADE FEDERAL DE UBERLANDIA
AVENIDA PARA 1720
CAMPUS UMUARAMA
UBERLANDIA 38400
Fax: +55 (34) 234 8022
Year instruction started: **1968**

■ **PARA**
FACULDADE ESTADUAL DE MEDICINA DO PARA
FUNDACAO EDUCACIONAL DO ESTADO DO PARA
TRAVESSA 14 DE ABRIL 1462
BELEM 66000
Fax: +55 (91) 229 9677
Year instruction started: **1971**

CENTRO DE CIENCIAS DA SAUDE
UNIVERSIDADE FEDERAL DO PARA
PRACA CAMILO SALGADO 1
BELEM 66000
Fax: +55 (91) 241 6201
Year instruction started: **1919**

■ **PARAIBA**
CENTRO DE CIENCIAS BIOLOGICAS E DA SAUDE
UNIVERSIDADE FEDERAL DA PARAIBA CAMPUS II
AVENIDA JUVENCIO ARRUDA 795
BODOCONGO
CAMPINA GRANDE 58100
Year instruction started: **1968**

CENTRO DE CIENCIAS DA SAUDE
UNIVERSIDADE FEDERAL DA PARAIBA
CIDADE UNIVERSITARIA
JOAO PESSOA 58000
Year instruction started: **1952**

■ **PARANA**
SIDADE ESTADUAL DO OESTE DO PARANA/UNIOESTE
AVENIDA BRASIL 1537
JARDIM UNIVERSITARIO
CP 711
CASCAVEL 81808
Fax: +55 (45) 223 4584

FACULDADE EVANGELICA DE MEDICINA DO PARANA
SOCIEDADE EVANGELICA BENEFICENTE DE CURITIBA
RUA ALAMEDA PRINCESA ISABEL 1580
CURITIBA 80730
Fax: +55 (41) 222 6494
Year instruction started: **1969**

CENTRO DE CIENCIAS DA SAUDE
UNIVERSIDADE CATOLICA DO PARANA
RUA IMACULADA CONCEICAO 1155
PRADO VELHO
CURITIBA 80215
Fax: +55 (41) 332 5588
Year instruction started: **1957**

SETOR DE CIENCIAS DA SAUDE
UNIVERSIDADE FEDERAL DO PARANA
RUA PADRE CAMARGO 280
CURITIBA 80060-240
Tel.: +55 (41) 264 2011
Fax: +55 (41) 262 2197
E-mail: coordmed@saude.ufpr.br
Year instruction started: **1912**
Language of instruction: **Portuguese**
Duration of basic medical degree course, including practical training: **9 years**
Entrance examination: **Yes**
Foreign students eligible: **Yes**

CENTRO DE CIENCIAS DA SAUDE
UNIVERSIDADE ESTADUAL DE LONDRINA
AVENIDA ROBERT KOCH 60
CP 1562
LONDRINA 86038-440
Tel.: +55 (43) 337 6574
Fax: +55 (43) 337 5100
Year instruction started: **1967**
Language of instruction: **Portuguese**
Duration of basic medical degree course, including practical training: **6 years**
Entrance examination: **Yes**
Foreign students eligible: **No**

CURSO DE MEDICINA
UNIVERSIDADE ESTADUAL DE MARINGA
AVENIDA COLOMBO 5790, ZONA 07
MARINGA 87020-900
Tel.: +55 (44) 224 8585
Fax: +55 (44) 222 754
Year instruction started: **1988**
Language of instruction: **Portuguese**
Duration of basic medical degree course, including practical training: **6 years**
Entrance examination: **Yes**
Foreign students eligible: **Yes**

■ PERNAMBUCO
FACULDADE DE CIENCIAS MEDICAS DE PERNAMBUCO
FUNDACAO DE ENSINO SUPERIOR DE PERNAMBUCO
RUA ARNOBIO MARQUES 310
CP 309
RECIFE 50040
Fax: +55 (81) 224 4623
Year instruction started: **1954**

CENTRO DE CIENCIAS DA SAUDE
UNIVERSIDADE FEDERAL DE PERNAMBUCO
AVENIDA PROFESSOR MORAES REGO S/N
RECIFE 50000
Fax: +55 (81) 271 8099
Year instruction started: **1915**

■ PIAUI
CENTRO DE CIENCIAS DA SAUDE
FUNDACAO UNIVERSIDADE FEDERAL DO PIAUI
AVENIDA FREI SERAFIM 2280
TERESINA 64000
Fax: +55 (86) 232 2812
Year instruction started: **1968**

■ RIO DE JANEIRO
FACULDADE DE MEDICINA DE CAMPOS
FUNDACAO BENEDITO PEREIRA NUNES
AVENIDA DR ALBERTO TORRES 217
CENTRO
CAMPOS 28035
Fax: +55 (247) 226 788
Year instruction started: **1967**

FACULDADE DE MEDICINA
CENTRO DE CIENCIAS MEDICAS
UNIVERSIDADE FEDERAL FLUMINENSE
RUA MARQUES DO PARANA S/N
NITEROI 24030
Fax: +55 (21) 717 4558
Year instruction started: **1926**

FACULDADE DE CIENCIAS MEDICAS DE NOVA IGUACU
SOCIEDADE DE ENSINO SUPERIOR DE NOVA IGUACU (SESNI)
AVENIDA ABILIO AUGUSTO TAVORA 2134
NOVA IGUACU 26260
Fax: +55 (21) 769 6627
Year instruction started: **1976**

FACULDADE DE MEDICINA DE PETROPOLIS
FUNDACAO OTACILIO GUALBERTO
RUA MACHADO FAGUNDES 326
CASCATINHA
PETROPOLIS 25716
Fax: +55 (242) 426 399
Year instruction started: **1967**

ESCOLA DE MEDICINA
FUNDACAO TECNICO-EDUCACIONAL SOUZA MARQUES
RUA DO CATETE 6
GLORIA
RIO DE JANEIRO 22220
Fax: +55 (21) 252 0817
Year instruction started: **1971**

FACULDADE DE CIENCIAS MEDICAS
UNIVERSIDADE DO ESTADO DO RIO DE JANEIRO
RUA PROFESSOR MANOEL DE ABREU 48
RIO DE JANEIRO 20550-170
Tel.: +55 (21) 204 2342/587 6105
Fax: +55 (21) 204 2343
Year instruction started: **1936**
Language of instruction: **Portuguese**
Duration of basic medical degree course, including practical training: **9 years**
Entrance examination: **Yes**
Foreign students eligible: **Yes**

ESCOLA DE MEDICINA E CIRURGIA
UNIVERSIDADE DO RIO DE JANEIRO
RUA SILVA RAMOS 32
RIO DE JANEIRO 20270-040
Tel.: +55 (21) 264 7175
Fax: +55 (21) 264 7175

Year instruction started: **1912**
Language of instruction: **Portuguese**
Duration of basic medical degree course, including practical training: **6 years**
Entrance examination: **Yes**
Foreign students eligible: **Yes**

FACULDADE DE MEDICINA
CENTRO DE CIENCIAS DA SAUDE
UNIVERSIDADE FEDERAL DO RIO DE JANEIRO
ILHA DA CIDADE UNIVERSITARIA
RIO DE JANEIRO 21910
Fax: +55 (21) 230 1957
Year instruction started: **1808**

CENTRO DE CIENCIAS BIOLOGICAS E DA SAUDE
UNIVERSIDADE GAMA FILHO
RUA MANOEL VITORINO 625
PIEDADE
RIO DE JANEIRO 20748-900
Tel.: +55 (21) 599 7153/599 7154
Fax: +55 (21) 591 4448
Year instruction started: **1965**
Language of instruction: **Portuguese**
Duration of basic medical degree course, including practical training: **6 years**
Entrance examination: **Yes**
Foreign students eligible: **Yes**

FACULDADE DE MEDICINA DE TERESOPOLIS
FUNDACAO EDUCACIONAL SERRA DOS ORGAOS
AVENIDA ALBERTO TORRES 111
CP 01
TERESOPOLIS 25964
Fax: +55 (21) 642 6170
Year instruction started: **1970**

FACULDADE DE MEDICINA DE VALENCA
FUNDACAO EDUCACIONAL DOM ANDRE ARCOVERDE
PRACA BALBINA FONSECA 186
VALENCA 27600
Fax: +55 (244) 521 888
Year instruction started: **1968**

FACULDADES INTEGRADAS SEVERINO SOMBRA CURSO DE MEDICINA
AVENIDA EXPEDICIONARIO OSWALDO DE ALMEIDA RAMOS 280
VASSOURAS 27700
Tel.: +55 (244) 711 326
Fax: +55 (244) 711 326
Year instruction started: **1969**
Language of instruction: **Portuguese**
Duration of basic medical degree course, including practical training: **6 years**
Entrance examination: **Yes**
Foreign students eligible: **Yes**

ESCOLA DE CIENCIAS MEDICAS DE VOLTA REDONDA
FUNDACAO OSWALDO ARANHA
AVENIDA PAULO DE FRONTIN 457
CENTRO
VOLTA REDONDA 27180
Fax: +55 (243) 423 836
Year instruction started: **1968**

■ **RIO GRANDE DO NORTE**
CENTRO DE CIENCIAS DA SAUDE
UNIVERSIDADE FEDERAL DO RIO GRANDE DO NORTE
AVENIDA NILO PECANHA S/N
PETROPOLIS
NATAL 59000
Fax: +55 (84) 231 4467
Year instruction started: **1956**

■ **RIO GRANDE DO SUL**
CENTRO DE CIENCIAS BIOLOGICAS E DA SAUDE
FUNDACAO UNIVERSIDADE DE CAXIAS DO SUL
RUA PINHEIRO MACHADO 3251
CAXIAS DO SUL 95100
Fax: +55 (54) 222 8223
Year instruction started: **1968**

FACULDADE DE MEDICINA
UNIVERSIDADE DE PASSO FUNDO
RUA TEIXEIRA SOARES 817
CP 566/567
PASSO FUNDO 99010-080
Tel.: +55 (54) 311 1177
Fax: +55 (54) 311 1307

Year instruction started: **1970**
Language of instruction: **Portuguese**
Duration of basic medical degree course, including practical training: **6 years**
Entrance examination: **Yes**
Foreign students eligible: **Yes**

CENTRO DE CIENCIAS DA SAUDE E BIOLOGICAS
UNIVERSIDADE CATOLICA DE PELOTAS
RUA GONCALVES CHAVES 373
PELOTAS 96100
Fax: +55 (53) 221 5023
Year instruction started: **1963**

FACULDADE DE MEDICINA
UNIVERSIDADE FEDERAL DE PELOTAS
AVENIDA DUQUE DE CAXIAS 250
FRAGATA
CP 464
PELOTAS 96030-001
Tel.: +55 (53) 221 3554
Fax: +55 (53) 221 3554
Year instruction started: **1963**
Language of instruction: **Portuguese**
Duration of basic medical degree course, including practical training: **6 years**
Entrance examination: **Yes**
Foreign students eligible: **Yes**

FUNDACAO FACULDADE FEDERAL DE CIENCIAS MEDICAS DE PORTO
    ALEGRE
RUA SARMENTO LEITE 245
PORTO ALEGRE 90050
Fax: +55 (51) 226 9756
Year instruction started: **1961**

FACULDADE DE MEDICINA
PONTIFICIA UNIVERSIDADE CATOLICA DO RIO GRANDE DO SUL
AVENIDA IPIRANGA 6690
PORTO ALEGRE 90610-000
Tel.: +55 (51) 339 1322
Fax: +55 (51) 339 1322
Year instruction started: **1970**
Language of instruction: **Portuguese**
Duration of basic medical degree course, including practical training: **6 years**
Entrance examination: **Yes**
Foreign students eligible: **Yes**

FACULDADE DE MEDICINA
UNIVERSIDADE FEDERAL DO RIO GRANDE DO SUL
RUA RAMIRO BARCELOS 2350
PORTO ALEGRE 90000
Fax: +55 (51) 221 2175
Year instruction started: **1897**

FACULDADE DE MEDICINA
FUNDACAO UNIVERSIDADE DO RIO GRANDE
RUA GENERAL OSORIO S/N
CP 503
RIO GRANDE 96200
Tel.: +55 (53) 231 1869
Fax: +55 (53) 231 9094
E-mail: comedici@super.furg.br
Year instruction started: **1966**
Language of instruction: **Portuguese**
Duration of basic medical degree course, including practical training: **6 years**
Entrance examination: **Yes**
Foreign students eligible: **Yes**

CURSO DE MEDICINA
UNIVERSIDADE FEDERAL DE SANTA MARIA
CAMOBI
SANTA MARIA 97119-900
Tel.: +55 (55) 226 1616
Fax: +55 (55) 226 2423
Year instruction started: **1954**
Language of instruction: **Portuguese**
Duration of basic medical degree course, including practical training: **6 years**
Entrance examination: **Yes**
Foreign students eligible: **Yes**

■ **RORAIMA**
CURSO DE MEDICINA
UNIVERSIDADE FEDERAL DE RORAIMA
BR 174 S/N
CAMPUS DO PARICARANA
BOA VISTA 69310-270
Tel.: +55 (95) 623 1120
Fax: +55 (95) 623 1120
E-mail: caio@technnet.com.br

Year instruction started: **1994**
Language of instruction: **Portuguese**
Duration of basic medical degree course, including practical training: **6 years**
Entrance examination: **Yes**
Foreign students eligible: **Yes**

■ **SANTA CATARINA**
CURSO DE MEDICINA DA FURB
UNIVERSIDADE REGIONAL DE BLUMENAU
RUA ANTONIO DA VEIGA 140
CP 1507
BLUMENAU 89010-971
Tel.: +55 (47) 321 0200
Fax: +55 (47) 322 8818
Year instruction started: **1990**
Language of instruction: **Portuguese**
Duration of basic medical degree course, including practical training: **6 years**
Entrance examination: **Yes**
Foreign students eligible: **Yes**

CURSO DE MEDICINA
UNIVERSIDADE FEDERAL DE SANTA CATARINA
CAMPUS UNIVERSITARIO
TRINDADE
FLORIANOPOLIS 88049-900
Tel.: +55 (48) 331 9499
Fax: +55 (48) 331 9542
Year instruction started: **1960**
Language of instruction: **Portuguese**
Duration of basic medical degree course, including practical training: **6 years**
Entrance examination: **Yes**
Foreign students eligible: **Yes**

■ **SAO PAULO**
FACULDADE MEDICINA, CAMPUS DE BOTUCATU
UNIVERSIDADE ESTADUAL PAULISTA (UNESP)
RUBIAO JUNIOR
CP 530
BOTUCATU 18618-970
Tel.: +55 (14) 821 2121
Fax: +55 (14) 822 0421
Telex: 142107 ujmf br
E-mail: vane@mb.unesp.br

Year instruction started: **1963**
Language of instruction: **Portuguese**
Duration of basic medical degree course, including practical training: **6 years**
Entrance examination: **Yes**
Foreign students eligible: **Yes**

FACULDADE DE CIENCIAS MEDICAS
UNIVERSIDADE SAO FRANCISCO
AVENIDA SAO FRANCISCO DE ASSIS 218
BRAGANCA PAULISTA 12900-000
Tel.: +55 (11) 784 482 34
Fax: +55 (11) 784 418 25
E-mail: usfbib@eu.ansp.br
Year instruction started: **1971**
Language of instruction: **Portuguese**
Duration of basic medical degree course, including practical training: **6 years**
Entrance examination: **Yes**
Foreign students eligible: **Yes**

FACULDADE DE CIENCIAS MEDICAS
PONTIFICIA UNIVERSIDADE CATOLICA DE CAMPINAS
AVENIDA JOHN BOYD DUNLOP S/N
CAMPINAS 13100
Tel.: +55 (19) 495 899
Year instruction started: **1976**
Language of instruction: **Portuguese**
Duration of basic medical degree course, including practical training: **6 years**
Entrance examination: **Yes**
Foreign students eligible: **Yes**

FACULDADE DE CIENCIAS MEDICAS
UNIVERSIDADE ESTADUAL DE CAMPINAS
CIDADE UNIVERSITARIA ZEFERINO VAZ
CP 6111
CAMPINAS 13081-970
Tel.: +55 (19) 239 4364/239 7765
Fax: +55 (19) 239 2512
E-mail: ceg15@head.fcm.unicamp.br
Year instruction started: **1963**
Language of instruction: **Portuguese**
Duration of basic medical degree course, including practical training: **6 years**
Entrance examination: **Yes**
Foreign students eligible: **Yes**

FACULDADE DE MEDICINA DE CATANDUVA
FUNDACAO PADRE ALBINO
AVENIDA SAO VICENTE DE PAULA 1455
VILA GUZZO
CATANDUVA 15800
Fax: +55 (175) 227 161
Year instruction started: **1970**

FACULDADE DE MEDICINA DE JUNDIAI
RUA FRANCISCO TELES 250
VILA ARENS
CP 1295
JUNDIAI 13202
Fax: +55 (11) 737 1376
Year instruction started: **1969**

FACULDADE DE MEDICINA DE MARILIA
RUA MONTE CARMELO 800
CP 451
MARILIA 17519-030
Tel.: +55 (144) 226 999
Fax: +55 (144) 221 079
E-mail: fmmb@eu.ansp.br
Year instruction started: **1967**
Language of instruction: **Portuguese**
Duration of basic medical degree course, including practical training: **6 years**
Entrance examination: **Yes**
Foreign students eligible: **Yes**

CENTRO DE CIENCIAS BIOMEDICAS
FACULDADE DE MEDICINA
UNIVERSIDADE DE MOGI DAS CRUZES
AVENIDA CANDIDO XAVIER DE ALMEIDA SOUZA 200
MOGI DAS CRUZES 08780
Fax: +55 (11) 469 5233
Year instruction started: **1968**

UNIVERSIDADE DO OESTE PAULISTA/UNOESTE
RUA BONGIOVANI 700
CIDADE UNIVERSITARIA
CP 1161
PRESIDENTE PRUDENTE 19050
Fax: +55 (182) 210 200

FACULDADE DE MEDICINA DE RIBEIRAO PRETO
UNIVERSIDADE DE SAO PAULO
AVENIDA BANDEIRANTES 3900
RIBEIRAO PRETO 14049-900
Tel.: +55 (16) 633 3035
Fax: +55 (16) 633 1586
E-mail: admin@fmrp.usp.br
Year instruction started: **1952**
Language of instruction: **Portuguese**
Duration of basic medical degree course, including practical training: **6 years**
Entrance examination: **Yes**
Foreign students eligible: **Yes**

FACULDADE DE MEDICINA DE SANTO AMARO
ORGANIZACAO SANTAMARENSE DE EDUCACAO E CULTURA (OSEC)
RUA PROFESSOR ENEAS DE SIQUEIRA NETO 340
SANTO AMARO 04829
Fax: +55 (11) 520 9160
Year instruction started: **1970**

FACULDADE DE MEDICINA DO ABC
FUNDACAO UNIVERSITARIA DO ABC
AVENIDA PRINCIPE DE GALES 821
SANTO ANDRE 09060
Fax: +55 (11) 449 3558
Year instruction started: **1969**

FACULDADE DE CIENCIAS MEDICAS DE SANTOS
FUNDACAO LUSIADA
RUA OSWALDO CRUZ 179
SANTOS 11100
Fax: +55 (11) 815 5665
Year instruction started: **1967**

FUNDACAO FACULDADE REGIONAL DE MEDICINA DE SAO JOSE DO RIO
    PRETO
AVENIDA BRIGADEIRO FARIA DE LIMA 5416
SAO JOSE DO RIO PRETO 15090
Fax: +55 (172) 271 277
Year instruction started: **1968**

FACULDADE DE CIENCIAS MEDICAS DA SANTA CASA DE SAO PAULO
FUNDACAO ARNALDO VIEIRA DE CARVALHO
RUA DR CESARIO MOTTA JUNIOR 112
SAO PAULO 01221
Year instruction started: **1963**

FACULDADE DE MEDICINA
UNIVERSIDADE DE SAO PAULO
AVENIDA DR ARNALDO 445
PACAEMBU
SAO PAULO 01246
Fax: +55 (11) 222 8649
Year instruction started: **1913**

ESCOLA PAULISTA DE MEDICINA
UNIVERSIDADE FEDERAL DE SAO PAULO
RUA BOTUCATU 740
SAO PAULO 04023-900
Tel.: +55 (11) 549 7699
Fax: +55 (11) 549 2127
E-mail: unifesp@epm.br
Year instruction started: **1933**
Language of instruction: **Portuguese**
Duration of basic medical degree course, including practical training: **6 years**
Entrance examination: **Yes**
Foreign students eligible: **Yes**

FACULDADE DE CIENCIAS MEDICAS
CENTRO DE CIENCIAS MEDICAS E BIOLOGICAS
PONTIFICIA UNIVERSIDADE CATOLICA DE SAO PAULO
PRACA DR JOSE ERMIRIO DE MORAES 290
SOROCABA 18030-230
Tel.: +55 (152) 312 773
Fax: +55 (152) 312 773
Year instruction started: **1951**
Language of instruction: **Portuguese**
Duration of basic medical degree course, including practical training: **6 years**
Entrance examination: **Yes**
Foreign students eligible: **Yes**

FACULDADE DE MEDICINA DE TAUBATE
IRMANDADE DE MISERICORDIA DE TAUBATE
AVENIDA TIRADENTES 500
TAUBATE 12100
Fax: +55 (122) 327 660
Year instruction started: **1967**

■ SERGIPE

CENTRO DE CIENCIAS BIOLOGICAS E DA SAUDE
FUNDACAO UNIVERSIDADE FEDERAL DE SERGIPE
AVENIDA DESEMBARGADOR MAYNARD 174
ARACAJU 49000
Fax: +55 (79) 241 3995
Year instruction started: **1961**

BULGARIA

Total population in 1995: **8 468 000**
Number of physicians per 100 000 population (1993): **333**
Number of medical schools: **5**
Duration of basic medical degree course, including practical training: **6 or 6.5
    years**
Title of degree awarded: *Magister* (**Physician**)
Medical registration/licence to practise: **Registration is obligatory with the
    Ministry of Health, Sveta Nedelia Square 5, Sofia 10000. The licence to
    practise medicine is granted to graduates of a recognized medical school.
    Foreigners must hold a residence permit.**
Work in government service after graduation: **Obligatory (2 years)**
Agreements with other countries: **Agreements exist with all countries of the
    newly independent states (NIS), countries of central and eastern Europe
    and former socialist countries.**

HIGHER MEDICAL INSTITUTE
1 CYRIL & METHODY STREET
PLEVEN 5800
Tel.: +359 (64) 291 05
Fax: +359 (64) 291 53
Year instruction started: **1974**
Language of instruction: **Bulgarian**
Duration of basic medical degree course, including practical training: **6 years**
Entrance examination: **Yes**
Foreign students eligible: **Yes**

I. P. PAVLOV HIGHER MEDICAL INSTITUTE
15A VASSIL APRILOV STREET
PLOVDIV 4002
Year instruction started: **1945**

MEDICAL UNIVERSITY
15 DIMITAR NESTOROV STREET
SOFIA 1400
Year instruction started: **1918**

MEDICAL FACULTY AT TRAKIA UNIVERSITY
11 ARMEJSKA STREET
STARA ZAGORA 6000
Tel.: +359 (42) 400 94
Fax: +359 (42) 470 00
Year instruction started: **1982**
Language of instruction: **Bulgarian**
Duration of basic medical degree course, including practical training: **6 years**
Entrance examination: **Yes**
Foreign students eligible: **Yes**

MEDICAL UNIVERSITY OF VARNA
55 MARIN DRINOV STREET
VARNA 9010
Tel.: +359 (52) 225 622
Fax: +359 (52) 222 584
Year instruction started: **1961**
Language of instruction: **Bulgarian**
Duration of basic medical degree course, including practical training: **6 years**
Entrance examination: **Yes**
Foreign students eligible: **Yes**

BURKINA FASO

Total population in 1995: **10 780 000**
Number of physicians per 100 000 population (1993): —
Number of medical schools: **1**
Duration of basic medical degree course, including practical training: **7 years**
Title of degree awarded: ***Doctorat d'État en Médecine*** (Doctor of Medicine)
Medical registration/licence to practise: **Registration is obligatory with the**
   ***Conseil national de l'Ordre du Burkina, 01 BP 403 Ouagadougou 01* and with**
   the government authorities. The licence to practise medicine is awarded by
   the Ministry of Health, Ouagadougou, following 10 years in government

service. Foreigners must hold a recognized degree and come from a country with which agreements exist.

Work in government service after graduation: **Obligatory (10 years)**

Agreements with other countries: **Agreements exist with France and with countries of the *Conseil Africain et Malagache de l'Enseignement Supérieur* (CAMES) and the former USSR.**

ECOLE SUPERIEURE DES SCIENCES DE LA SANTE
BP 7021
OUAGADOUGOU
Tel.: +226 307 543
Fax: +226 312 639
Year instruction started: **1981**
Language of instruction: **French**
Duration of basic medical degree course, including practical training: **7 years**
Entrance examination: **Yes**
Foreign students eligible: **Yes**

BURUNDI

Total population in 1995: **6 221 000**
Number of physicians per 100 000 population (1993): **6**
Number of medical schools: **1**
Duration of basic medical degree course, including practical training: **7 years**
Title of degree awarded: ***Docteur en Médecine* (Doctor of Medicine)**
Medical registration/licence to practise: —
Work in government service after graduation: —
Agreements with other countries: —

FACULTE DE MEDECINE DE BUJUMBURA
UNIVERSITE DU BURUNDI
IBARABARA RYA 28 MUNYONYO
BP 1020
BUJUMBURA
Tel.: +257 232 074
Fax: +257 232 267/232 268
Year instruction started: **1963**
Language of instruction: **French**
Duration of basic medical degree course, including practical training: **7 years**
Entrance examination: **No**
Foreign students eligible: **Yes**

CAMBODIA

Total population in 1995: **10 273 000**
Number of physicians per 100 000 population (1993): **58**
Number of medical schools: **1**
Duration of basic medical degree course, including practical training: **7 years**
Title of degree awarded: **Doctor of Medicine**
Medical registration/licence to practise: **Registration is obligatory with the Ministry of Health, Phnom Penh. The licence to practise medicine is granted to nationals who hold a degree from a recognized medical school.**
Work in government service: **Obligatory (1 year)**
Agreements with other countries: **None**

FACULTE MIXTE DE MEDECINE, DE PHARMACIE ET D'ODONTO-
    STOMATOLOGIE
BOULEVARD MONIVONG 73
PHNOM PENH
Tel.: +855 (23) 368 051
Year instruction started: **1980**
Language of instruction: **Khmer, French, English**
Duration of basic medical degree course, including practical training: **7 years**
Entrance examination: **Yes**
Foreign students eligible: **No**

CAMEROON

Total population in 1995: **13 560 000**
Number of physicians per 100 000 population (1993): **7**
Number of medical schools: **1**
Duration of basic medical degree course, including practical training: **7 years**
Title of degree awarded: ***Docteur en Médecine*** (Doctor of Medicine)
Medical registration/licence to practise: **Registration is obligatory with the *Ordre national des Médecins, BP 219, Yaoundé*. Graduates must provide full personal and legal details, together with a certified copy of their degree certificate, to obtain licensure from the Ministry of Health. Those who have qualified abroad must also provide a certificate of equivalence of their degree.**
Work in government service after graduation: **Not obligatory**
Agreements with other countries: **No formal agreements exist, but informal agreements exist with France and the United Kingdom.**

FACULTE DE MEDECINE ET DES SCIENCES BIOMEDICALES
UNIVERSITE DE YAOUNDE I
BP 1364
YAOUNDE
Tel.: +237 310 586
Fax: +237 311 224/315 178
Year instruction started: **1969**

CANADA

Total population in 1995: **29 680 000**
Number of physicians per 100 000 population (1993): **221**
Number of medical schools: **16**
Duration of basic medical degree course, including practical training: **3 or 4 years**
Title of degree awarded: **Doctor of Medicine (MD)**; *Docteur en Médecine*
Medical registration/licence to practise: **Registration is obligatory with the Medical Council of Canada, 2283 St Laurent Boulevard, Ottawa, Ontario K1G 3H7. The licence to practise medicine is granted by the Provincial Licensing Authorities to candidates who have at least 2 years' postgraduate training and who have passed parts 1 and 2 of the qualifying examination of the Medical Council of Canada. Foreigners may have to meet citizenship or permanent residence requirements.**
Work in government service after graduation: **Not obligatory**
Agreements with other countries: **An agreement between the Committee on Accreditation of Canadian Medical Schools and the Liaison Committee on Medical Education of the USA leads to mutual recognition of medical degrees awarded by universities in Canada and the USA.**

■ ALBERTA
FACULTY OF MEDICINE
UNIVERSITY OF CALGARY
HEALTH SCIENCES CENTRE
3330 HOSPITAL DRIVE N.W.
CALGARY T2N 4NI
Tel.: +1 (403) 220 4246
Fax: +1 (403) 270 1828
E-mail: psalo@acs.ucalgary.ca
Year instruction started: **1970**
Language of instruction: **English**
Duration of basic medical degree course, including practical training: **4 years**
Entrance examination: **Yes**
Foreign students eligible: **Yes**

FACULTY OF MEDICINE AND ORAL HEALTH SCIENCES
UNIVERSITY OF ALBERTA
2–45 MEDICAL SCIENCES BUILDING
EDMONTON T6G 2R7
Tel.: +1 (403) 492 6350
Fax: +1 (403) 492 9531
Year instruction started: **1913**
Language of instruction: **English**
Duration of basic medical degree course, including practical training: **4 years**
Entrance examination: **Yes**
Foreign students eligible: **Yes**

■ BRITISH COLUMBIA
FACULTY OF MEDICINE
UNIVERSITY OF BRITISH COLUMBIA
3250-910 WEST 10TH AVENUE
VANCOUVER V5T 4E3
Tel.: +1 (604) 875 4500
Fax: +1 (604) 875 5611
Year instruction started: **1950**
Language of instruction: **English**
Duration of basic medical degree course, including practical training: **4 years**
Entrance examination: **No**
Foreign students eligible: **No**

■ MANITOBA
FACULTY OF MEDICINE
UNIVERSITY OF MANITOBA
753 MCDERMOT AVENUE
WINNIPEG R3T 2N2
Tel.: +1 (204) 789 3569
Fax: +1 (204) 774 8941
E-mail: paraggebldghsc.lani@umanitoba.ca
Year instruction started: **1883**
Language of instruction: **English**
Duration of basic medical degree course, including practical training: **4 years**
Entrance examination: **Yes**

■ NEWFOUNDLAND
FACULTY OF MEDICINE
MEMORIAL UNIVERSITY OF NEWFOUNDLAND
300 PRINCE PHILLIP DRIVE
ST JOHN'S A1B 3V6

Tel.: +1 (709) 737 6602
Fax: +1 (709) 737 6746
Year instruction started: **1969**
Language of instruction: **English**
Duration of basic medical degree course, including practical training: **4 years**
Entrance examination: **Yes**
Foreign students eligible: **Yes**

■ **NOVA SCOTIA**
FACULTY OF MEDICINE
DALHOUSIE UNIVERSITY
5849 UNIVERSITY AVENUE
HALIFAX B2T 1E8
Tel.: +1 (902) 494 6592
Fax: +1 (902) 494 7119
Year instruction started: **1868**
Language of instruction: **English**
Duration of basic medical degree course, including practical training: **4 years**
Entrance examination: **Yes**
Foreign students eligible: **Yes**

■ **ONTARIO**
FACULTY OF HEALTH SCIENCES
MCMASTER UNIVERSITY
1200 MAIN STREET WEST
HAMILTON L8N 3Z5
Tel.: +1 (905) 525 9140
Fax: +1 (905) 528 4727
E-mail: martind@fhs.mcmaster.ca
Year instruction started: **1969**
Language of instruction: **English**
Duration of basic medical degree course, including practical training: **3 years**
Entrance examination: **No**
Foreign students eligible: **Yes**

FACULTY OF MEDICINE
QUEEN'S UNIVERSITY
BOTTERELL HALL
KINGSTON K7L 3N6
Tel.: +1 (613) 545 2544
Fax: +1 (613) 545 6884

Year instruction started: **1854**
Language of instruction: **English**
Duration of basic medical degree course, including practical training: **4 years**
Entrance examination: **Yes**
Foreign students eligible: **Yes**

FACULTY OF MEDICINE
UNIVERSITY OF WESTERN ONTARIO
HEALTH SCIENCES CENTER
LONDON N6A 5C1
Tel.: +1 (519) 661 3744
Fax: +1 (519) 661 3797
E-mail: admissions@do.med.uwo.ca
Year instruction started: **1882**
Language of instruction: **English**
Duration of basic medical degree course, including practical training: **4 years**
Foreign students eligible: **No**

FACULTY OF HEALTH SCIENCES
UNIVERSITY OF OTTAWA
451 SMYTH ROAD
OTTAWA K1H 8M5
Tel.: +1 (613) 562 5800
Year instruction started: **1945**
Language of instruction: **French, English**
Duration of basic medical degree course, including practical training: **4 years**
Entrance examination: **No**
Foreign students eligible: **No**

FACULTY OF MEDICINE
UNIVERSITY OF TORONTO
1 KING'S COLLEGE CIRCLE
TORONTO M5S 1A8
Tel.: +1 (416) 978 6585
Fax: +1 (416) 978 1774
E-mail: medicine.web@utoronto.ca
Year instruction started: **1887**
Language of instruction: **English**
Duration of basic medical degree course, including practical training: **4 years**
Entrance examination: **Yes**
Foreign students eligible: **Yes**

■ QUEBEC

FACULTY OF MEDICINE
MCGILL UNIVERSITY
MCINTYRE MEDICAL SCIENCES BUILDING
3655 DRUMMOND STREET
MONTREAL H3G 1Y6
Tel.: +1 (514) 398 3515
Fax: +1 (514) 398 3595
Year instruction started: **1829**
Language of instruction: **English**
Duration of basic medical degree course, including practical training: **4 years**
Entrance examination: **Yes**
Foreign students eligible: **Yes**

FACULTE DE MEDECINE
UNIVERSITE DE MONTREAL
CP 6128
SUCCURSALE A
MONTREAL H3C 3J7

FACULTE DE MEDECINE
UNIVERSITE LAVAL
PAVILLON FERDINAND-VANDRY
AVENUE DE LA MEDECINE
QUEBEC G1K 7P4
Tel.: +1 (418) 656 2331
Fax: +1 (418) 656 3442
E-mail: fmed@fmed.ulaval.ca
Year instruction started: **1854**
Language of instruction: **French**
Duration of basic medical degree course, including practical training: **4 years**
Entrance examination: **No**
Foreign students eligible: **Yes**

FACULTE DE MEDECINE
UNIVERSITE DE SHERBROOKE
3001 12 AVENUE NORD
FLEURIMONT
SHERBROOKE J1H 5N4
Tel.: +1 (819) 564 5203
Fax: +1 (819) 564 5444
Year instruction started: **1966**
Language of instruction: **French**
Duration of basic medical degree course, including practical training: **4 years**
Entrance examination: **No**
Foreign students eligible: **Yes**

■ **SASKATCHEWAN**
COLLEGE OF MEDICINE
UNIVERSITY OF SASKATCHEWAN
107 WIGGINS ROAD
SASKATOON S7N 5E5
Tel.: +1 (306) 966 6135
Fax: +1 (306) 966 6164
Year instruction started: **1953**
Language of instruction: **English**
Duration of basic medical degree course, including practical training: **4 years**
Entrance examination: **Yes**
Foreign students eligible: **No**

CENTRAL AFRICAN REPUBLIC

Total population in 1995: **3 344 000**
Number of physicians per 100 000 population (1993): **6**
Number of medical schools: **1**
Duration of basic medical degree course, including practical training: **6 years**
Title of degree awarded: *Docteur en Médecine* (*Diplôme d'État*) (**Doctor of Medicine (State Diploma)**)
Medical registration/licence to practise: —
Work in government service after graduation: —
Agreements with other countries: —

FACULTE DES SCIENCES DE LA SANTE
UNIVERSITE DE BANGUI
BP 1383
BANGUI
Year instruction started: **1976**

CHAD

Total population in 1995: **6 515 000**
Number of physicians per 100 000 population (1993): **2**
Number of medical schools: **1**
Duration of basic medical degree course, including practical training: **7 years**
Title of degree awarded: *Doctorat en Médecine* (**Doctor of Medicine**)
Medical registration/licence to practise: **Registration is obligatory with the *Ordre national des Médecins du Tchad, BP 1296, N'Djamena.***
Work in government service after graduation: **Not obligatory**
Agreements with other countries: **Agreements exist with Algeria, Cameroon, Central African Republic, Congo and Côte d'Ivoire.**

FACULTE DES SCIENCES DE LA SANTE
BP 1117
N'DJAMENA
Tel.: +235 517 144
Fax: +235 514 033
Year instruction started: **1990**
Language of instruction: **French**
Duration of basic medical degree course, including practical training: **7 years**
Entrance examination: **Yes**
Foreign students eligible: **Yes**

CHILE

Total population in 1995: **14 421 000**
Number of physicians per 100 000 population (1993): **108**
Number of medical schools: **6**
Duration of basic medical degree course, including practical training: **7 years**
Title of degree awarded: ***Médico Cirujano*** **(Physician and Surgeon)**
Medical registration/licence to practise: —
Obligation to work in government service: —
Agreements with other countries: —

FACULTAD DE MEDICINA
UNIVERSIDAD DE CONCEPCION
BARRIO UNIVERSITARIO S/N
CASILLA 60-C
CONCEPCION
Tel.: +56 (41) 228 353
Fax: +56 (41) 228 353
Year instruction started: **1924**
Language of instruction: **Spanish**
Duration of basic medical degree course, including practical training: **7 years**
Entrance examination: **Yes**
Foreign students eligible: **Yes**

FACULTAD DE MEDICINA
PONTIFICIA UNIVERSIDAD CATOLICA DE CHILE
LIRA 40
SANTIAGO
Year instruction started: **1833**

FACULTAD DE MEDICINA
UNIVERSIDAD DE CHILE
AVENIDA INDEPENDENCIA 1027
CASILLA 13898
SANTIAGO
Tel.: +56 (2) 678 6115
Fax: +56 (2) 737 4059/678 6436
Year instruction started: **1930**
Language of instruction: **Spanish**
Duration of basic medical degree course, including practical training: **7 years**
Entrance examination: **Yes**
Foreign students eligible: **Yes**

DEPARTAMENTO DE CIENCIAS DE LA SALUD
FACULTAD DE MEDICINA
UNIVERSIDAD DE LA FRONTERA
CASILLA 54-D
TEMUCO
Tel.: +56 (45) 212 108
Fax: +56 (45) 212 108
E-mail: decanmed@werken.ufro.cl
Year instruction started: **1971**
Language of instruction: **Spanish**
Duration of basic medical degree course, including practical training: **7 years**
Entrance examination: **No**
Foreign students eligible: **Yes**

FACULTAD DE MEDICINA
UNIVERSIDAD AUSTRAL DE CHILE
ISLA TEJA
CASILLA 567
VALDIVIA
Year instruction started: **1964**

FACULTAD DE MEDICINA
UNIVERSIDAD DE VALPARAISO
HONTANEDA 2653
CASILLA 92-V
VALPARAISO
Year instruction started: **1968**

CHINA

Total population in 1995: **1 232 083 000**
Number of physicians per 100 000 population (1993): **115**
Number of medical schools: **150**
Duration of basic medical degree course, including practical training: **3–8 years**
Title of degree awarded: **Bachelor of Medicine**
Medical registration/licence to practise: **Registration is obligatory with the health department of the local government. Graduates must undertake a 1-year internship and have working experience before receiving their final degree. Those who have graduated abroad must have their degree approved by the national education department. Foreigners may practise for short periods only with special authorization and must be registered with a medical institution in China.**

Information on the granting of a licence to practise medicine in Hong Kong Special Administrative Region (Hong Kong SAR) is available from the Medical Council of Hong Kong, Hong Kong Academy of Medicine Building, 99 Wong Chuk Hang Road, Aberdeen, Hong Kong SAR. All medical graduates wishing to register as a medical practitioner with the Medical Council of Hong Kong (with the exception of graduates of the University of Hong Kong and the Chinese University of Hong Kong, and Hong Kong Permanent Residents holding recognized United Kingdom, Irish and Commonwealth diplomas, subject to certain conditions), are required to pass the Council's Licensing Examination and successfully complete a period of pre-registration internship training in approved hospitals or institutions.
Work in government service after graduation: —
Agreements with other countries: —

■ ANHUI
BENGBU MEDICAL COLLEGE
108 ZHI HUAI ROAD
BENGBU 233003
Year instruction started: **1958**

ANHUI COLLEGE OF TRADITIONAL CHINESE MEDICINE
24 MEI SHAN ROAD
HEFEI 230038
Year instruction started: **1958**

ANHUI MEDICAL UNIVERSITY
MEISHAN ROAD
HEFEI 230032

Tel.: +86 (2) 813 965
Fax: +86 (2) 813 965
E-mail: aydxt@public.h.f.ah.cn
Year instruction started: **1949**
Language of instruction: **Chinese**
Duration of basic medical degree course, including practical training: **5 years**
Entrance examination: **Yes**
Foreign students eligible: **No**

SCHOOL OF MEDICINE
HUAINAN COLLEGE FOR THE COAL INDUSTRY
HUAINAN 232001
Year instruction started: **1985**

WANNAN MEDICAL COLLEGE
1 TIE SHAN
WUHU 241001
Year instruction started: **1958**

■ **BEIJING**
BEIJING COLLEGE OF ACUPUNCTURE–MOXIBUSTION AND
    ORTHOPAEDICS–TRAUMATOLOGY
6 WANG JING ZHONG HUAN NAN ROAD
DONG ZH1 MEN WAI CHAO YANG DISTRICT
BEIJING 100015
Year instruction started: **1986**

BEIJING MEDICAL UNIVERSITY
38 XUE YUAN ROAD
BEIJING 100083
Tel.: +86 (10) 201 7620
Fax: +86 (10) 201 5681
Year instruction started: 1912
Language of instruction: **Chinese**
Duration of basic medical degree course, including practical training: **5–7 years**
Entrance examination: **Yes**
Foreign students eligible: **Yes**

BEIJING SCHOOL OF MEDICINE
DA DONG ROAD
SHUNYI COUNTY
BEIJING 101300
Year instruction started: **1985**

COLLEGE OF TRADITIONAL CHINESE MEDICINE AND PHARMACY
BEIJING UNION UNIVERSITY
22 HUA YUAN STREET
JIANG ZHAI KOU
DONG CHENG DISTRICT
BEIJING 100013
Year instruction started: **1978**

BEIJING UNIVERSITY OF TRADITIONAL CHINESE MEDICINE (BUTCM)
11 BEI SAN HUAN DONG LU
BEIJING 100029
Tel.: +86 (10) 642 186 24
Fax: +86 (10) 642 208 67
E-mail: bucmpo@public.bta.net.cn
Year instruction started: **1956**
Language of instruction: **Chinese**
Duration of basic medical degree course, including practical training: **7 years**
Entrance examination: **Yes**
Foreign students eligible: **Yes**

TRAINING CENTRE OF GENERAL PRACTICE
CAPITAL UNIVERSITY OF MEDICAL SCIENCES
10 WEST TOU TIAO
YOU AN MEN WAI
BEIJING 100054
Tel.: +86 (10) 630 511 65
Fax: +86 (10) 630 587 89
E-mail: cumsfm@public.bta.net.cn
Year instruction started: **1960**

PEKING UNION MEDICAL COLLEGE
9 DONG DAN SAN TIAO
BEIJING 100730
Year instruction started: **1917**

SCHOOL OF MEDICINE OF GENERAL LOGISTICS DEPARTMENT
23 QI LI ZHUANG ROAD
FENG TAI DISTRICT
BEIJING 100017
Year instruction started: **1978**

■ FUJIAN

FUJIAN COLLEGE OF TRADITIONAL CHINESE MEDICINE
53 NORTH WU SI ROAD
FUZHOU 350003
Year instruction started: **1958**

FUJIAN MEDICAL COLLEGE
6 JIAO TONG ROAD
FUZHOU 350004
Year instruction started: **1937**

■ GANSU

GANSU COLLEGE OF TRADITIONAL CHINESE MEDICINE
35 EAST DING XI ROAD
LANZHOU 730000
Year instruction started: **1978**

LANZHOU MEDICAL COLLEGE
99 DONG GANGXI ROAD
LANZHOU 730000
Tel.: +86 (931) 861 7079
Fax: +86 (931) 861 7025
Year instruction started: **1954**
Language of instruction: **Chinese**
Duration of basic medical degree course, including practical training: **5 years**
Entrance examination: **Yes**
Foreign students eligible: **No**

DEPARTMENT OF MEDICINE
NORTHWEST COLLEGE FOR MINORITIES
1 NORTHWEST NEW VILLAGE
LANZHOU 730030
Year instruction started: **1958**

■ GUANGDONG

THE FIRST MILITARY MEDICAL UNIVERSITY
MEI HUA YUAN
GUANGZHOU 510515
Year instruction started: **1951**

GUANGDONG COLLEGE OF MEDICINE AND PHARMACY
40 BAO GANG GUANG HAN ZHI
GUANGZHOU 510224
Tel.: +86 (20) 844 290 40
Fax: +86 (20) 844 497 35
E-mail: pharna@gzsuns.edu.cn

Year instruction started: **1980**
Language of instruction: **Chinese**
Duration of basic medical degree course, including practical training: **5 years**
Entrance examination: **Yes**
Foreign students eligible: **No**

GUANGZHOU MEDICAL COLLEGE
195 DONG FENG ROAD WEST
GUANGZHOU 510182
Tel.: +86 (20) 813 634 81
Fax: +86 (20) 813 625 43
Year instruction started: **1958**
Language of instruction: **Chinese**
Duration of basic medical degree course, including practical training: **5 years**
Entrance examination: **Yes**
Foreign students eligible: **No**

GUANGZHOU UNIVERSITY OF TRADITIONAL CHINESE MEDICINE
10 JICHANG ROAD
GUANGZHOU 510407
Tel.: +86 (20) 865 912 33
Fax: +86 (20) 865 947 35
Year instruction started: **1956**
Language of instruction: **Chinese**
Duration of basic medical degree course, including practical training: **5 years**
Entrance examination: **Yes**
Foreign students eligible: **Yes**

MEDICAL COLLEGE
JINAN UNIVERSITY
SHI PAI
GUANGZHOU 510632
Tel.: +86 (20) 757 9343
Fax: +86 (20) 551 6941
Year instruction started: **1978**
Language of instruction: **Chinese**
Duration of basic medical degree course, including practical training: **6 years**
Entrance examination: **Yes**
Foreign students eligible: **Yes**

SUN YAT-SEN UNIVERSITY OF MEDICAL SCIENCES
74 ZHONG SHAN ROAD II
GUANGZHOU 510089
Tel.: +86 (20) 877 750 49
Fax: +86 (20) 877 656 79
E-mail: sums@gzsums.edu.cn

Year instruction started: **1866**
Language of instruction: **Chinese**
Duration of basic medical degree course, including practical training: **5 years**
Entrance examination: **Yes**
Foreign students eligible: **Yes**

MEDICAL COLLEGE
SHANTOU UNIVERSITY
12 RAO PING ROAD
SHANTOU 515031
Tel.: +86 (754) 855 1151
Fax: +86 (754) 855 7562
Telex: 45448 stuni cn
Year instruction started: **1977**
Language of instruction: **Chinese**
Duration of basic medical degree course, including practical training: **5 years**
Entrance examination: **Yes**
Foreign students eligible: **Yes**

DEPARTMENT OF MEDICINE
SHAOGUAN UNIVERSITY
SHAOGUAN 512005
Year instruction started: **1994**
Language of instruction: **Chinese**
Duration of basic medical degree course, including practical training: **3 years**
Entrance examination: **Yes**
Foreign students eligible: **No**

GUANGDONG MEDICAL COLLEGE
2 WENMINGDONG ROAD
ZHANJIANG 524023
Tel.: +86 (759) 228 1544
Fax: +86 (759) 228 4104
E-mail: gdmcpyes@letterbox.scut.edu.cn
Year instruction started: **1958**
Language of instruction: **Chinese**
Duration of basic medical degree course, including practical training: **5 years**
Entrance examination: **Yes**
Foreign students eligible: **Yes**

■ **GUANGXI**
YOUJIANG MEDICAL COLLEGE FOR NATIONALITIES OF GUANGXI
BAISE 533000
Year instruction started: **1958**

GUILIN MEDICAL COLLEGE
56 LE QUN ROAD
GUILIN 541001
Year instruction started: **1958**

GUANGXI COLLEGE OF TRADITIONAL CHINESE MEDICINE
21 EAST MING XIN ROAD
NANNING 530001
Year instruction started: **1956**

GUANGXI MEDICAL UNIVERSITY
6 BIN HU ROAD
NANNING 530021
Tel.: +86 (771) 531 1477
Fax: +86 (771) 531 2523
Year instruction started: **1934**
Language of instruction: **Chinese**
Duration of basic medical degree course, including practical training: **5 years**
Entrance examination: **Yes**
Foreign students eligible: **Yes**

■ GUIZHOU
QIANNAN SCHOOL OF MEDICINE FOR MINORITIES
QUIN YI STREET
DUYUN 558003
Tel.: +86 (854) 222 496
Year instruction started: **1985**
Language of instruction: **Chinese**
Duration of basic medical degree course, including practical training: **3 years**
Entrance examination: **Yes**
Foreign students eligible: **No**

GUIYANG COLLEGE OF TRADITIONAL CHINESE MEDICINE
1 EAST ROAD
GUIYANG 550002
Year instruction started: **1965**

GUIYANG MEDICAL COLLEGE
4 BEIJING ROAD
GUIYANG 550004
Year instruction started: **1938**

ZUNYI MEDICAL COLLEGE
WAI HUAN ROAD
ZUNYI 563003
Year instruction started: **1949**

■ HAINAN

HAINAN MEDICAL COLLEGE
33 LONG HUA ROAD
HAIKOU 570005
Year instruction started: **1952**

■ HEBEI

CHENGDE MEDICAL COLLEGE
CUI QIAO ROAD
CHENGDE 067000
Tel.: +86 (314) 206 4592
Fax: +86 (314) 206 4089
Year instruction started: **1945**
Language of instruction: **Chinese**
Duration of basic medical degree course, including practical training: **5 years**
Entrance examination: **Yes**
Foreign students eligible: **No**

HANDAN MEDICAL SCHOOL
HANDAN 056002
Tel.: +86 (310) 301 4817
Year instruction started: **1958**
Language of instruction: **Chinese**
Duration of basic medical degree course, including practical training: **3 years**
Entrance examination: **Yes**
Foreign students eligible: **No**

HEBEI MEDICAL UNIVERSITY
5 WEST CHANG AN ROAD
SHIJIAZHUANG 050017
Year instruction started: **1970**

NORTH CHINA MEDICAL COLLEGE FOR THE COAL INDUSTRY
JIAN SHE ROAD
TANGSHAN 063000
Year instruction started: **1958**

ZHANGJIAKOU MEDICAL COLLEGE
14 CHANG QING ROAD
ZHANGJIAKOU 075000
Year instruction started: **1949**

■ HEILONGJIANG
HARBIN MEDICAL UNIVERSITY
157 BAOJIAN ROAD
NANGANG DISTRICT
HARBIN 150086
Tel.: +86 (451) 666 9485
Fax: +86 (451) 667 5769
E-mail: pub@hrbmu.edu.cn
Year instruction started: **1926**
Language of instruction: **Chinese**
Duration of basic medical degree course, including practical training: **5–7 years**
Entrance examination: **Yes**
Foreign students eligible: **No**

HEILONGJIANG COLLEGE OF TRADITIONAL CHINESE MEDICINE
14 HE PING ROAD
HARBIN 150040
Tel.: +86 (451) 211 2786
Fax: +86 (451) 211 2786
Year instruction started: **1959**
Language of instruction: **Chinese**
Duration of basic medical degree course, including practical training: **5 years**
Entrance examination: **Yes**
Foreign students eligible: **Yes**

JIAMUSI MEDICAL COLLEGE
DEXIANG STREET
JIAMUSI 154002
Year instruction started: **1958**

JIXI MEDICAL SCHOOL FOR THE COAL INDUSTRY
JIXI 158100

MUDANJIANG MEDICAL COLLEGE
TONG XIANG ROAD
MUDANJIANG 157001
Year instruction started: **1958**

QIQIHAR MEDICAL COLLEGE
24 XIANG YANG STREET
QIQIHAR 161041
Year instruction started: **1978**

■ **HENAN**
KAIFENG SCHOOL OF MEDICINE
65 QIAN YING MEN STREET
KAIFENG 475001
Tel.: +86 (378) 595 8866
Year instruction started: **1929**
Language of instruction: **Chinese**
Duration of basic medical degree course, including practical training: **3 years**
Entrance examination: **Yes**
Foreign students eligible: **No**

LUOYANG SCHOOL OF MEDICINE
6 ANHUI ROAD
LUOYANG 471003
Year instruction started: **1958**

ZHANG ZHONGJING SCHOOL OF TRADITIONAL CHINESE MEDICINE
COLLEGE OF SCIENCE AND ENGINEERING
WO LONG GANG
NANYANG
Year instruction started: **1985**

XINXIANG MEDICAL COLLEGE
XINYAN ROAD
XINXIANG 453003
Tel.: +86 (373) 305 3410
Fax: +86 (373) 304 1119
Year instruction started: **1950**
Language of instruction: **Chinese**
Duration of basic medical degree course, including practical training: **5 years**
Entrance examination: **Yes**
Foreign students eligible: **No**

HENAN COLLEGE OF TRADITIONAL CHINESE MEDICINE
EAST JIN SHUI ROAD
ZHENGZHOU 450003
Year instruction started: **1958**

HENAN MEDICAL UNIVERSITY
40 UNIVERSITY ROAD
ZHENGZHOU 450052
Year instruction started: **1953**

■ **HONG KONG SAR**
FACULTY OF MEDICINE
THE CHINESE UNIVERSITY OF HONG KONG
SHATIN
NEW TERRITORIES
HONG KONG SAR
Tel.: +852 260 968 70
Fax: +852 260 369 58
Telex: 50301 cuhk hx
Year instruction started: **1981**
Language of instruction: **English**
Duration of basic medical degree course, including practical training: **5 years**
Entrance examination: **Yes**
Foreign students eligible: **Yes**

FACULTY OF MEDICINE
UNIVERSITY OF HONG KONG
7 SASSOON ROAD
HONG KONG SAR
Tel.: +852 281 992 14
Fax: +852 285 597 42
Telex: 71919 cereb hx
Year instruction started: **1887**
Language of instruction: **English**
Duration of basic medical degree course, including practical training: **5 years**
Entrance examination: **No**
Foreign students eligible: **Yes**

■ **HUBEI**
ENSHI SCHOOL OF MEDICINE
61 FOUTH LANE
WU YANG STREET
ENSHI 445000
Year instruction started: **1958**

YUNYANG MEDICAL COLLEGE
SHIYAN 442000
Tel.: +86 (719) 889 1088
Fax: +86 (719) 889 1080
Year instruction started: **1971**
Language of instruction: **Chinese**
Duration of basic medical degree course, including practical training: **5 years**
Entrance examination: **Yes**
Foreign students eligible: **No**

HUBEI COLLEGE OF TRADITIONAL CHINESE MEDICINE
110 YUN JIA QIAO
WUHAN 430061
Year instruction started: **1958**

HUBEI MEDICAL UNIVERSITY
39 DONG HU ROAD
WUCHANG
WUHAN 430071
Tel.: +86 (27) 736 0602
Fax: +86 (27) 736 0601
E-mail: rong@public.wh.hb.cn
Year instruction started: **1943**
Language of instruction: **Chinese, English**
Duration of basic medical degree course, including practical training: **5 years**
Entrance examination: **Yes**
Foreign students eligible: **Yes**

TONGJI MEDICAL UNIVERSITY
13 HANGKONG ROAD
WUHAN 430030
Tel.: +86 (27) 362 2600
Fax: +86 (27) 586 1050/585 8920
Year instruction started: **1907**
Language of instruction: **Chinese**
Duration of basic medical degree course, including practical training: **3 years**
Entrance examination: **Yes**
Foreign students eligible: **Yes**

WUHAN SCHOOL OF MEDICINE FOR THE METALLURGICAL INDUSTRY
25 YE JIN STREET
WUHAN
Year instruction started: **1965**

XIANNING MEDICAL COLLEGE
XIANNING 437100
Tel.: +86 (715) 826 0538
Fax: +86 (715) 826 0538
Year instruction started: **1965**
Language of instruction: **Chinese**
Duration of basic medical degree course, including practical training: **5 years**
Entrance examination: **Yes**
Foreign students eligible: **No**

MEDICAL SCHOOL OF THE THREE GORGE COLLEGE
159 YI LING ROAD
YICHANG 443003
Year instruction started: **1958**

■ **HUNAN**
HUNAN COLLEGE OF TRADITIONAL CHINESE MEDICINE
107 SHAO SHAN ROAD
CHANGSHA 410007
Tel.: +86 (731) 555 6660
Fax: +86 (731) 553 2948
Year instruction started: **1960**
Language of instruction: **Chinese**
Duration of basic medical degree course, including practical training: **5 years**
Entrance examination: **Yes**
Foreign students eligible: **Yes**

HUNAN MEDICAL SCHOOL
CHANGSHA 410006
Tel.: +86 (731) 880 2644
Year instruction started: **1985**
Language of instruction: **Chinese**
Duration of basic medical degree course, including practical training: **3 years**
Entrance examination: **Yes**
Foreign students eligible: **No**

HUNAN MEDICAL UNIVERSITY
22 BEI ZHAN ROAD
PO BOX 46
CHANGSHA 410078
Tel.: +86 (731) 447 2685
Fax: +86 (731) 447 1339
Year instruction started: **1914**
Language of instruction: **Chinese**
Duration of basic medical degree course, including practical training: **5 years**
Entrance examination: **Yes**
Foreign students eligible: **Yes**

CHENZHOU MEDICAL COLLEGE
25 RENMIN WEST ROAD
CHENZHOU 423000
Tel.: +86 (735) 222 4561

Year instruction started: **1958**
Language of instruction: **Chinese**
Duration of basic medical degree course, including practical training: **3 years**
Entrance examination: **Yes**
Foreign students eligible: **No**

HENGYANG MEDICAL COLLEGE
WEST COLLEGE VILLAGE
HENGYANG 421001
Year instruction started: **1958**

■ INNER MONGOLIA AUTONOMOUS REGION
BAOTOU MEDICAL COLLEGE
GANG TIE STREET
BAOTOU 024010
Year instruction started: **1958**

INNER MONGOLIA MEDICAL COLLEGE
5 XIN HUA STREET
HOHHOT 100059
Tel.: +86 (471) 696 3300
Fax: +86 (471) 696 5120
Year instruction started: **1956**
Language of instruction: **Chinese**
Duration of basic medical degree course, including practical training: **5 years**
Entrance examination: **Yes**
Foreign students eligible: **Yes**

INNER MONGOLIA COLLEGE OF TRADITIONAL MONGOLIAN MEDICINE
16 CUI LIN HE STREET
TONGLIAO 028041
Year instruction started: **1978**

■ JIANGSU
NANJING COLLEGE OF TRADITIONAL CHINESE MEDICINE
282 HAN ZHONG ROAD
NANJING 210029
Tel.: +86 (25) 661 2904
Fax: +86 (25) 661 2904
Year instruction started: **1955**
Language of instruction: **Chinese**
Duration of basic medical degree course, including practical training: **3–7 years**
Entrance examination: **Yes**
Foreign students eligible: **Yes**

NANJING MEDICAL UNIVERSITY
140 HAN ZHONG ROAD
NANJING 210029
Tel.: +86 (25) 661 2696
Fax: +86 (25) 650 8960
Year instruction started: **1934**
Language of instruction: **Chinese**
Duration of basic medical degree course, including practical training: **5 years**
Entrance examination: **Yes**
Foreign students eligible: **Yes**

NANJING RAILWAY MEDICAL COLLEGE
DIN JIA QIAO ROAD
NANJING 210009
Year instruction started: **1958**

NANJING UNIVERSITY SCHOOL OF MEDICINE
22 HAN KOU ROAD
NANJING 210093
Tel.: +86 (25) 663 7551
Fax: +86 (25) 330 2728
Telex: 34151 prcnu cn
Year instruction started: **1987**
Language of instruction: **Chinese**
Duration of basic medical degree course, including practical training: **7 years**
Entrance examination: **Yes**
Foreign students eligible: **Yes**

NAVY SCHOOL OF MEDICINE
2 MA QUN STREET
NANJING 210049
Year instruction started: **1973**

NANTONG MEDICAL COLLEGE
19 QI XIN ROAD
NANTONG 226001
Tel.: +86 (513) 551 7191
Fax: +86 (513) 551 7359
E-mail: nmcl@public.nt.js.cn
Year instruction started: **1912**
Language of instruction: **Chinese**
Duration of basic medical degree course, including practical training: **3–5 years**
Entrance examination: **Yes**
Foreign students eligible: **No**

SUZHOU MEDICAL COLLEGE
48 REN MIN ROAD
SUZHOU 215007
Year instruction started: **1957**

MEDICAL DEPARTMENT OF JIANGNAN COLLEGE
WUXI 214063
Tel.: +86 (510) 551 1263
Fax: +86 (510) 551 2506
Year instruction started: **1985**
Language of instruction: **Chinese**
Duration of basic medical degree course, including practical training: **3 years**
Entrance examination: **Yes**
Foreign students eligible: **No**

XUZHOU MEDICAL COLLEGE
84 WEST HUAI HAI ROAD
XUZHOU 221002
Year instruction started: **1958**

MEDICAL COLLEGE OF YANGZHOU UNIVERSITY
HUBEI ROAD
YANGZHOU
Year instruction started: **1979**

ZHENJIANG MEDICAL COLLEGE
3 YI ZHENG ROAD
ZHENJIANG 212001
Year instruction started: **1980**

■ **JIANGXI**
GANNAN COLLEGE OF MEDICINE
QINGNIAN ROAD
GANZHOU
Year instruction started: **1958**

JINGGANGSHAN MEDICAL SCHOOL
JIAN 343000
Tel.: +86 (796) 822 4771
Year instruction started: **1978**
Language of instruction: **Chinese**
Duration of basic medical degree course, including practical training: **3 years**
Entrance examination: **Yes**
Foreign students eligible: **No**

JIUJIANG SCHOOL OF MEDICINE
17 LU FENG ROAD
JIUJIANG 332000
Tel.: +86 (792) 822 6155
Fax: +86 (792) 822 6303
Year instruction started: **1951**
Language of instruction: **Chinese**
Duration of basic medical degree course, including practical training: **3 years**
Entrance examination: **Yes**
Foreign students eligible: **No**

JIANGXI COLLEGE OF TRADITIONAL CHINESE MEDICINE
56 YANG MING ROAD
NANCHANG 330006
Tel.: +86 (791) 621 0664
Fax: +86 (791) 621 0664
Year instruction started: **1959**
Language of instruction: **Chinese**
Duration of basic medical degree course, including practical training: **3–5 years**
Entrance examination: **Yes**
Foreign students eligible: **Yes**

JIANGXI MEDICAL COLLEGE
161 BA YI STREET
NANCHANG 330006
Year instruction started: **1952**

YICHUN SCHOOL OF MEDICINE
57 WEST ZHONG SHAN ROAD
YICHUN 336000
Year instruction started: **1958**

■ JILIN
BETHUNE MEDICAL UNIVERSITY
6 XINMIN STREET
CHANGCHUN
Year instruction started: **1938**

CHANGCHUN COLLEGE OF TRADITIONAL CHINESE MEDICINE
15 GONG NONG ROAD
CHANGCHUN 130021
Year instruction started: **1958**

CHANGCHUN MEDICAL SCHOOL
CHANGCHUN 130031
Tel.: +86 (431) 484 1362
Year instruction started: **1993**
Language of instruction: **Chinese**
Duration of basic medical degree course, including practical training: **3 years**
Entrance examination: **Yes**
Foreign students eligible: **No**

AIR FORCE SCHOOL OF MEDICINE
100 JIANG NAN STREET
JILIN 132011
Year instruction started: **1975**

JILIN MEDICAL COLLEGE
1 BEIJING ROAD
JILIN 132001
Year instruction started: **1951**

YANBIAN MEDICAL COLLEGE
121 JUZI STREET
YANJI 133000
Year instruction started: **1948**

■ LIAONING
DALIAN MEDICAL UNIVERSITY
465 ZHONG SHAN LU
DALIAN 116027
Tel.: +86 (411) 469 1802/467 1241
Fax: +86 (411) 467 2546
Year instruction started: **1947**
Language of instruction: **Chinese**
Duration of basic medical degree course, including practical training: **5 years**
Entrance examination: **Yes**
Foreign students eligible: **Yes**

SCHOOL OF MEDICINE OF DALIAN UNIVERSITY
26 WU SI ROAD
XI GANG DISTRICT
DALIAN
Year instruction started: **1986**

JINZHOU MEDICAL COLLEGE
JINZHOU
Year instruction started: **1946**

CHINA MEDICAL UNIVERSITY
92 BEI ER ROAD
HEPING DISTRICT
SHENYANG 110001
Tel.: +86 (24) 386 3731
Fax: +86 (24) 387 5539
Year instruction started: **1931**
Language of instruction: **Japanese, Chinese, English**
Duration of basic medical degree course, including practical training: **5 years**
Entrance examination: **Yes**
Foreign students eligible: **Yes**

LIAONING COLLEGE OF TRADITIONAL CHINESE MEDICINE
79 CONGSHUN BEI LING STREET
SHENYANG 110032
Year instruction started: **1958**

SHENYANG MEDICAL COLLEGE
HUANGHE SOUTH STREET
SHENYANG 110031
Tel.: +86 (246) 842 619
Fax: +86 (246) 228 565
Year instruction started: **1978**
Language of instruction: **Chinese**
Duration of basic medical degree course, including practical training: **5 years**
Entrance examination: **Yes**
Foreign students eligible: **No**

■ **NINGXIA HUI AUTONOMOUS REGION**
NINGXIA MEDICAL COLLEGE
SOUTH SHENG LI STREET
YINCHUAN 750004
Tel.: +86 (951) 409 1158
Year instruction started: **1958**
Language of instruction: **Chinese**
Duration of basic medical degree course, including practical training: **5 years**
Entrance examination: **Yes**
Foreign students eligible: **No**

■ **QINGHAI**
QINGHAI MEDICAL COLLEGE
84 KUN LUN ROAD
XINING 810001
Year instruction started: **1958**

■ SHAANXI
THE FOURTH MILITARY MEDICAL UNIVERSITY
CHANG LE ROAD
XIAN 310033
Year instruction started: **1954**

SHAANXI MEDICAL SCHOOL
XIAN 710068
Tel.: +86 (29) 522 0726
Fax: +86 (29) 522 0723
Year instruction started: **1994**
Language of instruction: **Chinese**
Duration of basic medical degree course, including practical training: **3 years**
Entrance examination: **Yes**
Foreign students eligible: **No**

XIAN MEDICAL UNIVERSITY
WEST XIAO ZHAI ROAD
XIAN 710061
Year instruction started: **1937**

SHAANXI COLLEGE OF TRADITIONAL CHINESE MEDICINE
1 WEI YANG ROAD
XIANYANG 712083
Year instruction started: **1958**

MEDICAL DEPARTMENT
XIZANG NATIONAL COLLEGE
XIANYANG 712082
Tel.: +86 (891) 376 3078
Year instruction started: **1964**

YAN'AN MEDICAL COLLEGE
DU PU CHUAN
YAN'AN 716000
Year instruction started: **1978**

■ SHANDONG
BINZHOU MEDICAL COLLEGE
522 YELLOW RIVER THIRD ROAD
BINZHOU 256603
Year instruction started: **1974**

HEZE SCHOOL OF MEDICINE
WEST KAO PENG STREET
HEZE 274030
Year instruction started: **1958**

SHANDONG COLLEGE OF TRADITIONAL CHINESE MEDICINE
JING ROAD
JINAN 250014
Year instruction started: **1958**

SHANDONG MEDICAL UNIVERSITY
44 WEST WENHUA ROAD
JINAN
Year instruction started: **1948**

JINING MEDICAL COLLEGE
38 JIAN SHE ROAD
JINING 272113
Year instruction started: **1974**

LINYI SCHOOL OF MEDICINE
QING NIAN ROAD
LINYI 276002
Year instruction started: **1966**

QINGDAO MEDICAL COLLEGE
38 DENGZHOU ROAD
QINGDAO 266021
Tel.: +86 (532) 380 1514
Fax: +86 (532) 380 1449
Year instruction started: **1946**
Language of instruction: **Chinese, Japanese, English**
Duration of basic medical degree course, including practical training: **5 years**
Entrance examination: **Yes**
Foreign students eligible: **Yes**

TAISHAN MEDICAL COLLEGE
2 EAST YING SHENG ROAD
TAI'AN
Year instruction started: **1974**

WEIFANG MEDICAL COLLEGE
12 SHENG LI STREET
WEIFANG 261042
Year instruction started: **1950**

■ **SHANGHAI**
SHANGHAI SCHOOL OF MEDICINE
42 NAN FENG ROAD
NAN QIAO TOWN
FENGXIAN 201400
Year instruction started: **1985**

THE SECOND MILITARY MEDICAL UNIVERSITY
594 XIANG YIN ROAD
SHANGHAI 200433
Year instruction started: **1949**

SHANGHAI MEDICAL UNIVERSITY
138 MEDICAL COLLEGE ROAD
SHANGHAI 200032
Year instruction started: **1926**

MEDICAL COLLEGE
SHANGHAI RAILWAY UNIVERSITY
1238 GONG HE XIN ROAD
SHANGHAI 200070
Tel.: +86 (56) 626 087
Fax: +86 (56) 901 123
Year instruction started: **1958**
Language of instruction: **Chinese, Japanese, English**
Duration of basic medical degree course, including practical training: **5 years**
Entrance examination: **Yes**

SHANGHAI SECOND MEDICAL UNIVERSITY
280 SOUTH CHONG QING ROAD
SHANGHAI 200025
Tel.: +86 (21) 632 008 79
Fax: +86 (21) 632 029 16
Year instruction started: **1952**
Language of instruction: **Chinese, French, English**
Duration of basic medical degree course, including practical training: **3–7 years**
Entrance examination: **Yes**
Foreign students eligible: **Yes**

SHANGHAI UNIVERSITY OF TRADITIONAL CHINESE MEDICINE
530 LINGLING ROAD
SHANGHAI 200032
Tel.: +86 (21) 641 746 00
Fax: +86 (21) 641 782 90

Year instruction started: **1956**
Language of instruction: **Chinese**
Duration of basic medical degree course, including practical training: **3–7 years**
Entrance examination: **Yes**
Foreign students eligible: **Yes**

■ SHANXI
DATONG SCHOOL OF MEDICINE
4 YIWEI STREET
DATONG 037008
Tel.: +86 (352) 502 2195
Fax: +86 (352) 502 6174
Year instruction started: **1958**
Language of instruction: **Chinese**
Entrance examination: **Yes**
Foreign students eligible: **No**

CHANGZHI MEDICAL COLLEGE
46 SOUTH YANAN ROAD
SHANGZHI 046000
Year instruction started: **1958**

SHANXI COLLEGE OF TRADITIONAL CHINESE MEDICINE
19 JI CI ROAD
TAIYUAN 030024
Year instruction started: **1982**

SHANXI MEDICAL COLLEGE
XIAN JIAN ROAD
TAIYUAN 030001
Year instruction started: **1950**

■ SICHUAN
CHENGDU COLLEGE OF TRADITIONAL CHINESE MEDICINE
15 SHI ER QIAO STREET
CHENGDU 610075
Tel.: +86 (28) 778 4542
Fax: +86 (28) 776 3471
Year instruction started: **1956**
Language of instruction: **Chinese**
Duration of basic medical degree course, including practical training: **5 years**
Entrance examination: **Yes**
Foreign students eligible: **Yes**

WEST CHINA UNIVERSITY OF MEDICAL SCIENCES
17 SECTION 3
SOUTH REN MIN ROAD
CHENGDU 610044
Tel.: +86 (28) 550 1002
Fax: +86 (28) 558 3252
Year instruction started: **1910**
Language of instruction: **Chinese, English**
Duration of basic medical degree course, including practical training: **5–7 years**
Entrance examination: **Yes**
Foreign students eligible: **No**

CHONGQING MEDICAL UNIVERSITY
1 YIXUEYUAN LU
YU ZHONG QU
CHONGQING 630046
Tel.: +86 (811) 880 9229
Fax: +86 (811) 881 2985
Year instruction started: **1956**
Language of instruction: **Chinese, English**
Duration of basic medical degree course, including practical training: **5 years**
Entrance examination: **Yes**
Foreign students eligible: **Yes**

THE THIRD MILITARY MEDICAL UNIVERSITY
GAO TAN YAN
SHA PING BA
CHONGQING 630038
Year instruction started: **1954**

DEPARTMENT OF TRADITIONAL MEDICINE
YUZHOU UNIVERSITY
CHONGQING 630000

LUZHOU MEDICAL COLLEGE
ZHONG SHAN
LUZHOU 646000
Year instruction started: **1958**

NORTH SICHUAN MEDICAL COLLEGE
20 FUJIANG ROAD
NANCHONG 637007
Tel.: +86 (817) 222 6611
Fax: +86 (817) 222 5475

Year instruction started: **1951**
Language of instruction: **Chinese**
Duration of basic medical degree course, including practical training: **5 years**
Entrance examination: **Yes**
Foreign students eligible: **No**

■ **TAIWAN**
No information available

■ **TIANJIN**
MEDICAL COLLEGE FOR ARMED POLICE
TIANJIN 300162

COLLEGE OF MEDICINE
NANKAI UNIVERSITY
94 WEIJIN ROAD
TIANJIN 300071
Tel.: +86 (22) 235 098 42
Fax: +86 (22) 235 098 42
E-mail: nkdxyxy@public1.tpt.tj.cn
Year instruction started: **1989**
Language of instruction: **Chinese**
Duration of basic medical degree course, including practical training: **7 years**
Entrance examination: **Yes**
Foreign students eligible: **Yes**

TIANJIN COLLEGE OF TRADITIONAL CHINESE MEDICINE
20 YU QUAN ROAD
TIANJIN 300319
Year instruction started: **1978**
Language of instruction: **Chinese**
Duration of basic medical degree course, including practical training: **5 years**
Entrance examination: **Yes**
Foreign students eligible: **No**

TIANJIN MEDICAL UNIVERSITY
22 QI XIANG TAI ROAD
TIANJIN 300070
Year instruction started: **1952**
Language of instruction: **Chinese**
Duration of basic medical degree course, including practical training: **5–7 years**
Entrance examination: **Yes**
Foreign students eligible: **No**

■ TIBET AUTONOMOUS REGION
YANWANGSHAN SCHOOL OF TRADITIONAL TIBET MEDICINE
LHASA 850003
Year instruction started: **1987**
Language of instruction: **Zang**
Duration of basic medical degree course, including practical training: **3 years**
Entrance examination: **Yes**
Foreign students eligible: **No**

■ XINJIANG UYGUR AUTONOMOUS REGION
XINJIANG SCHOOL OF TRADITIONAL URGUR MEDICINE
HETIAN 848000
Year instruction started: **1988**
Language of instruction: **Urgur**
Duration of basic medical degree course, including practical training: **3 years**
Entrance examination: **Yes**
Foreign students eligible: **No**

SHIHEZI MEDICAL COLLEGE
SECOND ROAD (NORTH)
SHIHEZI 832002
Tel.: +86 (993) 201 2036
Fax: +86 (993) 201 5620
Year instruction started: **1949**
Language of instruction: **Chinese**
Duration of basic medical degree course, including practical training: **5 years**
Entrance examination: **Yes**
Foreign students eligible: **No**

XINJIANG COLLEGE OF TRADITIONAL CHINESE MEDICINE
10 XINYI ROAD
URUMQI 830000
Year instruction started: **1986**

XINJIANG MEDICAL COLLEGE
8 XINYI ROAD
URUMQI 830054
Tel.: +86 (991) 484 3398
Fax: +86 (991) 484 3398
Year instruction started: **1956**
Language of instruction: **Chinese**
Duration of basic medical degree course, including practical training: **3–8 years**
Entrance examination: **Yes**
Foreign students eligible: **Yes**

■ YUNNAN
DALI MEDICAL COLLEGE
SOUTH REN MIN ROAD
DALI 671000
Year instruction started: **1982**

KUNMING MEDICAL COLLEGE
84 WEST REN MIN ROAD
KUNMING 650031
Year instruction started: **1956**

YUNNAN COLLEGE OF TRADITIONAL CHINESE MEDICINE
6 BAI TA ROAD
KUNMING 650011
Year instruction started: **1956**

■ ZHEJIANG
HANGZHOU MEDICAL SCHOOL
HANGZHOU 310012
Tel.: +86 (571) 571 8858
Year instruction started: **1994**
Language of instruction: **Chinese**
Duration of basic medical degree course, including practical training: **3 years**
Entrance examination: **Yes**
Foreign students eligible: **No**

ZHEJIANG COLLEGE OF TRADITIONAL CHINESE MEDICINE
QING CHUN STREET
HANGZHOU 310009
Year instruction started: **1959**

ZHEJIANG MEDICAL UNIVERSITY
157 YAN AN ROAD
HANGZHOU 310006
Tel.: +86 (571) 702 2700
Fax: +86 (571) 707 1571/707 7389
Year instruction started: **1912**
Language of instruction: **Chinese, English**
Duration of basic medical degree course, including practical training: **5 years**
Entrance examination: **Yes**
Foreign students eligible: **No**

WENZHOU MEDICAL COLLEGE
82 XUE YUAN ROAD
WENZHOU 325003
Tel.: +86 (577) 833 4941
Fax: +86 (577) 834 1041
Year instruction started: **1958**
Language of instruction: **Chinese**
Duration of basic medical degree course, including practical training: **5 years**
Entrance examination: **Yes**
Foreign students eligible: **Yes**

COLOMBIA

Total population in 1995: **36 444 000**
Number of physicians per 100 000 population (1993): **105**
Number of medical schools: **26**
Duration of basic medical degree course, including practical training: **6–7 years**
Title of degree awarded: ***Médico, Médico Cirujano* (Physician, Physician and Surgeon)**
Medical registration/licence to practise: **The licence to practise medicine is granted by the Ministry of Health, Carrera 13 No. 32–76, Bogotá. Graduates must provide the original degree certificate, authenticated citizenship or identity papers and an attestation of the completion of the compulsory year of social service in a duly approved post. Those who have graduated abroad must have their degree validated by the *Instituto Colombiano para el Fomento de la Educación Superior, Calle 17 No. 3–40, Zona Postal No. 1, Santafé de Bogotá.***
Work in government service after graduation: **Obligatory (1 year)**
Agreements with other countries: —

■ ANTIOQUIA
FACULTAD DE MEDICINA
INSTITUTO DE CIENCIAS DE LA SALUD "CES"
CALLE 10A NO. 22-04
APDO 054591
MEDELLIN
Tel.: +57 (4) 268 3711
Fax: +57 (4) 266 6046
E-mail: ces@medellincetcol.net.co.
Year instruction started: **1973**
Language of instruction: **Spanish, English**
Duration of basic medical degree course, including practical training: **6 years**
Entrance examination: **Yes**
Foreign students eligible: **Yes**

FACULTAD DE MEDICINA
UNIVERSIDAD DE ANTIOQUIA
CIUDAD UNIVERSITARIA
CALLE 67 NO. 5–108
APDO 1226
MEDELLIN
Year instruction started: **1872**

FACULTAD DE MEDICINA
UNIVERSIDAD PONTIFICIA BOLIVARIANA
CALLE 78B NO. 72–109
APDO 56006
MEDELLIN
Tel.: +57 (4) 441 5544
Fax: +57 (4) 257 2428
Year instruction started: **1976**
Language of instruction: **Spanish**
Duration of basic medical degree course, including practical training: **6 years**
Entrance examination: **Yes**
Foreign students eligible: **Yes**

■ **ATLANTICO**
DIVISION CIENCIAS DE LA SALUD
UNIVERSIDAD DEL NORTE
KM 5 CARRETERA A PUERTO COLOMBIA
APDO 1569
BARRANQUILLA
Tel.: +57 (58) 359 8957
Fax: +57 (58) 359 8852
E-mail: webmaster@uninorte.edu.co
Year instruction started: **1975**
Language of instruction: **Spanish, English**
Duration of basic medical degree course, including practical training: **7 years**
Entrance examination: **No**
Foreign students eligible: **Yes**

FACULTAD DE MEDICINA
UNIVERSIDAD LIBRE DE COLOMBIA
SECCIONAL ATLANTICO
CARRETERA 46 NO. 48–170
APDO 1752
BARRANQUILLA
Year instruction started: **1974**

FACULTAD DE MEDICINA
UNIVERSIDAD METROPOLITANA
CARRERA 42-F NO. 75B–169
APDO 50576
BARRANQUILLA
Tel.: +57 (95) 358 7889
Fax: +57 (95) 358 3378
Year instruction started: **1975**
Language of instruction: **Spanish**
Duration of basic medical degree course, including practical training: **7 years**
Entrance examination: **No**
Foreign students eligible: **Yes**

■ BOLIVAR

DIVISION DE CIENCIAS DE LA SALUD
UNIVERSIDAD DE CARTAGENA
CALLE DE LA UNIVERSIDAD 36–100
APDO 1382
CARTAGENA
Year instruction started: **1828**

■ BOYACA

FACULTAD DE MEDICINA
FUNDACION UNIVERSITARIA DE BOYACA
CARRERA 2 ESTE NO. 64–169
APDO 1118
TUNJA

FACULTAD DE MEDICINA
UNIVERSIDAD PEDAGOGICA Y TECNOLOGICA DE COLOMBIA
CALLE 24
ANTIGUO HOSPITAL SAN RAFAEL
TUNJA
Tel.: +57 (987) 424 577/437 173
Fax: +57 (987) 424 577
Year instruction started: **1994**
Language of instruction: **Spanish, English**
Duration of basic medical degree course, including practical training: **6 years**
Entrance examination: **Yes**
Foreign students eligible: **Yes**

■ CALDAS
FACULTAD DE MEDICINA
UNIVERSIDAD DE CALDAS
CALLE 65 NO. 26-10
APDO 275
MANIZALES
Year instruction started: **1952**

■ CAUCA
FACULTAD DE CIENCIAS DE LA SALUD
UNIVERSIDAD DEL CAUCA
CARRERA 6
CALLE 13 NORTE
POPAYAN
Tel.: +57 (28) 234 118
Fax: +57 (28) 236 251
Year instruction started: **1950**
Language of instruction: **Spanish, English**
Duration of basic medical degree course, including practical training: **6.5 years**
Entrance examination: **Yes**
Foreign students eligible: **Yes**

■ CUNDINAMARCA
FACULTAD DE MEDICINA
UNIVERSIDAD DE LA SABANA
CAMPUS UNIVERSITARIO
PUENTE DEL COMUN
VIA CHIA
CHIA
Tel.: +57 (1) 760 377
Year instruction started: **1994**
Language of instruction: **Spanish**
Duration of basic medical degree course, including practical training: **7 years**
Entrance examination: **Yes**
Foreign students eligible: **Yes**

FACULTAD DE MEDICINA
COLEGIO MAYOR DE NUESTRA SENORA DEL ROSARIO
CALLE 10 NO. 18–75
APDO 24743
SANTA FE DE BOGOTA
Tel.: +57 (1) 247 0752
Fax: +57 (1) 277 3110

Year instruction started: **1966**
Language of instruction: **Spanish, French, English**
Duration of basic medical degree course, including practical training: **6 years**
Entrance examination: **Yes**
Foreign students eligible: **Yes**

ESCUELA COLOMBIANA DE MEDICINA
TRANSVERSAL 9A BIS NO. 133-25
APDO 100998
SANTA FE DE BOGOTA
Tel.: +57 (1) 258 3723
Fax: +57 (1) 625 2030
Year instruction started: **1979**
Language of instruction: **Spanish, English**
Duration of basic medical degree course, including practical training: **6 years**
Entrance examination: **Yes**
Foreign students eligible: **Yes**

ESCUELA DE MEDICINA "JUAN N. CORPAS"
AVENIDA CORPAS KILOMETRO 3
CP 2787
SANTA FE DE BOGOTA
Tel.: +57 (1) 681 5612
Fax: +57 (1) 681 3558/683 4378
Year instruction started: **1971**
Language of instruction: **Spanish**
Duration of basic medical degree course, including practical training: **6 years**
Entrance examination: **Yes**
Foreign students eligible: **Yes**

FACULTAD DE MEDICINA
FUNDACION UNIVERSITARIA SAN MARTIN
CARRERA 19 NO. 80-72
SANTA FE DE BOGOTA
Tel.: +57 (1) 616 8071/621 1353
Fax: +57 (1) 235 8356
Year instruction started: **1994**
Language of instruction: **Spanish**
Duration of basic medical degree course, including practical training: **6 years**
Entrance examination: **Yes**
Foreign students eligible: **Yes**

FACULTAD DE MEDICINA
PONTIFICIA UNIVERSIDAD JAVERIANA
CARRERA 7A NO. 40–62
APDO 56710
SANTA FE DE BOGOTA
Tel.: +57 (1) 288 2166
Fax: +57 (1) 288 9273
E-mail: fmedicina@javercol.javeriana.edu.co
Year instruction started: **1942**
Language of instruction: **Spanish**
Duration of basic medical degree course, including practical training: **6 years**
Entrance examination: **Yes**
Foreign students eligible: **Yes**

FACULTAD DE MEDICINA
UNIVERSIDAD MILITAR "NUEVA GRANADA"
TRANSVAL 5 NO. 49-00
SANTA FE DE BOGOTA
Tel.: +57 (91) 285 3405
Fax: +57 (91) 285 3405/232 7281
Year instruction started: **1978**
Language of instruction: **Spanish**
Duration of basic medical degree course, including practical training: **6 years**
Entrance examination: **Yes**
Foreign students eligible: **Yes**

FACULTAD DE MEDICINA
UNIVERSIDAD NACIONAL DE COLOMBIA
CIUDAD UNIVERSITARIA
APDO 14490
SANTA FE DE BOGOTA
Year instruction started: **1867**

■ **HUILA**
FACULTAD DE MEDICINA Y CIENCIAS DE LA SALUD
UNIVERSIDAD SURCOLOMBIANA
AVENIDA PASTRANA BORRERO, CARRERA 1
APDO 385
NEIVA
Year instruction started: **1983**

■ QUINDIO
FACULTAD DE CIENCIAS DE LA SALUD
UNIVERSIDAD DEL QUINDIO
CARRERA 15
CALLE 12 NORTE
APDO 460
ARMENIA
Tel.: +57 (967) 493 897
Fax: +57 (967) 462 563
Year instruction started: **1980**
Language of instruction: **Spanish**
Duration of basic medical degree course, including practical training: **7 years**
Entrance examination: **Yes**
Foreign students eligible: **Yes**

■ RISARALDA
FACULTAD DE MEDICINA
UNIVERSIDAD TECNOLOGICA DE PEREIRA
APDO 97
PEREIRA
Tel.: +57 (963) 350 722
Fax: +57 (963) 350 722
Year instruction started: **1977**
Language of instruction: **Spanish, English**
Duration of basic medical degree course, including practical training: **6 years**
Entrance examination: **Yes**
Foreign students eligible: **Yes**

■ SANTANDER
FACULTAD DE MEDICINA
CORPORACION UNIVERSITARIA DE SANTANDER (UDES)
CAMPUS UNIVERSITARIO—LAGOS DEL CACIQUE
APDO 40223
BUCARAMANGA
Tel.: +57 (76) 651 6500
Fax: +57 (76) 651 6492
Year instruction started: **1996**
Duration of basic medical degree course, including practical training: **6 years**

ESCUELA DE MEDICINA FACULTAD DE SALUD
UNIVERSIDAD INDUSTRIAL DE SANTANDER
CARRERA 27
CALLE 9
APDO 678
BUCARAMANGA
Year instruction started: **1967**
Language of instruction: **Spanish**
Duration of basic medical degree course, including practical training: **6 years**
Entrance examination: **Yes**
Foreign students eligible: **Yes**

ESCUELA DE MEDICINA
UNIVERSIDAD DEL VALLE
HOSPITAL UNIVERSITARIO DEL VALLE 1007
CALI 25360
Tel.: +57 (23) 554 3019
Fax: +57 (23) 557 6914
Year instruction started: **1951**
Language of instruction: **Spanish**
Duration of basic medical degree course, including practical training: **6 years**
Entrance examination: **Yes**
Foreign students eligible: **Yes**

FACULTAD DE MEDICINA
UNIVERSIDAD LIBRE
DIAGONAL 37A NO. 3–29
APDO 1040
CALI
Year instruction started: **1976**

CONGO

Total population in 1995: **2 668 000**
Number of physicians per 100 000 population (1993): **27**
Number of medical schools: **1**
Duration of basic medical degree course, including practical training: **7 years**
Title of degree awarded: ***Docteur en Médecine*** (**Doctor of Medicine**)
Medical registration/licence to practise: —
Obligation to work in government service: —
Agreements with other countries: —

INSTITUT SUPERIEUR DES SCIENCES DE LA SANTE (INSSSA)
BP 2672
BRAZZAVILLE
Tel.: +242 813 931
Telex: 5331 kg
Year instruction started: **1975**
Language of instruction: **French**
Duration of basic medical degree course, including practical training: **7 years**
Entrance examination: **Yes**
Foreign students eligible: **Yes**

COOK ISLANDS

Total population in 1995: —
Number of physicians per 100 000 population (1993): **111**
Number of medical schools: **1**
Duration of basic medical degree course, including practical training: —
Title of degree awarded: —
Medical registration/licence to practise: **Registration is obligatory with the Cook Islands Medical Council. The licence to practise medicine is granted to holders of a degree from a recognized medical institution.**
Work in government service after graduation: **Obligatory (3 years)**
Agreements with other countries: **None**

ST MARY'S SCHOOL OF MEDICINE
COOK ISLANDS
Tel.: +682 (1) 533 6603
Fax: +682 (1) 532 1655
Year instruction started: **1998**

COSTA RICA

Total population in 1995: **3 500 000**
Number of physicians per 100 000 population (1993): **126**
Number of medical schools: **4**
Duration of basic medical degree course, including practical training: **5 or 6 years (a further year of supervised clinical practice is required before the degree is awarded)**
Title of degree awarded: ***Médico Cirujano* (Physician and Surgeon)**
Medical registration/licence to practise: **Registration is obligatory with the *Colegio de Médicos y Cirujanos de Costa Rica, Sabana Sur, San José*. The licence to practise medicine is granted to graduates who have completed**

1 year of social service. Graduates of foreign medical schools must have their degree validated. Foreigners must have been resident in Costa Rica for at least 5 years to obtain a licence to practise.

Work in government service after graduation: **Obligatory (1 year)**
Agreements with other countries: —

ESCUELA AUTONOMA DE CIENCIAS MEDICAS DE CENTRO AMERICA
SABANA OESTE
CARRETERA ESCAZU
APDO 638-1007
CENTRO COLON
SAN JOSE
Tel.: +506 296 3944
Fax: +506 231 4368
Year instruction started: **1978**
Language of instruction: **Spanish**
Duration of basic medical degree course, including practical training: **5 years**
Entrance examination: **Yes**
Foreign students eligible: **Yes**

FACULTAD DE MEDICINA
UNIVERSIDAD DE COSTA RICA
CIUDAD UNIVERSITARIA "RODRIGO FACIO"
SAN PEDRO DE MONTES DE OCA
SAN JOSE
Tel.: +506 207 4570
Fax: +506 207 5667
Year instruction started: **1963**
Language of instruction: **Spanish**
Duration of basic medical degree course, including practical training: **6 years**
Entrance examination: **Yes**
Foreign students eligible: **Yes**

ESCUELA DE MEDICINA
UNIVERSIDAD DE IBEROAMERICA (UNIBE)
APDO 11870
SAN JOSE 1000
Year instruction started: **1995**
Language of instruction: **Spanish**
Duration of basic medical degree course, including practical training: **5 years**
Entrance examination: **Yes**
Foreign students eligible: **Yes**

ESCUELA DE MEDICINA
UNIVERSIDAD INTERNACIONAL DE LAS AMERICAS
APDO 1447-1002
SAN JOSE 1002
Tel.: +506 233 5304
Fax: +506 222 3216
Year instruction started: **1992**
Language of instruction: **Spanish, English**
Duration of basic medical degree course, including practical training: **5 years**
Entrance examination: **Yes**
Foreign students eligible: **Yes**

CÔTE D'IVOIRE

Total population in 1995: **14 015 000**
Number of physicians per 100 000 population (1993): —
Number of medical schools: **1**
Duration of basic medical degree course, including practical training: **8 years**
Title of degree awarded: ***Doctorat d'État en Médecine* (Doctor of Medicine)**
Medical registration/licence to practise: **Registration is obligatory with the
    Conseil national de l'Ordre des Médecins, Abidjan 01. The licence to practise
    medicine is awarded by the President of the *Conseil national de l'Ordre des
    Médecins* and the *Ministère de la Santé publique* to graduates of a recog-
    nized medical school on presentation of their citizenship papers.
    Foreigners require special authorization to practise.**
Work in government service after graduation: —
Agreements with other countries: —

FACULTE DE MEDECINE
UNIVERSITE D'ABIDJAN
BP V 166
ABIDJAN
Year instruction started: **1966**

CROATIA

Total population in 1995: **4 501 000**
Number of physicians per 100 000 population (1993): **201**
Number of medical schools: **2**
Duration of basic medical degree course, including practical training: **6 years**
Title of degree awarded: —
Medical registration/licence to practise: —
Work in government service after graduation: —
Agreements with other countries: —

MEDICINSKI FAKULTET
SVEUCILISTA U RIJECI
UL. BRACE BRANCHETTA 20
RIJEKA 51000
Tel.: +385 (51) 514 790
Fax: +385 (51) 514 790/227 856
Year instruction started: **1955**
Language of instruction: **Croatian, Italian, English**
Duration of basic medical degree course, including practical training: **6 years**
Entrance examination: **Yes**
Foreign students eligible: **Yes**

MEDICINSKI FAKULTET
SVEUCILISTA U ZAGREBU
SALATA 3
ZAGREB 10000
Tel.: +385 (1) 456 6909
Fax: +385 (1) 456 6724
Year instruction started: **1917**
Language of instruction: **Croatian**
Duration of basic medical degree course, including practical training: **6 years**
Entrance examination: **Yes**
Foreign students eligible: **Yes**

CUBA

Total population in 1995: **11 018 000**
Number of physicians per 100 000 population (1993): **518**
Number of medical schools: **13**
Duration of basic medical degree course, including practical training: **6 years**
Title of degree awarded: *Doctor en Medicina* (Doctor of Medicine)
Medical registration/licence to practise: **Registration is obligatory with the
    Ministerio de Salud Pública, Calle 23 y N, Vedado, Habana. Physicians
    should provide a copy of their qualifications from the university con-
    cerned. Those who have qualified abroad must have their degree validated
    by the competent authorities. Foreigners must receive authorization from
    the Ministry of Public Health to practise.**
Work in government service after graduation: **Obligatory**
Agreements with other countries: —

INSTITUTO SUPERIOR DE CIENCIAS MEDICAS "CARLOS J. FINLAY"
CARRETERA CENTRAL OESTE Y MADAME CURIE
CAMAGUEY 70100
Tel.: +53 (7) 989 10
Fax: +53 (7) 615 87
E-mail: cpinf@finlay.sld.cu
Year instruction started: **1968**
Language of instruction: **Spanish**
Duration of basic medical degree course, including practical training: **6 years**
Entrance examination: **Yes**

FACULTAD DE CIENCIAS MEDICAS CIEGO DE AVILA
CIRCUNVALACION Y CARRETERA DE MORON
CIEGO DE AVILA 65100

FACULTAD DE CIENCIAS MEDICAS CIENFUEGOS
CALLE 51 ENTRE 36 Y 38
CIENFUEGOS 55100

FACULTAD DE CIENCIAS MEDICAS GUANTANAMO
CALLE 5 OESTE ENTRE 8 Y 9 NORTE
GUANTANAMO 95100

INSTITUTO SUPERIOR DE CIENCIAS MEDICAS DE LA HABANA
CALLE 146 Y AVENIDA 31
PLAYA
HABANA 11600
Tel.: +53 (7) 218 545
Fax: +53 (7) 336 257
Year instruction started: **1726**
Language of instruction: **Spanish**, **English**
Duration of basic medical degree course, including practical training: **6 years**
Entrance examination: **Yes**
Foreign students eligible: **Yes**

FACULTAD DE CIENCIAS MEDICAS HOLGUIN
AVENIDA LENIN NO. 4 ESQUINA A AGUILERA
HOLGUIN 80100

FACULTAD DE CIENCIAS MEDICAS LAS TUNAS
AVENIDA DE LA JUVENTUD S/N
LAS TUNAS 75100

FACULTAD DE CIENCIAS MEDICAS GRANMA "CELIA SANCHEZ MANDULAY"
AVENIDA CAMILO CIENFUEGAS
ESQUINA CARRETERA CAMPECHUELA
MANZANILLO 87510
E-mail: dec@golfo.grm.sld.cu, vdoc@golfo.grm.sld.cu
Year instruction started: **1982**
Language of instruction: **Spanish**
Duration of basic medical degree course, including practical training: **6 years**
Entrance examination: **Yes**
Foreign students eligible: **Yes**

FACULTAD DE CIENCIAS MEDICAS MATANZAS
CARRETERA DE QUINTANILLA KM 101
MATANZAS 40100

FACULTAD DE CIENCIAS MEDICAS PINAR DEL RIO
CARRETERA CENTRAL KM 89
PINAR DEL RIO 20100

FACULTAD DE CIENCIAS MEDICAS SANCTI SPIRITUS
CARRETERA CIRCUNVALACION NORTE
BANDA
SANCTI SPIRITUS 60100

INSTITUTO SUPERIOR DE CIENCIAS MEDICAS DE VILLA CLARA
CARRETERA DE ACUEDUCTO Y CIRCUNVALACION
SANTA CLARA 50200
Year instruction started: **1966**

INSTITUTO SUPERIOR DE CIENCIAS MEDICAS DE SANTIAGO DE CUBA
AVENIDA DE LAS AMERICAS Y CALLE E
SANTIAGO DE CUBA 90100
Year instruction started: **1962**

CZECH REPUBLIC

Total population in 1995: **10 251 000**
Number of physicians per 100 000 population (1993): **293**
Number of medical schools: 7
Duration of basic medical degree course, including practical training: **6 years**
Title of degree awarded: ***Doktor Vseobecné Medicíny, Zkratka (M.U.Dr.)*** **(General Practitioner)**

Medical registration/licence to practise: **The licence to practise medicine is granted by the Czech Medical Chamber to medical graduates who have completed the first- and second-level postgraduate professional examination. Graduates of foreign medical schools must have their degree validated and may be required to take a further examination and a language examination.**

Work in government service after graduation: **Obligatory (2 years)**

Agreements with other countries: **Bilateral and multilateral agreements exist with a number of countries.**

LEKARSKA FAKULTA
MASARYKOVY UNIVERZITY V BRNO
KOMENSKEHO NAM. 2
662 43 BRNO
Tel.: +420 (5) 421 264 90
Fax: +420 (5) 421 262 00
E-mail: dmala@med.muni.cz
Year instruction started: **1919**
Language of instruction: **Czech, English**
Duration of basic medical degree course, including practical training: **6 years**
Entrance examination: **Yes**
Foreign students eligible: **Yes**

LEKARSKA FAKULTA
UNIVERZITY KARLOVY V HRADCI KRALOVE
SIMKOVA 870
500 38 HRADEC KRALOVE
Tel.: +420 (49) 581 6242
Fax: +420 (49) 551 3597
Year instruction started: **1945**
Language of instruction: **Czech, English**
Duration of basic medical degree course, including practical training: **6 years**
Entrance examination: **Yes**
Foreign students eligible: **Yes**

LEKARSKA FAKULTA
UNIVERSITA PALACKEHO
TR SVOBODY 8
771 26 OLOMOUC
Tel.: +420 (68) 522 3907
Fax: +420 (68) 522 3907
E-mail: dekan@risc.upol.cz

Year instruction started: **1573**
Language of instruction: **Czech, English**
Duration of basic medical degree course, including practical training: **6 years**
Entrance examination: **Yes**
Foreign students eligible: **Yes**

LEKARSKA FAKULTA
UNIVERZITY KARLOVY V PLZNI
HUSOVA 13
306 05 PLZEN
Tel.: +420 (19) 722 1200
Fax: +420 (19) 722 1460
E-mail: veda@lfp.cuni.cz
Year instruction started: **1945**
Language of instruction: **Czech, English**
Duration of basic medical degree course, including practical training: **6 years**
Entrance examination: **Yes**
Foreign students eligible: **Yes**

LEKARSKA FAKULTA 1
UNIVERZITY KARLOVY
KATERINSKA 32
121 08 PRAHA 2
Tel.: +420 (2) 295 270
Fax: +420 (2) 295 270
E-mail: studij@lf1.cuni.cz
Year instruction started: **1348**
Language of instruction: **Czech, English**
Duration of basic medical degree course, including practical training: **6 years**
Entrance examination: **Yes**
Foreign students eligible: **Yes**

LEKARSKA FAKULTA 2
UNIVERZITY KARLOVY
V UVALU 84
150 18 PRAHA 5
Tel.: +420 (2) 244 311 11/244 358 00/244 358 01
Fax: +420 (2) 244 358 20
E-mail: dean.office@lfmotol.cuni.cz
Year instruction started: **1953**
Language of instruction: **Czech, English**
Duration of basic medical degree course, including practical training: **6 years**
Entrance examination: **Yes**
Foreign students eligible: **Yes**

LEKARSKA FAKULTA 3
UNIVERZITY KARLOVY
RUSKA 87
100 00 PRAHA 10
Tel.: +420 (2) 673 118 12/673 167 10/673 122 33
Fax: +420 (2) 673 118 12/671 022 33
Year instruction started: **1348**
Language of instruction: **Czech, English**
Duration of basic medical degree course, including practical training: **6 years**
Entrance examination: **Yes**
Foreign students eligible: **Yes**

DEMOCRATIC PEOPLE'S REPUBLIC OF KOREA

Total population in 1995: **22 466 000**
Number of physicians per 100 000 population (1993): —
Number of medical schools: **10**
Duration of basic medical degree course, including practical training: **6 years**
Title of degree awarded: **Doctor**
Medical registration/licence to practise: —
Work in government service after graduation: —
Agreements with other countries: —

CHONGJIN MEDICAL UNIVERSITY
SUBUKDONG
POHANG DISTRICT
CHONGJIN
Year instruction started: **1948**

HAEJU MEDICAL UNIVERSITY
KWANGSOKDONG
HAEJU
Year instruction started: **1959**

HAMHUNG MEDICAL UNIVERSITY
RIHWADONG
HOESANG DISTRICT
HAMHUNG
Year instruction started: **1946**

HYESAN MEDICAL UNIVERSITY
SINAMDONG
HYESAN
Year instruction started: **1971**

KANGGYE MEDICAL UNIVERSITY
SOCHONDONG
KANGGYE
Year instruction started: **1969**

PYONGSONG MEDICAL UNIVERSITY
OKJONDONG
PYONGSONG
Year instruction started: **1972**

PYONGYANG MEDICAL UNIVERSITY
RYONHWADONG
CENTRAL DISTRICT
PYONGYANG
Year instruction started: **1948**

SARIWON MEDICAL UNIVERSITY
UNHADONG
SARIWON
Year instruction started: **1971**

SINUIJU MEDICAL UNIVERSITY
PYONGHWADONG
SINUIJU
Year instruction started: **1969**

WONSAN MEDICAL UNIVERSITY
WAUDONG
WONSAN
Year instruction started: **1971**

DEMOCRATIC REPUBLIC OF THE CONGO

Total population in 1995: **46 812 000**
Number of physicians per 100 000 population (1993): —
Number of medical schools: **3**
Duration of basic medical degree course, including practical training: **6 or 7 years**
Title of degree awarded: ***Docteur en Medécine, Chirurgie et Accouchement***
      (Doctor of Medicine, Surgery and Midwifery)
Medical registration/licence to practise: —
Work in government service after graduation: —
Agreements with other countries: —

FACULTE DE MEDECINE
UNIVERSITE DE KINSHASA
BP 834
KINSHASA
Year instruction started: **1954**

FACULTE DE MEDECINE
UNIVERSITE DE KISANGANI
BP 2012
KISANGANI
Year instruction started: **1983**

FACULTE DE MEDECINE
UNIVERSITE DE LUBUMBASHI
BP 1825
LUBUMBASHI
Tel.: +243 (222) 3315
Year instruction started: **1956**
Language of instruction: **French, English**
Duration of basic medical degree course, including practical training: **7 years**
Entrance examination: **Yes**
Foreign students eligible: **Yes**

DENMARK

Total population in 1995: **5 237 000**
Number of physicians per 100 000 population (1993): **283**
Number of medical schools: **3**
Duration of basic medical degree course, including practical training: **6.5 years**
Title of degree awarded: *Candidatus medicinae* **(cand. med.); Doctor of Medicine**
Medical registration/licence to practise: **The licence to practise medicine is granted by the National Board of Health, PO Box 2020, DK-1012 Copenhagen K.**
Work in government service after graduation: **Not obligatory**
Agreements with other countries: **An agreement exists with other countries of the European Union (Directive 93/16/EEC governing the employment of doctors).**

DET SUNDHEDSVIDENSKABELIGE FAKULTET
AARHUS UNIVERSITET
VENNELYST BOULEVARD 9
DK-8000 AARHUS C
Year instruction started: **1934**

DET SUNDHEDSVIDENSKABELIGE FAKULTET
KOBENHAVNS UNIVERSITET
PANUM INSTITUTET
BLEGDAMSVEJ 3 C
DK-2200 KOBENHAVN N
Year instruction started: **1736**

DET SUNDHEDSVIDENSKABELIGE FAKULTET
ODENSE UNIVERSITET
WINSLOWPARKEN 15, 1 SAL
DK-5230 ODENSE C
Year instruction started: **1966**

DJIBOUTI

Total population in 1995: **617 000**
Number of physicians per 100 000 population (1993): **20**
Number of medical schools: **None**
Medical registration/licence to practise: **Registration is obligatory with the** *Ordre des Médecins, Djibouti.* **The licence to practise medicine is issued by the** *Ministère de la Santé publique et des Affaires sociales, BP 1974, Djibouti,* **to graduates of a recognized medical school. Foreigners must receive authorization to practise.**
Work in government service after graduation: **Not obligatory**
Agreements with other countries: —

DOMINICA

Total population in 1995: **71 000**
Number of physicians per 100 000 population (1993): **46**
Number of medical schools: **1**
Duration of basic medical degree course, including practical training: **5 years**
Title of degree awarded: **Doctor of Medicine**
Medical registration/licence to practise: **Registration is obligatory with the Dominica Medical Board, Ministry of Health, Roseau. The licence to practise medicine is granted to graduates of a recognized medical school who have completed an additional 18-month internship after graduation. Foreigners must have evidence of an offer of employment.**
Work in government service after graduation: **Obligatory (18 months)**
Agreements with other countries: **None**

SCHOOL OF MEDICINE
ROSS UNIVERSITY
PO BOX 266
ROSEAU
Tel.: +1 (767) 445 5355/(212) 279 5500
Fax: +1 (767) 445 5583/(212) 629 3147
Year instruction started: **1978**
Language of instruction: **English**
Duration of basic medical degree course, including practical training: **5 years**
Entrance examination: **No**
Foreign students eligible: **Yes**

DOMINICAN REPUBLIC

Total population in 1995: **7 961 000**
Number of physicians per 100 000 population (1993): **77**
Number of medical schools: **10**
Duration of basic medical degree course, including practical training: **4–7 years (a
    further 2 years of supervised clinical practice is required before the degree
    is awarded)**
Title of degree awarded: *Doctor en Medicina* (Doctor of Medicine)
Medical registration/licence to practise: **The licence to practise medicine is
    granted by the *Secretaria de Estado de Salud Pública, Avenida San Cristóbal
    esquina Avenida Tiradentes, Santo Domingo*. All graduates must complete 1
    year of social service in a rural area and have their degree validated by a
    recognized university in the Dominican Republic.**
Work in government service after graduation: **Obligatory (1 year in a rural area)**
Agreements with other countries: —

ESCUELA DE MEDICINA
UNIVERSIDAD TECNOLOGICA DEL CIBAO (UTECI)
LA VEGA
Year instruction started: **1983**

FACULTAD DE CIENCIAS MEDICAS
UNIVERSIDAD NORDESTANA (UNNE)
27 DE FEBRERO ESO. RESTAURACION
APDO 239
SAN FRANCISCO DE MACORIS
Tel.: +1809 588 3239/588 3505/588 3151
Fax: +1809 244 1647

Year instruction started: **1978**
Language of instruction: **Spanish**
Duration of basic medical degree course, including practical training: **5 years**
Entrance examination: **Yes**
Foreign students eligible: **Yes**

ESCUELA DE MEDICINA
FACULTAD DE CIENCIAS MEDICAS
UNIVERSIDAD CENTRAL DEL ESTE (UCE)
AVENIDA DE CIRCUNVALACION
SAN PEDRO DE MACORIS
Year instruction started: **1970**

DEPARTAMENTO DE MEDICINA
FACULTAD DE CIENCIAS DE LA SALUD
PONTIFICIA UNIVERSIDAD CATOLICA MADRE Y MAESTRA (PUCMM)
AUTOPISTO DUARTE KM 1 1/2
APDO 822
SANTIAGO DE LOS CABALLEROS
Tel.: +1809 580 1962
Fax: +1809 582 4549
Year instruction started: **1976**
Language of instruction: **Spanish**
Duration of basic medical degree course, including practical training: **5 years**
Entrance examination: **No**
Foreign students eligible: **Yes**

ESCUELA DE MEDICINA
UNIVERSIDAD TECNOLOGICA DE SANTIAGO (UTESA)
EDIFICIO CURIEL
AVENIDA CENTRAL
SANTIAGO DE LOS CABALLEROS
Year instruction started: **1982**

ESCUELA DE MEDICINA
FACULTAD DE CIENCIAS DE LA SALUD
INSTITUTO TECNOLOGICO DE SANTO DOMINGO (INTEC)
AVENIDA DE LOS PROCERES
GALA
APDO 342-9/249-2
SANTO DOMINGO

Tel.: +1809 567 9271
Fax: +1809 566 3200
Telex: 4184 intec dr
E-mail: intecl!lucero@redid.edu.do
Year instruction started: **1972**
Language of instruction: **Spanish**
Duration of basic medical degree course, including practical training: **5 years**
Entrance examination: **No**
Foreign students eligible: **Yes**

DEPARTAMENTO DE MEDICINA
FACULTAD DE CIENCIAS DE LA SALUD
UNIVERSIDAD AUTONOMA DE SANTO DOMINGO (UASD)
CIUDAD UNIVERSITARIA
SANTO DOMINGO
Year instruction started: **1600**

ESCUELA DE MEDICINA
UNIVERSIDAD IBEROAMERICANA (UNIBE)
AVENIDA FRANCIA 129
APDO 22233
SANTO DOMINGO
Tel.: +1809 689 4111
Fax: +1809 686 5533
E-mail: unibe!castagnoc@redid.edu.do
Year instruction started: **1982**
Language of instruction: **Spanish, English**
Duration of basic medical degree course, including practical training: **7 years**
Entrance examination: **Yes**
Foreign students eligible: **Yes**

ESCUELA DE MEDICINA
UNIVERSIDAD NACIONAL "PEDRO HENRIQUEZ URENA" (UNPHU)
AVENIDA JOHN F. KENNEDY KM 5 1/2
APDO 1423
SANTO DOMINGO
Tel.: +1809 562 6601
Fax: +1809 563 2254
Year instruction started: **1966**
Language of instruction: **Spanish**
Duration of basic medical degree course, including practical training: **4 years**
Entrance examination: **Yes**
Foreign students eligible: **Yes**

ESCUELA DE MEDICINA
FACULTAD DE CIENCIAS DE LA SALUD
UNIVERSIDAD TECNOLOGICA DE SANTIAGO (UTESA)
ISABEL AGUIAR 61
HERRERA
APDO 21243
SANTO DOMINGO
Tel.: +1809 530 1080/221 6221
Fax: +1809 682 0200
Year instruction started: **1981**
Language of instruction: **Spanish, English**
Duration of basic medical degree course, including practical training: **4 years**
Entrance examination: **No**
Foreign students eligible: **Yes**

ECUADOR

Total population in 1995: **11 699 000**
Number of physicians per 100 000 population (1993): **111**
Number of medical schools: **8**
Duration of basic medical degree course, including practical training: **6–8 years**
Title of degree awarded: ***Doctor en Medicina y Cirugía* (Doctor of Medicine and Surgery)**
Medical registration/licence to practise: **Registration is obligatory with the *Colegio Médico de Pichincha*. The licence to practise medicine is granted by the Ministry of Public Health, *Juan Larrea 446 entre Checa y Riofrio*, Quito, to graduates who have completed 1 year of service in a rural area. Those who have qualified abroad must also have their degree validated by a university in Ecuador.**
Work in government service after graduation: **Obligatory (1 year in a rural area)**
Agreements with other countries: **Agreements exist with Argentina, China and Spain.**

FACULTAD DE MEDICINA Y CIENCIAS DE LA SALUD
UNIVERSIDAD CATOLICA DE CUENCA
PIO BRAVO 2-52 Y MANUEL VEGA
CASILLA 19A
CUENCA
Tel.: +593 (7) 830 752
Fax: +593 (7) 838 011

Year instruction started: **1977**
Language of instruction: **Spanish, English**
Duration of basic medical degree course, including practical training: **7 years**
Entrance examination: **No**
Foreign students eligible: **Yes**

FACULTAD DE CIENCIAS MEDICAS
UNIVERSIDAD DE CUENCA
AVENIDA EL PARAISO S/N
C.P. 01 01 1891
CUENCA
Tel.: +593 (7) 811 002
Fax: +593 (7) 881 406
Year instruction started: **1870**

FACULTAD DE MEDICINA
UNIVERSIDAD CATOLICA DE SANTIAGO DE GUAYAQUIL
AVENIDA CARLOS JULIO AROSEMENA KM 1.5
CASILLA 09-01-4671
GUAYAQUIL
Tel.: +593 (4) 200 906/286 265
Fax: +593 (4) 200 127
Year instruction started: **1968**
Language of instruction: **Spanish**
Duration of basic medical degree course, including practical training: **7 years**
Entrance examination: **Yes**
Foreign students eligible: **Yes**

FACULTAD DE CIENCIAS MEDICAS
UNIVERSIDAD DE GUAYAQUIL
CIUDAD UNIVERSITARIA SALVADOR ALLENDE
CASILLA 5852
GUAYAQUIL
Tel.: +593 (4) 281 047
Fax: +593 (4) 281 047
Year instruction started: **1867**

FACULTAD CIENCIAS MEDICAS
UNIVERSIDAD NACIONAL DE LOJA
CASILLA 349
LOJA
Tel.: +593 (7) 571 379
Fax: +593 (7) 573 478
Year instruction started: **1969**

FACULTAD CIENCIAS DE LA SALUD
UNIVERSIDAD TECNICA DE MANABI
AVENIDA UNIVERSITARIA
PORTOVIEJO
MANABI
Tel.: +593 (5) 631 291
Fax: +593 (5) 631 291
Year instruction started: **1992**
Language of instruction: **Spanish**
Duration of basic medical degree course, including practical training: **8 years**
Entrance examination: **Yes**
Foreign students eligible: **Yes**

FACULTAD DE CIENCIAS MEDICAS
UNIVERSIDAD CENTRAL DEL ECUADOR
SODIRO Y IQUIQUE
CASILLA 6120
QUITO
Tel.: +593 (2) 526 024
Fax: +593 (2) 526 530
E-mail: red@bicme.ecx.ec
Year instruction started: **1826**
Language of instruction: **Spanish**
Duration of basic medical degree course, including practical training: **7 years**
Entrance examination: **No**
Foreign students eligible: **Yes**

COLEGIO DE CIENCIAS DE LA SALUD
UNIVERSIDAD SAN FRANCISCO DE QUITO
CAMPUS CUMBAYA
VIA INTEROCEANICA Y ENTRADA A JARDINES DEL ESTE
CASILLA 17-12-841
QUITO
Tel.: +593 (2) 895 723
Fax: +593 (2) 890 070
E-mail: med@mail.usfq.edu.ec
Year instruction started: **1994**
Language of instruction: **Spanish, English**
Duration of basic medical degree course, including practical training: **6 years**
Entrance examination: **Yes**
Foreign students eligible: **Yes**

EGYPT

Total population in 1995: **63 271 000**
Number of physicians per 100 000 population (1993): **202**
Number of medical schools: **12**
Duration of basic medical degree course, including practical training: **6 or 7 years
(a further year of supervised clinical practice is required before the degree
is awarded)**
Title of degree awarded: **Bachelor of Medicine and Surgery**
Medical registration/licence to practise: **Registration is obligatory with the
General Medical Association and the Ministry of Health and Population,
Cairo. The licence to practise medicine is granted to graduates who have
obtained a diploma or a Master's degree in a specialization. Graduates of
foreign medical schools must also have their degree validated. Foreigners
are not entitled to practise.**
Work in government service after graduation: **Obligatory (2 years)**
Agreements with other countries: **Agreements exist with a number of African,
Arab and European countries.**

FACULTY OF MEDICINE
UNIVERSITY OF ALEXANDRIA
ALEXANDRIA
Tel.: +20 (3) 482 7426
Fax: +20 (3) 483 3076
Year instruction started: **1942**
Language of instruction: **English**
Duration of basic medical degree course, including practical training: **7 years**
Entrance examination: **No**
Foreign students eligible: **Yes**

FACULTY OF MEDICINE
UNIVERSITY OF ASYUT
ASYUT
Year instruction started: **1960**

BENHA FACULTY OF MEDICINE
ZAGAZIG UNIVERSITY
BENHA 13518
Tel.: +20 (213) 227 518
Fax: +20 (213) 227 518
Year instruction started: **1986**
Language of instruction: **English**
Duration of basic medical degree course, including practical training: **6 years**
Entrance examination: **No**
Foreign students eligible: **Yes**

FACULTY OF MEDICINE
AIN SHAMS UNIVERSITY
ABBASSIA
CAIRO
Year instruction started: **1948**

FACULTY OF MEDICINE
AL-AZHAR UNIVERSITY
MADINET NASR
ABBASSIA
CAIRO
Year instruction started: **1965**

FACULTY OF MEDICINE
UNIVERSITY OF CAIRO
CAIRO
Year instruction started: **1827**

FACULTY OF MEDICINE
SUEZ CANAL UNIVERSITY
CIRCULAR ROAD
EZ EL-DIN
ISMAILIA 41522
Tel.: +20 (64) 226 539/381 496
Fax: +20 (64) 328 543
Year instruction started: **1980**
Language of instruction: **English**
Duration of basic medical degree course, including practical training: **6 years**
Entrance examination: **No**
Foreign students eligible: **No**

FACULTY OF MEDICINE
UNIVERSITY OF MANSURA
MANSURA
Year instruction started: **1962**

FACULTY OF MEDICINE
UNIVERSITY OF MINYA
MINYA
Year instruction started: **1984**

FACULTY OF MEDICINE
MENOUFIA UNIVERSITY
SHIBIN EL KOM
Year instruction started: **1984**

TANTA FACULTY OF MEDICINE
TANTA
Year instruction started: **1962**

FACULTY OF MEDICINE
ZAGAZIG UNIVERSITY
ZAGAZIG
Tel.: +20 (55) 322 809
Fax: +20 (55) 327 830
Year instruction started: **1970**
Language of instruction: **English**
Duration of basic medical degree course, including practical training: **6 years**
Entrance examination: **Yes**
Foreign students eligible: **No**

EL SALVADOR

Total population in 1995: **5 796 000**
Number of physicians per 100 000 population (1993): **91**
Number of medical schools: **6**
Duration of basic medical degree course, including practical training: **7 or 8 years
(a further year of supervised clinical practice is required before the degree
is awarded)**
Title of degree awarded: ***Doctor en Medicina*** (Doctor of Medicine)
Medical registration/licence to practise: **The licence to practise medicine is
granted by the *Junta de Vigilancia de la Profesión Médica, Avenida España
736, San Salvador*. Nationals and foreigners who have qualified in El
Salvador must have completed 1 year of social service before the degree is
awarded. Foreigners must have a residence permit and be officially linked
to a university.**
Work in government service after graduation: **Obligatory (1 year)**
Agreements with other countries: —

FACULTAD DE MEDICINA
UNIVERSIDAD EVANGELICA DE EL SALVADOR
63 AVENIDA SUR Y PASAJE 138
APDO 1789
SAN SALVADOR
Tel.: +503 223 7378/245 1988/245 1992
Fax: +503 223 7378/245 1988/245 1992

Year instruction started: **1981**
Language of instruction: **Spanish**
Duration of basic medical degree course, including practical training: **7 years**
Entrance examination: **Yes**
Foreign students eligible: **Yes**

FACULTAD DE MEDICINA
UNIVERSIDAD NACIONAL
PEDRO HENRIQUEZ URENA HOSPITAL ROSALES
FINAL C. ARCE
SAN SALVADOR

ESCUELA DE MEDICINA
FACULTAD DE CIENCIAS DE LA SALUD
UNIVERSIDAD NUEVA SAN SALVADOR
CALLE ARCE Y 23 AVENIDA SUR 1243
APDO 2596
SAN SALVADOR
Tel.: +503 221 2288
Fax: +503 221 2729
Year instruction started: **1982**
Language of instruction: **Spanish**
Duration of basic medical degree course, including practical training: **7 years**
Entrance examination: **No**
Foreign students eligible: **Yes**

FACULTAD DE MEDICINA Y CIRUGIA
UNIVERSIDAD SALVADORENA ALBERTO MASFERRER
19A AVENIDA NORTE ENTRE 3A C/PONIENTE Y ALAMEDA JUAN PABLO II
APDO 2053
SAN SALVADOR
Tel.: +503 221 1136/221 1137
Fax: +503 222 8006
Year instruction started: **1981**
Language of instruction: **Spanish**
Duration of basic medical degree course, including practical training: **7 years**
Entrance examination: **Yes**
Foreign students eligible: **Yes**

FACULTAD DE MEDICINA
UNIVERSIDAD AUTONOMA DE SANTA ANA
SANTA ANA

UNIVERSIDAD DR JOSE MATIAS DELGADO
CARRETERA A SANTA TECLA
KM 8.5 CIUDAD MERLIOT
SANTA TECLA

ESTONIA

Total population in 1995: **1 471 000**
Number of physicians per 100 000 population (1993): **312**
Number of medical schools: **1**
Duration of basic medical degree course, including practical training: **6 years**
Title of degree awarded: —
Medical registration/licence to practise: —
Work in government service after graduation: —
Agreements with other countries: —

TARTU ULIKOOL ARSTITEADUSKOND
VESKI 63
TARTU 2400
Tel.: +372 (7) 465 320
Fax: +372 (7) 465 326
Year instruction started: **1632**
Language of instruction: **Estonian, Russian, English**
Duration of basic medical degree course, including practical training: **6 years**
Entrance examination: **Yes**
Foreign students eligible: **Yes**

ETHIOPIA

Total population in 1995: **58 243 000**
Number of physicians per 100 000 population (1993): **4**
Number of medical schools: **3**
Duration of basic medical degree course, including practical training: **6 years (a
    further period of 1 year of supervised clinical practice is required before
    the degree is awarded)**
Title of degree awarded: **Doctor of Medicine**
Medical registration/licence to practise: **Registration is obligatory with the
    Ministry of Health, PO Box 1234, Addis Ababa.**
Work in government service after graduation: **Obligatory**
Agreements with other countries: **None**

FACULTY OF MEDICINE
ADDIS ABABA UNIVERSITY
PO BOX 1176
ADDIS ABABA
Year instruction started: **1965**

GONDAR COLLEGE OF MEDICAL SCIENCES
ADDIS ABABA UNIVERSITY
GONDAR
Year instruction started: **1978**

JIMMA TENA SAYNS ENSTITUTE
PO BOX 378
JIMMA
Tel.: +251 (7) 111 457/111 458
Fax: +251 (7) 110 575
Year instruction started: **1984**
Language of instruction: **English**
Duration of basic medical degree course, including practical training: **6 years**

FIJI

Total population in 1995: **797 000**
Number of physicians per 100 000 population (1993): **38**
Number of medical schools: **1**
Duration of basic medical degree course, including practical training: **6 years**
Title of degree awarded: **Bachelor of Medicine and Surgery (MB, BS)**
Medical registration/licence to practise: **Registration is obligatory with the Fiji Medical Council, Ministry of Health, Suva. The licence to practise medicine is granted to graduates of a recognized medical school who have completed a 1-year internship. Those who have graduated abroad must hold a contract with the Government.**
Work in government service after graduation: **Obligatory**
Agreements with other countries: —

FIJI SCHOOL OF MEDICINE
BROWN STREET
PRIVATE MAIL BAG
SUVA GPO
Tel.: +679 311 00
Fax: +679 303 69

Year instruction started: **1885**
Language of instruction: **English**
Duration of basic medical degree course, including practical training: **6 years**
Entrance examination: **Yes**
Foreign students eligible: **No**

FINLAND

Total population in 1995: **5 126 000**
Number of physicians per 100 000 population (1993): **269**
Number of medical schools: **5**
Duration of basic medical degree course, including practical training: **6 years**
Title of degree awarded: ***Lääketieteen lisensiaatti*** (Licenciate in Medicine)
Medical registration/licence to practise: **Registration is obligatory with the National Board of Medicolegal Affairs, Siltasaarenkatu 18 C, FIN-00530 Helsinki 53. The licence to practise medicine is granted to medical graduates on completion of 2 years of practical training. Graduates of foreign medical schools must pass 3 examinations (theoretical, clinical and administrative) and undergo an additional 6 months of training.**
Work in government service after graduation: —
Agreements with other countries: **Agreements exist with other countries of the European Union (Directive 93/16/EEC governing the employment of doctors) and with other Nordic countries.**

LAAKETIETEELLINEN TIEDEKUNTA
HELSINGIN YLIOPISTO
TOOLONTULLINKATU 8
PO BOX 20
FIN-00014 HELSINKI
Tel.: +358 (9) 434 61
Fax: +358 (9) 434 6629
Year instruction started: **1640**
Language of instruction: **Finnish, Swedish, English**
Duration of basic medical degree course, including practical training: **6 years**
Entrance examination: **Yes**
Foreign students eligible: **Yes**

LAAKETIETEELLINEN TIEDEKUNTA
KUOPION YLIOPISTO
SAVILAHDENTIG 9 JA HARJULANTIE 1
PO BOX 6
FIN-70210 KUOPIO
Year instruction started: **1972**

LAAKETIETEELLINEN TIEDEKUNTA
OULUN YLIOPISTO
KAJAANINTIE 52A
FIN-90230 OULU
Year instruction started: **1960**

LAAKETIETEELLINEN TIEDEKUNTA
TAMPEREEN YLIOPISTO
PO BOX 607
FIN-33101 TAMPERE
Year instruction started: **1972**

LAAKETIETEELLINEN TIEDEKUNTA
TURUN YLIOPISTO
KIINAMYLLYNKATU 13
PO BOX 25
FIN-20520 TURKU
Tel.: +358 (2) 333 51
Fax: +358 (2) 333 8413
Year instruction started: **1943**
Language of instruction: **Finnish**
Duration of basic medical degree course, including practical training: **6 years**
Entrance examination: **Yes**
Foreign students eligible: **Yes**

FRANCE

Total population in 1995: **58 333 000**
Number of physicians per 100 000 population (1993): **280**
Number of medical schools: **45**
Duration of basic medical degree course, including practical training: **8 or 8.5 years**
Title of degree awarded: ***Diplôme d'État de Docteur en Médecine*** (Doctor of Medicine (State Diploma)); ***Diplôme d'Université de Docteur en Médecine*** (Doctor of Medicine (University Diploma)) (awarded to foreign students who do not hold the French *Baccalauréat*)
Medical registration/licence to practise: —
Work in government service after graduation: —
Agreements with other countries: **An agreement exists with other countries of the European Union (Directive 93/16/EEC governing the employment of doctors).**

FACULTE DE MEDECINE
UNIVERSITE DE PICARDIE
3 RUE DES LOUVELS
F-80036 AMIENS CEDEX 1
Fax: +33 (3) 228 277 60
Year instruction started: **1804**

FACULTE DE MEDECINE
UNIVERSITE D'ANGERS
1 RUE HAUTE DE RECULEE
F-49045 ANGERS CEDEX
Fax: +33 (2) 417 358 81
Year instruction started: **1432**

UFR DE SCIENCES MEDICALES ET PHARMACEUTIQUES
UNIVERSITE DE BESANCON
4 PLACE SAINT JACQUES
F-25030 BESANCON CEDEX
Fax: +33 (3) 816 655 27
Year instruction started: **1806**

UFR DE MEDECINE ET DE BIOLOGIE HUMAINE "LEONARD DE VINCI"
UNIVERSITE DE PARIS XIII
74 RUE MARCEL CACHIN
F-93012 BOBIGNY CEDEX
Tel.: +33 (1) 483 876 08
Fax: +33 (1) 483 877 77
Year instruction started: **1968**
Language of instruction: **French**
Duration of basic medical degree course, including practical training: **8 years**
Entrance examination: **No**
Foreign students eligible: **Yes**

FACULTE DE MEDECINE HYACINTHES-VINCENT
UNIVERSITE DE BORDEAUX
146 RUE LEO SAIGNAT
F-33076 BORDEAUX CEDEX
Tel.: +33 (5) 575 713 13
Fax: +33 (5) 575 715 89
Year instruction started: **1878**

FACULTE DE MEDECINE PAUL BROCA
UNIVERSITE DE BORDEAUX
146 RUE LEO SAIGNAT
F-33076 BORDEAUX CEDEX
Tel.: +33 (5) 575 711 51
Fax: +33 (5) 575 715 89
Year instruction started: **1878**

FACULTE DE MEDECINE VICTOR PACHON
UNIVERSITE DE BORDEAUX
146 RUE LEO SAIGNAT
F-33076 BORDEAUX CEDEX
Tel.: +33 (5) 575 713 13
Fax: +33 (5) 575 715 89
Year instruction started: **1878**

FACULTE DE MEDECINE
UNIVERSITE DE BREST
22 AVENUE CAMILLE DESMOULINS
BP 815
F-29285 BREST CEDEX
Tel.: +33 (2) 980 164 20
Fax: +33 (2) 980 164 74
Year instruction started: **1966**
Language of instruction: **French**
Duration of basic medical degree course, including practical training: **at least 8
    years**
Entrance examination: **No**
Foreign students eligible: **Yes**

FACULTE DE MEDECINE
UNIVERSITE DE CAEN
AVENUE DE LA COTE DE NACRE
F-14032 CAEN CEDEX
Tel.: +33 (2) 310 682 22
Fax: +33 (2) 310 682 05
Year instruction started: **1437**
Language of instruction: **French**
Duration of basic medical degree course, including practical training: **8 years**
Entrance examination: **No**
Foreign students eligible: **Yes**

FACULTE DE MEDECINE
UNIVERSITE DE CLERMONT-FERRAND
28 PLACE HENRI-DUNANT
BP 38
F-63001 CLERMONT-FERRAND CEDEX
Fax: +33 (4) 732 779 05
Year instruction started: **1681**

UFR DE CRETEIL
UNIVERSITE PARIS XII VAL-DE-MARNE
8 RUE DU GENERAL SARRAIL
F-94010 CRETEIL CEDEX
Tel.: +33 (1) 498 136 12/498 136 02
Fax: +33 (1) 498 136 81
Year instruction started: **1968**
Language of instruction: **French, English**
Duration of basic medical degree course, including practical training: **8 years**
Entrance examination: **Yes**
Foreign students eligible: **Yes**

FACULTE DE MEDECINE
UNIVERSITE DE BOURGOGNE
7 BOULEVARD JEANNE D'ARC
BP 138
F-21033 DIJON CEDEX
Tel.: +33 (3) 803 933 08
Fax: +33 (3) 803 933 00
Year instruction started: **1772**
Language of instruction: **French**
Duration of basic medical degree course, including practical training: **8 years**
Entrance examination: **No**
Foreign students eligible: **Yes**

FACULTE DE MEDECINE PARIS-OUEST
UNIVERSITE RENE DESCARTES
104 BOULEVARD RAYMOND POINCARE
F-92380 GARCHES
Tel.: +33 (1) 474 108 37
Fax: +33 (1) 474 168 83
Year instruction started: **1969**

FACULTE DE MEDECINE
UFR DE MEDECINE KREMLIN-BICETRE
UNIVERSITE PARIS-SUD XI
63 RUE GABRIEL PERI
F-94276 KREMLIN-BICETRE CEDEX
Tel.: +33 (1) 495 966 00
Fax: +33 (1) 495 967 00
E-mail: fac.medecine@kb.4-psud.fr
Year instruction started: **1969**
Language of instruction: **French**
Duration of basic medical degree course, including practical training: **8 years**
Entrance examination: **Yes**
Foreign students eligible: **Yes**

FACULTE DE MEDECINE
UNIVERSITE SCIENTIFIQUE ET MEDICALE DE GRENOBLE
DOMAINE DE "LA MERCI"
F-38706 LA TRONCHE CEDEX
Tel.: +33 (4) 766 371 22
Fax: +33 (4) 766 371 70
Year instruction started: **1369**

FACULTE DE MEDECINE
HENRI WAREMBOURG UNIVERSITE DE LILLE II
1 PLACE DE VERDUN
F-59045 LILLE CEDEX
Tel.: +33 (3) 206 269 03
Fax: +33 (3) 206 268 68
Year instruction started: **1875**
Language of instruction: **French**
Duration of basic medical degree course, including practical training: **8 years**
Entrance examination: **No**
Foreign students eligible: **Yes**

FACULTE LIBRE DE MEDECINE DE LILLE
UNIVERSITE CATHOLIQUE DE LILLE
56 RUE DU PORT
F-59046 LILLE CEDEX
Tel.: +33 (3) 201 341 40
Fax: +33 (3) 201 341 31

Year instruction started: **1876**
Language of instruction: **French**
Duration of basic medical degree course, including practical training: **8 years**
Entrance examination: **No**
Foreign students eligible: **Yes**

FACULTE DE MEDECINE ET DE PHARMACIE
UNIVERSITE DE LIMOGES
2 RUE DU DOCTEUR MARCLAND
F-87025 LIMOGES CEDEX
Tel.: +33 (5) 554 358 03
Fax: +33 (5) 554 358 01
Year instruction started: **1841**

FACULTE DE MEDECINE ALEXIS CARREL
12 RUE GUILLAUME PARRADIN
F-69372 LYON CEDEX 08
Tel.: +33 (4) 787 786 05
Fax: +33 (4) 787 787 37

FACULTE DE MEDECINE GRANGE BLANCHE
UNIVERSITE CLAUDE BERNARD
8 AVENUE ROCKEFELLER
F-69373 LYON CEDEX 08
Tel.: +33 (4) 787 770 90
Fax: +33 (4) 787 772 11
Year instruction started: **1877**

FACULTE DE MEDECINE LYON-NORD
UNIVERSITE CLAUDE BERNARD
8 AVENUE ROCKEFELLER
F-69373 LYON CEDEX 08
Tel.: +33 (4) 787 770 79
Fax: +33 (4) 787 772 11
Year instruction started: **1877**

FACULTE DE MEDECINE-MARSEILLE
UNIVERSITE D'AIX-MARSEILLE
27 BOULEVARD JEAN MOULIN
F-13385 MARSEILLE CEDEX 05
Tel.: +33 (4) 918 345 11
Fax: +33 (4) 918 344 96

Year instruction started: **1557**
Language of instruction: **French**
Duration of basic medical degree course, including practical training: **8 years**
Entrance examination: **No**
Foreign students eligible: **Yes**

FACULTE DE MEDECINE
UNIVERSITE DE MONTPELLIER
2 RUE DE L'ECOLE DE MEDECINE
F-34060 MONTPELLIER CEDEX
Tel.: +33 (4) 676 010 04
Fax: +33 (4) 676 617 57
Year instruction started: **1180**

FACULTE DE MEDECINE
UNIVERSITE DE NANTES
1 RUE GASTON VEIL
BP 1024
F-44035 NANTES CEDEX
Tel.: +33 (2) 404 120 01
Fax: +33 (2) 404 128 09
Year instruction started: **1834**

FACULTE DE MEDECINE PASTEUR
UNIVERSITE DE NICE
AVENUE DE VALLOMBROSE
F-06107 NICE CEDEX 02
Tel.: +33 (4) 933 776 03
Fax: +33 (4) 933 776 03
Year instruction started: **1968**

FACULTE DE MEDECINE PIERRE BENITE
UNIVERSITE LYON-SUD
BP 12
F-69921 OULLINS CEDEX
Tel.: +33 (4) 788 631 03/788 631 05
Fax: +33 (4) 788 631 01

FACULTE DE MEDECINE NECKER-ENFANTS MALADES
UNIVERSITE DE PARIS
156 RUE DE VAUGIRARD
F-75730 PARIS CEDEX 15
Tel.: +33 (1) 406 153 53
Fax: +33 (1) 422 265 23

FACULTE DE MEDECINE SAINT-ANTOINE
UNIVERSITE DE PARIS
27 RUE DE CHALIGNY
F-75571 PARIS CEDEX 12
Tel.: +33 (1) 400 114 47
Fax: +33 (1) 400 114 99

UFR DE MEDECINE BIOMEDICALE
UNIVERSITE DE PARIS V
45 RUE DES SAINTS PERES
F-75270 PARIS CEDEX 06
Tel.: +33 (1) 428 622 22
Fax: +33 (1) 428 622 00

FACULTE DE MEDECINE LARIBOISIERE-SAINT-LOUIS
UNIVERSITE DE PARIS VII
10 AVENUE DE VERDUN
F-75010 PARIS
Tel.: +33 (1) 448 977 96
Fax: +33 (1) 408 978 00
Year instruction started: **1970**
Language of instruction: **French**
Duration of basic medical degree course, including practical training: **8 years**
Entrance examination: **Yes**
Foreign students eligible: **Yes**

FACULTE DE MEDECINE XAVIER BICHAT
UNIVERSITE DE PARIS VII
16 RUE HENRI HUCHARD
BP 416
F-75870 PARIS CEDEX 18
Tel.: +33 (1) 448 561 00
Fax: +33 (1) 422 651 81
Year instruction started: **1968**

FACULTE DE MEDECINE BROUSSAIS HOTEL-DIEU
UNIVERSITE DE PIERRE ET MARIE CURIE (PARIS VI)
15 RUE DE L'ECOLE DE MEDECINE
F-75270 PARIS CEDEX 06
Tel.: +33 (1) 432 928 00
Fax: +33 (1) 432 591 14

Year instruction started: **1969**
Language of instruction: **French**
Duration of basic medical degree course, including practical training: **at least 8 years**
Entrance examination: **No**
Foreign students eligible: **Yes**

FACULTE DE MEDECINE PITIE-SALPETRIERE
UNIVERSITE DE PIERRE ET MARIE CURIE (PARIS VI)
91 BOULEVARD DE L'HOPITAL
F-75634 PARIS CEDEX 13
Tel.: +33 (1) 407 795 60
Fax: +33 (1) 407 798 22
Year instruction started: **1966**

FACULTE DE MEDECINE COCHIN-PORT ROYAL
UNIVERSITE RENE DESCARTES (PARIS V)
24 RUE DU FAUBOURG SAINT-JACQUES
F-75674 PARIS CEDEX 14
Tel.: +33 (1) 444 122 01
Fax: +33 (1) 444 122 23
Year instruction started: **1967**

FACULTE DE MEDECINE DE GUADELOUPE
UNIVERSITE DES ANTILLES ET DE LA GUYANNE
BOULEVARD LEGITIMUS
BP 145
F-97154 POINTE-A-PITRE CEDEX
Tel.: +33 (590) 916 490
Fax: +33 (590) 914 259

FACULTE DE MEDECINE ET DE PHARMACIE
UNIVERSITE DE POITIERS
34 RUE DU JARDIN DES PLANTES
BP 199
F-86005 POITIERS CEDEX
Tel.: +33 (5) 494 543 02
Fax: +33 (5) 494 543 05
Year instruction started: **1431**
Language of instruction: **French**
Duration of basic medical degree course, including practical training: **8 years**
Entrance examination: **No**
Foreign students eligible: **Yes**

FACULTE DE MEDECINE
UNIVERSITE DE REIMS
51 RUE COGNACQ-JAY
F-51095 REIMS CEDEX
Tel.: +33 (3) 260 535 02
Fax: +33 (3) 260 587 06
Year instruction started: **1605**

FACULTE DE MEDECINE
UFR DES SCIENCES MEDICALES
UNIVERSITE DE RENNES
2 AVENUE PROFESSEUR LEON-BERNARD
F-35043 RENNES CEDEX
Tel.: +33 (2) 993 368 02
Fax: +33 (2) 995 413 96
E-mail: clauderioux@uni-rennes1.fr
Year instruction started: **1803**
Language of instruction: **French**
Duration of basic medical degree course, including practical training: **8 years**
Entrance examination: **Yes**
Foreign students eligible: **Yes**

FACULTE DE MEDECINE J LISFRANC
UNIVERSITE DE SAINT-ETIENNE
15 RUE AMBROISE PARE
F-42023 SAINT-ETIENNE CEDEX 2
Tel.: +33 (4) 774 214 03/774 214 04
Fax: +33 (4) 774 214 89
Year instruction started: **1969**

FACULTE DE MEDECINE
UFR DE MEDECINE ET DE PHARMACIE
UNIVERSITE DE ROUEN
AVENUE DE L'UNIVERSITE
BP 97
F-76803 SAINT-ETIENNE-DU-ROUVRAY
Tél.: +33 (2) 356 652 01
Fax: +33 (2) 356 655 75
Year instruction started: **1605**

FACULTE DE MEDECINE
UFR DE SCIENCES MEDICALES
UNIVERSITE DE LOUIS PASTEUR
4 RUE KIRSCHLEGER
F-67085 STRASBOURG CEDEX
Tel.: +33 (3) 883 587 02/883 587 03
Fax: +33 (3) 882 433 25
Year instruction started: **1538**

FACULTE DE MEDECINE PURPAN
UNIVERSITE DE TOULOUSE
37 ALLEE J GUESDES
F-31073 TOULOUSE CEDEX
Fax: +33 (5) 612 520 55

FACULTE DE MEDECINE DE RANGUEIL
UNIVERSITE PAUL SABATIER
133 ROUTE DE NARBONNE
F-31062 TOULOUSE CEDEX
Tel.: +33 (5) 615 323 13
Fax: +33 (5) 621 718 18
Year instruction started: **16th century**

FACULTE DE MEDECINE DE TOURS
UNIVERSITE FRANCOIS-RABELAIS
2 BIS BOULEVARD TONNELLE
BP 3223
F-37032 TOURS CEDEX
Tel.: +33 (2) 473 660 04
Fax: +33 (2) 473 660 99
Year instruction started: **13th century**
Language of instruction: **French**
Duration of basic medical degree course, including practical training: **8.5 years**
Entrance examination: **No**
Foreign students eligible: **Yes**

FACULTE DES SCIENCES MEDICALES
UNIVERSITE DE NANCY I
9 AVENUE DE LA FORET DE HAYE
BP 184
F-54505 VANDOEUVRE-LES-NANCY CEDEX
Tel.: +33 (3) 835 925 01
Fax: +33 (3) 835 925 03
Year instruction started: **1872**

GABON

Total population in 1995: **1 106 000**
Number of physicians per 100 000 population (1993): **19**
Number of medical schools: **1**
Duration of basic medical degree course, including practical training: **7 years**
Title of degree awarded: ***Docteur d'État en Médecine* (Doctor of Medicine)**
Medical registration/licence to practise: **Information on registration is available from the *Ordre des Médecins, Libreville.***
Work in government service after graduation: **Not obligatory**
Agreements with other countries: —

CENTRE UNIVERSITAIRE DES SCIENCES DE LA SANTE (CUSS)
BP 4009
LIBREVILLE
Year instruction started: **1973**

GAMBIA

Total population in 1995: **1 141 000**
Number of physicians per 100 000 population (1993): **2**
Number of medical schools: **None**
Medical registration/licence to practise: **Registration is obligatory with the Gambia Medical and Dental Council, Kanifing (next to the Post Office), Kombo St Mary's Division (KSMD). The licence to practise medicine is renewed annually and is granted to graduates who have completed a 2-year internship. Foreigners may be granted a temporary licence.**
Work in government service after graduation: **Not obligatory**
Agreements with other countries: **None**

GEORGIA

Total population in 1995: **5 442 000**
Number of physicians per 100 000 population (1993): **436**
Number of medical schools: **2**
Duration of basic medical degree course, including practical training: **6 or 7 years**
Title of degree awarded: —
Medical registration/licence to practise: —
Work in government service after graduation: —
Agreements with other countries: —

"AIETI" HIGHEST MEDICAL SCHOOL
29 VAZHA PSHAVELA AVENUE
TBILISI 380109
Tel.: +995 (32) 395 509
Fax: +995 (32) 932 396
Telex: 212280 aieti su
E-mail: tsk@who.ge
Year instruction started: **1991**
Language of instruction: **Georgian, English**
Duration of basic medical degree course, including practical training: **6 years**
Entrance examination: **Yes**
Foreign students eligible: **Yes**

TBILISI STATE MEDICAL UNIVERSITY
7 ASIATIANI STREET
TBILISI 380077
Tel.: +995 (32) 333 801
Telex: 212223 lazer su
E-mail: rima@ridmu.kheta.ge
Year instruction started: **1921**
Language of instruction: **Georgian, Russian, English**
Duration of basic medical degree course, including practical training: **7 years**
Entrance examination: **Yes**
Foreign students eligible: **Yes**

GERMANY

Total population in 1995: **81 922 000**
Number of physicians per 100 000 population (1993): **319**
Number of medical schools: **39**
Duration of basic medical degree course, including practical training: **6 or 6.5 years (a further 1.5 years of practical training is required before the degree is awarded)**
Title of degree awarded: ***Staatsexamen und Arzt im Praktikum*** **(State examination and completion of compulsory practical training)**
Medical registration/licence to practise: **Registration is obligatory with the** *Arztekammern der Länder* **(General Medical Council of the respective provinces). The licence to practise medicine is granted to graduates of recognized medical schools who have completed 18 months of practical training. They must be of good character and in good health. Foreigners from countries outside the European Union may be granted a temporary licence only.**
Work in government service after graduation: **Not obligatory**
Agreements with other countries: **An agreement exists with other countries of the European Union (Directive 93/16/EEC governing the employment of doctors).**

MEDIZINISCHE FAKULTAET
RHEINISCH-WESTFAELISCHE TECHNISCHE HOCHSCHULE AACHEN
PAUWELSSTRASSE 30
D-52062 AACHEN
Tel.: +49 (241) 808 9168
Fax: +49 (241) 888 8470
Year instruction started: **1966**
Language of instruction: **German**
Duration of basic medical degree course, including practical training: **6 years**
Entrance examination: **Yes**
Foreign students eligible: **Yes**

FACHBEREICH HUMANMEDIZIN
FREIE UNIVERSITAET BERLIN
UNIVERSITAETSKLINIKUM BENJAMIN FRANKLIN
HINDENBURGDAMM 30
D-12200 BERLIN
Year instruction started: **1948**

BEREICH MEDIZIN (CHARITE)
HUMBOLDT UNIVERSITAET ZU BERLIN
SCHUMANNSTRASSE 20/21
D-10117 BERLIN
Year instruction started: **1710**

MEDIZINISCHE FACULTAET VIRCHOW KLINIKUM
HUMBOLDT UNIVERSITAET ZU BERLIN
AUGUSTENBURGERPLATZ 1
D-13353 BERLIN

MEDIZINISCHE FAKULTAET
RUHR-UNIVERSITAET BOCHUM
UNIVERSITAETSSTRASSE 150
D-44780 BOCHUM
Tel.: +49 (234) 700 4960
Fax: +49 (234) 709 4190
Year instruction started: **1969**
Language of instruction: **German**
Duration of basic medical degree course, including practical training: **6 years**
Entrance examination: **No**
Foreign students eligible: **Yes**

MEDIZINISCHE FAKULTAET
RHEINISCHE FRIEDRICH-WILHELMS-UNIVERSITAET BONN
AM HOF 1B
D-53113 BONN
Tel.: +49 (228) 737 246/737 298
Fax: +49 (228) 737 077
Year instruction started: **1818**
Language of instruction: **German**
Duration of basic medical degree course, including practical training: **6 years**
Entrance examination: **Yes**
Foreign students eligible: **No**

MEDIZINISCHE FAKULTAET "CARL-GUSTAV CARUS"
TECHNISCHE UNIVERSITAET DRESDEN
FETSCHERSTRASSE 74
D-01307 DRESDEN
Year instruction started: **1954**
Language of instruction: **German**
Duration of basic medical degree course, including practical training: **6 years**
Entrance examination: **Yes**
Foreign students eligible: **Yes**

MEDIZINISCHE FAKULTAET
HEINRICH-HEINE UNIVERSITAET DUESSELDORF
UNIVERSITAETSSTRASSE 1
D-40225 DUESSELDORF
Tel.: +49 (211) 811 2242
Fax: +49 (211) 811 2285
Year instruction started: **1923**
Language of instruction: **German**
Duration of basic medical degree course, including practical training: **6 years**
Entrance examination: **Yes**
Foreign students eligible: **Yes**

MEDIZINISCHE FAKULTAET
FRIEDRICH-ALEXANDER-UNIVERSITAET ERLANGEN-NUERNBERG
UNIVERSITAETSSTRASSE 40
D-91054 ERLANGEN
Year instruction started: **1743**

MEDIZINISCHE FAKULTAET
UNIVERSITAET-GESAMTHOCHSCHULE ESSEN
HUFELANDSTRASSE 55
D-45122 ESSEN

Tel.: +49 (201) 723 4696
Fax: +49 (201) 723 5914
Year instruction started: **1971**
Language of instruction: **German**
Duration of basic medical degree course, including practical training: **6 years**
Entrance examination: **No**
Foreign students eligible: **Yes**

FACHBEREICH HUMANMEDIZIN
JOHANN-WOLFGANG-GOETHE-UNIVERSITAET FRANKFURT
THEODOR-STERN-KAI 7
D-60590 FRANKFURT AM MAIN
Tel.: +49 (69) 630 162 89
Fax: +49 (69) 630 159 22
E-mail: dekanat@ddm.klinik.uni-frankfurt.de
Year instruction started: **1914**
Language of instruction: **German**
Duration of basic medical degree course, including practical training: **6 years**
Entrance examination: **Yes**
Foreign students eligible: **Yes**

MEDIZINISCHE FAKULTAET
ALBERT-LUDWIGS-UNIVERSITAET FREIBURG
WERTHMANNPLATZ
D-79098 FREIBURG IM BREISGAU
Year instruction started: **1457**

FACHBEREICH HUMANMEDIZIN
JUSTUS-LIEBIG-UNIVERSITAET GIESSEN
RUDOLF-BUCHHEIM-STRASSE 8
D-35385 GIESSEN
Year instruction started: **1607**

MEDIZINISCHE FAKULTAET
GEORG-AUGUST-UNIVERSITAET GOETTINGEN
ROBERT-KOCH-STRASSE 40
D-37075 GOETTINGEN
Tel.: +49 (551) 395 328
Fax: +49 (551) 396 994
Telex: 96703 unigoe d
E-mail: ghahne@uni-goettingen.de

Year instruction started: **1737**
Language of instruction: **German**
Duration of basic medical degree course, including practical training: **6 years**
Entrance examination: **No**
Foreign students eligible: **Yes**

BEREICH MEDIZIN
ERNST-MORITZ-ARNDT UNIVERSITAET
FLEISCHMANNSTRASSE 8
D-17487 GREIFSWALD
Year instruction started: **1456**

BEREICH MEDIZIN
MARTIN-LUTHER-UNIVERSITAET HALLE-WITTENBERG
MAGDEBURGERSTRASSE 3
D-06907 HALLE/SAALE
Year instruction started: **1717**

FACHBEREICH MEDIZIN
UNIVERSITAET HAMBURG
UNIVERSITAETS-KRANKENHAUS EPPENDORF
MARTINISTRASSE 52
D-20246 HAMBURG
Year instruction started: **1919**

MEDIZINISCHE HOCHSCHULE HANNOVER
KONSTANTY-GUTSCHOW-STRASSE 8
D-30623 HANNOVER
Year instruction started: **1965**

MEDIZINISCHE FAKULTAET
RUPRECHT-KARLS-UNIVERSITAET HEIDELBERG
IM NEUENHEIMER FELD 346
D-69120 HEIDELBERG
Tel.: +49 (6221) 562 702
Fax: +49 (6221) 564 365
Year instruction started: **1387**
Language of instruction: **German**
Duration of basic medical degree course, including practical training: **6 years**
Entrance examination: **Yes**
Foreign students eligible: **Yes**

FACHBEREICH MEDIZIN
UNIVERSITAET DES SAARLANDES/SAARBRUECKEN
ANLAGENGEBAUEDE
D-66424 HOMBURG
Year instruction started: **1946**

MEDIZINISCHE FAKULTAET
FRIEDRICH-SCHILLER-UNIVERSITAET JENA
BACHSTRASSE 18
D-07740 JENA
Tel.: +49 (3641) 633 017
Fax: +49 (3641) 633 013
Year instruction started: **1558**
Language of instruction: **German**
Duration of basic medical degree course, including practical training: **6 years**
Entrance examination: **Yes**
Foreign students eligible: **Yes**

FACHBEREICH MEDIZIN
CHRISTIAN-ALBRECHTS-UNIVERSITAET KIEL
OLSHAUSENSTRASSE 40–60
D-24098 KIEL
Tel.: +49 (431) 880 2126
Fax: +49 (431) 880 2072
Year instruction started: **1665**
Language of instruction: **German**
Duration of basic medical degree course, including practical training: **6 years**
Entrance examination: **No**
Foreign students eligible: **Yes**

MEDIZINISCHE FAKULTAET
UNIVERSITAET ZU KOELN
JOSEPH-STELZMANN-STRASSE 9
D-50931 KOELN
Tel.: +49 (221) 478 6039
Fax: +49 (221) 478 6276
Year instruction started: **1393**
Language of instruction: **German**
Duration of basic medical degree course, including practical training: **6 years**
Entrance examination: **Yes**
Foreign students eligible: **Yes**

MEDIZINISCHE FAKULTAET
UNIVERSITAET LEIPZIG
LIEBIGSTRASSE 27
D-04103 LEIPZIG
Tel.: +49 (341) 971 5930
Fax: +49 (341) 971 5939
Year instruction started: **1475**
Language of instruction: **German**
Duration of basic medical degree course, including practical training: **6 years**
Entrance examination: **No**
Foreign students eligible: **Yes**

MEDIZINISCHE FAKULTAET
UNIVERSITAET LUEBECK
RATZEBURGER ALLEE 160
D-23538 LUEBECK
Tel.: +49 (451) 5000
Fax: +49 (451) 500 3016
Telex: 26492 ul d
Year instruction started: **1964**
Language of instruction: **German**
Duration of basic medical degree course, including practical training: **6 years**
Entrance examination: **No**
Foreign students eligible: **Yes**

MEDIZINISCHE FAKULTAET
OTTO-VON-GUERUERICKE UNIVERSITAET
LEIPZIGERSTRASSE 44
D-39120 MAGDEBURG
Year instruction started: **1954**

FACHBEREICH MEDIZIN
JOHANNES-GUTENBERG-UNIVERSITAET MAINZ
OBERE ZAHLBACHERSTRASSE 63
D-55131 MAINZ
Year instruction started: **1946**

FAKULTAET FUER KLINISCHE MEDIZIN MANNHEIM
UNIVERSITAET HEIDELBERG
THEODOR-KUTZER-UFER 1–3
D-68135 MANNHEIM
Tel.: +49 (621) 383 2527
Fax: +49 (621) 383 3802

Year instruction started: **1965**
Language of instruction: **German**
Duration of basic medical degree course, including practical training: **6 years**
Entrance examination: **No**
Foreign students eligible: **Yes**

FACHBEREICH HUMANMEDIZIN
PHILIPPS-UNIVERSITAET MARBURG
BALDINGERSTRASSE
D-35033 MARBURG
Year instruction started: **1527**

FACHBEREICH MEDIZIN
LUDWIG-MAXIMILIANS-UNIVERSITAET MUENCHEN
BAUARIARING 19
D-80336 MUENCHEN
Year instruction started: **1826**

FAKULTAET FUER MEDIZIN
TECHNISCHE UNIVERSITAET MUENCHEN
ISMANINGERSTRASSE 22
D-81675 MUENCHEN
Tel.: +49 (89) 414 040 21
Fax: +49 (89) 414 049 35
Year instruction started: **1967**
Language of instruction: **German**
Duration of basic medical degree course, including practical training: **6 years**
Entrance examination: **Yes**
Foreign students eligible: **Yes**

MEDIZINISCHE FAKULTAET
WESTFAELISCHE WILHELMS-UNIVERSITAET MUENSTER
DOMAGKSTRASSE 3
D-48129 MUENSTER
Year instruction started: **1925**

MEDIZINISCHE FAKULTAET
UNIVERSITAET REGENSBURG
FRANZ-JOSEF-STRASSE-ALLEE 11
D-93042 REGENSBURG
Tel.: +49 (941) 944 6084
Fax: +49 (941) 944 6079

Year instruction started: **1970**
Language of instruction: **German**
Duration of basic medical degree course, including practical training: **6 years**
Entrance examination: **Yes**
Foreign students eligible: **Yes**

NATURWISSENSCHAFTLICHE FAKULTAET III (BIOLOGIE UND
   VORKLINISCHE MEDIZIN)
UNIVERSITAET REGENSBURG
UNIVERSITAETSSTRASSE 31
D-93040 REGENSBURG
Year instruction started: **1970**

MEDIZINISCHE FAKULTAET
UNIVERSITAET ROSTOCK
SCHILLINGALLEE 35
D-18055 ROSTOCK
Tel.: +49 (381) 494 5001
Fax: +49 (381) 494 5002
Year instruction started: **1419**
Language of instruction: **German**
Duration of basic medical degree course, including practical training: **6 years**
Entrance examination: **No**
Foreign students eligible: **Yes**

MEDIZINISCHE FACULTAET
EBERHARD-KARLS-UNIVERSITAET TUEBINGEN
GEISSWEG 5
D-72076 TUEBINGEN
Tel.: +49 (7071) 297 3663
Fax: +49 (7071) 296 864
Year instruction started: **1477**
Language of instruction: **German**
Duration of basic medical degree course, including practical training: **6.5 years**
Entrance examination: **Yes**
Foreign students eligible: **Yes**

MEDIZINISCHE FAKULTAET
UNIVERSITAET ULM
ALBERT-EINSTEIN-ALLEE
D-89069 ULM
Tel.: +49 (731) 502 01
Fax: +49 (731) 502 2038

Year instruction started: **1969**
Language of instruction: **German**
Duration of basic medical degree course, including practical training: **6 years**
Entrance examination: **No**
Foreign students eligible: **Yes**

MEDIZINISCHE FAKULTAET
UNIVERSITAET WITTEN-HERDECKE
ALFRED-HERRHAUSEN-STRASSE 50
D-58448 WITTEN
Tel.: +49 (2302) 926 700
Fax: +49 (2302) 926 701
Year instruction started: **1983**
Language of instruction: **German**
Duration of basic medical degree course, including practical training: **6 years**
Entrance examination: **No**
Foreign students eligible: **Yes**

MEDIZINISCHE FAKULTAET
JULIUS-MAXIMILIANS-UNIVERSITAET WUERZBURG
JOSEF-SCHNEIDER-STRASSE 2
D-97080 WUERZBURG
Tel.: +49 (931) 201 3856
Fax: +49 (931) 201 3860
Year instruction started: **1583**
Language of instruction: **German**
Duration of basic medical degree course, including practical training: **6 years**
Entrance examination: **Yes**
Foreign students eligible: **Yes**

GHANA

Total population in 1995: **17 832 000**
Number of physicians per 100 000 population (1993): **4**
Number of medical schools: **2**
Duration of basic medical degree course, including practical training: **6 years**
Title of degree awarded: **Bachelor of Medicine and Bachelor of Surgery (MB, ChB)**
Medical registration/licence to practise: **Registration is obligatory with the Ghana Medical and Dental Council, PO Box 10586, Accra. The licence to practise medicine is granted to graduates who have completed a 1-year internship. Foreigners who have graduated abroad must hold a certificate of temporary**

registration and complete a 1-year internship in a recognized hospital
before obtaining full registration.
Work in government service after graduation: **Obligatory (1 year)**
Agreements with other countries: **An agreement exists with the United Kingdom.**

UNIVERSITY OF GHANA MEDICAL SCHOOL
PO BOX 4236
ACCRA
Tel.: +233 (21) 666 987
Fax: +233 (21) 663 062
E-mail: library@gha.healthnet.org
Year instruction started: **1963**
Language of instruction: **English**
Duration of basic medical degree course, including practical training: **6 years**
Entrance examination: **No**
Foreign students eligible: **Yes**

SCHOOL OF MEDICAL SCIENCES
UNIVERSITY OF SCIENCE AND TECHNOLOGY
UNIVERSITY POST OFFICE
KUMASI
Tel.: +233 (51) 603 03
Fax: +233 (51) 603 02
Telex: 2555 ust gh
Year instruction started: **1975**
Language of instruction: **English**
Duration of basic medical degree course, including practical training: **6 years**
Entrance examination: **Yes**
Foreign students eligible: **Yes**

GREECE

Total population in 1995: **10 490 000**
Number of physicians per 100 000 population (1993): **387**
Number of medical schools: **7**
Duration of basic medical degree course, including practical training: **6 years**
Title of degree awarded: *Ptychion latrikis* **(Diploma of Medicine)**
Medical registration/licence to practise: **Registration is obligatory with the
competent Medical Board. The licence to practise medicine is granted by
the Division of Health and Hygiene of the provincial authorities to gradu-
ates of a recognized medical school. Foreigners must provide full legal
details to obtain a licence.**

Work in government service after graduation: **Obligatory (1 year in a rural area)**
Agreements with other countries: **An agreement exists with other countries of the European Union (Directive 93/16/EEC governing the employment of doctors).**

MEDICAL SECTION
UNIVERSITY OF THRAKI
ALEXANDROUPOLIS
Year instruction started: **1984**

MEDICAL DEPARTMENT
SCHOOL OF HEALTH SCIENCES
NATIONAL AND KAPODISTRIAN UNIVERSITY OF ATHENS
ATHENS
Year instruction started: **1836**

MEDICAL SCHOOL
UNIVERSITY OF IOANNINA
UNIVERSITY CAMPUS
PO BOX 1186
IOANNINA 45110
Tel.: +30 (651) 418 02/405 77
Fax: +30 (651) 405 77
Year instruction started: **1977**
Language of instruction: **Greek**
Duration of basic medical degree course, including practical training: **6 years**
Entrance examination: **Yes**
Foreign students eligible: **Yes**

MEDICAL DEPARTMENT
SCHOOL OF HEALTH SCIENCES
UNIVERSITY OF CRETE
ELEFTERIAS SQUARE
IRAKLION
Year instruction started: **1984**

MEDICAL SCHOOL
UNIVERSITY OF THESSALY
22 PAPAKIRIAZI
LARISSA 41222
Tel.: +30 (41) 259 974
Fax: +30 (41) 255 420

Year instruction started: **1990**
Language of instruction: **Greek**
Duration of basic medical degree course, including practical training: **6 years**
Entrance examination: **Yes**
Foreign students eligible: **Yes**

FACULTY OF MEDICINE
SCHOOL OF HEALTH SCIENCES
UNIVERSITY OF PATRAS
PATRAS 26500
Tel.: +30 (61) 992 942
Fax: +30 (61) 996 103
Language of instruction: **Greek**
Duration of basic medical degree course, including practical training: **6 years**
Entrance examination: **No**
Foreign students eligible: **Yes**

MEDICAL SCHOOL
ARISTOTLE UNIVERSITY OF THESSALONIKI
THESSALONIKI 54006
Tel.: +30 (31) 999 283
Fax: +30 (31) 999 293
Year instruction started: **1942**
Language of instruction: **Greek**
Duration of basic medical degree course, including practical training: **6 years**
Entrance examination: **Yes**
Foreign students eligible: **Yes**

GRENADA

Total population in 1995: **—**
Number of physicians per 100 000 population (1993): **50**
Number of medical schools: **1**
Duration of basic medical degree course, including practical training: **4.5 years**
Title of degree awarded: **Doctor of Medicine (MD)**
Medical registration/licence to practise: **Registration is obligatory with the Medical Registration Board, Ministry of Health, St George's. The licence to practise medicine is granted to graduates from St George's University School of Medicine or an acceptable equivalent.**
Work in government service after graduation: **Not obligatory (except for those who have studied with a government grant, who must complete 3 years in the service of the state)**
Agreements with other countries: **Agreements exist with British Commonwealth countries, Eastern Caribbean countries and the USA.**

ST GEORGE'S UNIVERSITY SCHOOL OF MEDICINE[1]
UNIVERSITY CENTRE
PO BOX 7
ST GEORGE'S
Tel.: +1473 444 4357
Fax: +1473 444 4823
E-mail: sgu-info@mssl.com
Year instruction started: **1977**
Language of instruction: **English**
Duration of basic medical degree course, including practical training: **4.5 years**
Entrance examination: **Yes**
Foreign students eligible: **Yes**

GUATEMALA

Total population in 1995: **10 928**
Number of physicians per 100 000 population (1993): **90**
Number of medical schools: **2**
Duration of basic medical degree course, including practical training: **6 or 7 years**
Title of degree awarded: ***Médico y Cirujano* (Physician and Surgeon)**
Medical registration/licence to practise: —
Work in government service after graduation: —
Agreements with other countries: —

FACULTAD DE CIENCIAS MEDICAS
UNIVERSIDAD DE SAN CARLOS
CIUDAD UNIVERSITARIA
ZONA 1
GUATEMALA
Tel.: +502 (2) 476 7370
Fax: +502 (2) 476 9639
Year instruction started: **1676**
Language of instruction: **Spanish**
Duration of basic medical degree course, including practical training: **6 years**
Entrance examination: **No**
Foreign students eligible: **Yes**

---

[1] Students study at St George's University School of Medicine from the first to fourth and seventh to eleventh terms. The fifth and sixth terms are spent at Kingstown Medical College, Saint Vincent and the Grenadines.

FACULTAD DE MEDICINA
UNIVERSIDAD FRANCISCO MARROQUIN
6A AVENIDA 7-55
ZONA 10
GUATEMALA 01010
Tel.: +502 (2) 348 327/348 328
Fax: +502 (2) 348 329
Year instruction started: **1978**
Language of instruction: **Spanish**
Duration of basic medical degree course, including practical training: **7 years**
Entrance examination: **Yes**
Foreign students eligible: **Yes**

GUINEA

Total population in 1995: **7 518 000**
Number of physicians per 100 000 population (1993): **15**
Number of medical schools: **1**
Duration of basic medical degree course, including practical training: **8 years**
Title of degree awarded: ***Docteur en Médecine*** **(Doctor of Medicine)**
Medical registration/licence to practise: —
Work in government service after graduation: —
Agreements with other countries: —

FACULTE DE MEDECINE, PHARMACIE ET ODONTO-STOMATOLOGIE
UNIVERSITE DE CONAKRY
ROUTE DE DIXINN
BP 1017
CONAKRY
Year instruction started: **1967**
Language of instruction: **French**
Duration of basic medical degree course, including practical training: **8 years**
Entrance examination: **Yes**
Foreign students eligible: **Yes**

GUINEA-BISSAU

Total population in 1995: **1 091 000**
Number of physicians per 100 000 population (1993): **18**
Number of medical schools: **1**
Duration of basic medical degree course, including practical training: **6 years**
Title of degree awarded: ***Doctor en Medicina*** **(Doctor of Medicine)**

Medical registration/licence to practise: **Registration is obligatory with the Ministry of Public Health, BP 50, Bissau. The licence to practise medicine is granted by the Ministry on receipt of information from the Dean of the Faculty of Medicine and a certified copy of the medical diploma. Graduates of foreign medical schools must have their degree certified. Foreigners must be in possession of a work and a residence permit.**

Work in government service after graduation: **Not obligatory**

Agreements with other countries: **Agreements exist with countries to which medical students are sent for training, mainly Brazil, Cuba and countries of Europe and North America.**

ESCOLA SUPERIOR DE MEDICINA
EDUARDO MONDLANE
BP 427
BISSAU
Tel.: +245 203 089
Fax: +245 201 107
Year instruction started: **1986**
Language of instruction: **Spanish, Portuguese**
Duration of basic medical degree course, including practical training: **6 years**

GUYANA

Total population in 1995: **838 000**
Number of physicians per 100 000 population (1993): **33**
Number of medical schools: **1**
Duration of basic medical degree course, including practical training: **5 years**
Title of degree awarded: **Doctor of Medicine**
Medical registration/licence to practise: —
Work in government service after graduation: —
Agreements with other countries: —

FACULTY OF HEALTH SCIENCES
SCHOOL OF MEDICINE
UNIVERSITY OF GUYANA
TURKEYEN CAMPUS
PO BOX 101110
GEORGETOWN
Tel.: +592 (2) 254 04
Fax: +592 (2) 235 96

Year instruction started: **1985**
Language of instruction: **English**
Duration of basic medical degree course, including practical training: **5 years**
Entrance examination: **No**
Foreign students eligible: **Yes**

HAITI

Total population in 1995: **7 259 000**
Number of physicians per 100 000 population (1993): **16**
Number of medical schools: **1**
Duration of basic medical degree course, including practical training: **6 years**
Title of degree awarded: *Docteur en Médecine* (Doctor of Medicine)
Medical registration/licence to practise: **Registration is obligatory with the**
   Ministère de la Santé publique et de la Population, Palais des Ministères, Port-
   ***au-Prince*. The licence to practise medicine is granted to medical graduates**
   who have completed 1 year of social service. Those who have qualified
   abroad must have their degree validated by the Faculty of Medicine in
   Haiti. Foreigners require special authorization to practise.
Work in government service after graduation: **Not obligatory**
Agreements with other countries: **None**

ECOLE DE MEDECINE ET DE PHARMACIE
UNIVERSITE D'ETAT D'HAITI
RUE OSWALD DURAND 89
PORT-AU-PRINCE
Tel.: +509 220 488/221 131/221 132
Fax: +509 573 974
Year instruction started: **1867**
Language of instruction: **French**
Duration of basic medical degree course, including practical training: **6 years**
Entrance examination: **Yes**
Foreign students eligible: **Yes**

HONDURAS

Total population in 1995: **5 816 000**
Number of physicians per 100 000 population (1993): **22**
Number of medical schools: **1**
Duration of basic medical degree course, including practical training: **8 years (a**
   further 2 years of practice is required before the degree is awarded)
Title of degree awarded: *Doctor en Medicina y Cirugía* (Doctor of Medicine and
   Surgery)

Medical registration/licence to practise: **Registration is obligatory with the**
   Colegio Médico de Honduras, Tegucigalpa. **The licence to practise medicine**
   is granted to graduates who have completed 1 year of social service and 1
   year as an intern on a rotating basis. Those who have qualified abroad
   must have their degree validated. Foreigners must hold a residence permit.
Work in government service after graduation: **Not obligatory**
Agreements with other countries: **Agreements exist with El Salvador and**
   Guatemala.

FACULTAD DE CIENCIAS MEDICAS
UNIVERSIDAD NACIONAL AUTONOMA DE HONDURAS
ATRAS DEL HOSPITAL ESCUELA
TEGUCIGALPA
Year instruction started: **1907**

HUNGARY

Total population in 1995: **10 049 000**
Number of physicians per 100 000 population (1993): **337**
Number of medical schools: **4**
Duration of basic medical degree course, including practical training: **6 years**
Title of degree awarded: *Orvosdoktor* **(Doctor of Medicine)**
Medical registration/licence to practise: —
Work in government service after graduation: —
Agreements with other countries: —

SEMMELWEIS ORVOSTUDOMANYI EGYETEM
ULLOI UT 26
H-1085 BUDAPEST
Tel.: +36 (1) 210 0245
Fax: +36 (1) 118 1660
Year instruction started: **1769**
Language of instruction: **Hungarian, German, English**
Duration of basic medical degree course, including practical training: **6 years**
Entrance examination: **Yes**
Foreign students eligible: **Yes**

DEBRECENI ORVOSTUDOMANYI EGYETEM
NAGYERDEI KRT 98
H-4012 DEBRECEN
Tel.: +36 (52) 417 571
Fax: +36 (52) 419 807
E-mail: edu.office@jaguar.dote.hu

Year instruction started: **1912**
Language of instruction: **Hungarian, English**
Duration of basic medical degree course, including practical training: **6 years**
Entrance examination: **Yes**
Foreign students eligible: **Yes**

PECSI ORVOSTUDOMANYI EGYETEM
SZIGETI UT 12
H-7624 PECS
Tel.: +36 (72) 324 122
Fax: +36 (72) 326 244
Year instruction started: **1923**
Language of instruction: **Hungarian, English**
Duration of basic medical degree course, including practical training: **6 years**
Entrance examination: **Yes**
Foreign students eligible: **Yes**

ALBERT SZENT–GYORGYI ORVOSTUDOMANYI EGYETEM
PO BOX 481
ZRINYI UTCA 9
H-6701 SZEGED
Tel.: +36 (62) 312 529
Fax: +36 (62) 312 529
E-mail: lednitzky@medea.szote.u-szeged.hu
Year instruction started: **1872**
Language of instruction: **Hungarian, English**
Duration of basic medical degree course, including practical training: **6 years**
Entrance examination: **Yes**
Foreign students eligible: **Yes**

ICELAND

Total population in 1995: **271 000**
Number of physicians per 100 000 population (1993): —
Number of medical schools: **1**
Duration of basic medical degree course, including practical training: **6 years**
Title of degree awarded: ***Candidatus Medicinae et Chirurgiae* (Candidate of Medicine and Surgery)**
Medical registration/licence to practise: —
Work in government service after graduation: —
Agreements with other countries: —

HASKOLI ISLANDS LAEKNADEILD
VATNSMYRARVEGI 16
IS-101 REYKJAVIK
Tel.: +354 525 4880/525 4881
Fax: +354 525 4884
E-mail: annah@rhi.hi.is
Year instruction started: **1876**
Language of instruction: **Icelandic**
Duration of basic medical degree course, including practical training: **6 years**
Entrance examination: **Yes**
Foreign students eligible: **Yes**

INDIA

Total population in 1995: **944 580 000**
Number of physicians per 100 000 population (1993): **48**
Number of medical schools: **140**
Duration of basic medical degree course, including practical training: **4–6 years (followed by 1 year's internship before the degree is awarded)**
Title of degree awarded: **Bachelor of Medicine and Bachelor of Surgery (MB, BS)**
Medical registration/licence to practise: **Registration is obligatory with the Medical Council of India, Temple Lane, Lotla Road, New Delhi. The licence to practise medicine is granted to graduates who have completed 1 year as an intern in an approved hospital on a rotating basis or 1 year in the Armed Forces Medical Service. Foreigners with qualifications recognized by the Medical Council of India may be granted a licence to practise for a limited period.**
Work in government service after graduation: **Not obligatory**
Agreements with other countries: —

■ ANDRA PRADESH
GUNTUR MEDICAL COLLEGE
VIJAYAWADA UNIVERSITY OF HEALTH SCIENCES
GUNTUR 522001
Year instruction started: **1946**

DECCAN COLLEGE OF MEDICAL SCIENCES
VIJAYAWADA UNIVERSITY OF HEALTH SCIENCES
NAWAB LUTFUD DOWLAH PALACE
ZAFARGARH
KANCHANBAGH POST OFFICE
HYDERABAD 500258
Tel.: +91 (40) 239 547/239 225
Fax: +91 (40) 239 235

Year instruction started: **1985**
Language of instruction: **English**
Duration of basic medical degree course, including practical training: **4 years**
Entrance examination: **Yes**
Foreign students eligible: **Yes**

GANDHI MEDICAL COLLEGE
VIJAYAWADA UNIVERSITY OF HEALTH SCIENCES
BASHEERBAGH
HYDERABAD 500001
Year instruction started: **1954**

OSMANIA MEDICAL COLLEGE
VIJAYAWADA UNIVERSITY OF HEALTH SCIENCES
HYDERABAD 500001
Year instruction started: **1946**

RANGARAYA MEDICAL COLLEGE
VIJAYAWADA UNIVERSITY OF HEALTH SCIENCES
EAST GODAVARY DISTRICT
KAKINADA 533003
Year instruction started: **1958**

KURNOOL MEDICAL COLLEGE
VIJAYAWADA UNIVERSITY OF HEALTH SCIENCES
KURNOOL 518001
Year instruction started: **1957**

SRI VENKATESVARA MEDICAL COLLEGE
VIJAYAWADA UNIVERSITY OF HEALTH SCIENCES
TIRUPATI 517501
Year instruction started: **1960**

SIDDHARTHA MEDICAL COLLEGE
VIJAYAWADA UNIVERSITY OF HEALTH SCIENCES
VIJAYAWADA 520008
Tel.: +91 (866) 540 390
Fax: +91 (866) 540 463
Telex: 475269 uhs in
Year instruction started: **1981**
Language of instruction: **English**
Duration of basic medical degree course, including practical training: **5 years**
Entrance examination: **Yes**
Foreign students eligible: **No**

ANDHRA MEDICAL COLLEGE
VIJAYAWADA UNIVERSITY OF HEALTH SCIENCES
VISAKHAPATNAM 530001
Year instruction started: **1923**

KAKATIYA MEDICAL COLLEGE
VIJAYAWADA UNIVERSITY OF HEALTH SCIENCES
WARANGAL 506002
Year instruction started: **1959**

■ **ASSAM**
ASSAM MEDICAL COLLEGE
DIBRUGARH UNIVERSITY
DIBRUGARH 786002
Tel.: +91 (373) 200 80
Year instruction started: **1947**
Language of instruction: **English**
Duration of basic medical degree course, including practical training: **4 years**
Entrance examination: **Yes**
Foreign students eligible: **No**

GUWAHATI MEDICAL COLLEGE
GUWAHATI UNIVERSITY
GUWAHATI 781001
Year instruction started: **1960**

SILCHAR MEDICAL COLLEGE AND HOSPITAL
ASSAM UNIVERSITY
GHUNGOOR
SILCHAR 788001
Year instruction started: **1968**

■ **BIHAR**
JAWAHARLAL NEHRU MEDICAL COLLEGE
BHAGALPUR UNIVERSITY
BHAGALPUR 812001
Year instruction started: **1971**

ANUGRAH NARAIN MAGADH MEDICAL COLLEGE
MAGADH UNIVERSITY
BODHGAYA
GAYA 823001
Year instruction started: **1970**

MAHATMA GANDHI MEMORIAL MEDICAL COLLEGE
RANCHI UNIVERSITY
MANGO POST OFFICE
JAMSHEDPUR 831001
Year instruction started: **1961**

DARBHANGA MEDICAL COLLEGE
L.N. MITHILA UNIVERSITY
LAHERIASARAI 846001
Year instruction started: **1946**

SRI KRISHNA MEDICAL COLLEGE
BABASAHEB BHIMRAO AMBEDKAR BIHAR UNIVERSITY
UMANAGAR POST OFFICE
MUZAFFARPUR 842001
Year instruction started: **1970**

NALANDA MEDICAL COLLEGE
MAGADH UNIVERSITY
PATNA 800001
Year instruction started: **1970**

PATNA MEDICAL COLLEGE
PATNA UNIVERSITY
PATNA 800004
Year instruction started: **1925**

RAJENDRA MEDICAL COLLEGE
RANCHI UNIVERSITY
BARIATU
RANCHI 834009
Tel.: +91 (651) 301 533/301 566
Year instruction started: **1960**
Language of instruction: **English**
Duration of basic medical degree course, including practical training: **4 years**
Entrance examination: **Yes**
Foreign students eligible: **No**

■ CHANDIGARH
MEDICAL COLLEGE[1]
PUNJAB UNIVERSITY
CHANDIGARH
Year instruction started: **1991**

---

[1] Recognized to 31 August 1998.

■ **DELHI**
ALL-INDIA INSTITUTE OF MEDICAL SCIENCES
ANSARI NAGAR
NEW DELHI 110016
Year instruction started: **1956**

LADY HARDINGE MEDICAL COLLEGE
DELHI UNIVERSITY
NEW DELHI 110000
Year instruction started: **1916**

MAULANA AZAD MEDICAL COLLEGE
DELHI UNIVERSITY
NEW DELHI 110000
Year instruction started: **1958**

UNIVERSITY COLLEGE OF MEDICAL SCIENCES
DELHI UNIVERSITY
SHAHDARA
NEW DELHI 110095
Tel.: +91 (11) 228 2971/228 2972/228 2973
Fax: +91 (11) 229 0495
E-mail: hdbmi@ucms.ernet.in
Year instruction started: **1971**
Language of instruction: **English**
Duration of basic medical degree course, including practical training: **5 years**
Entrance examination: **Yes**
Foreign students eligible: **No**

■ **GOA**
GOA MEDICAL COLLEGE
GOA UNIVERSITY
PANAJI 403001
Year instruction started: **1963**

■ **GUJARAT**
B.J. MEDICAL COLLEGE
GUJARAT UNIVERSITY
AHMEDABAD 380016
Year instruction started: **1946**

N.H.L. MUNICIPAL MEDICAL COLLEGE
GUJARAT UNIVERSITY
ELLIS BRIDGE
AHMEDABAD 380006
Tel.: +91 (79) 657 6275
Year instruction started: **1963**
Language of instruction: **English**
Duration of basic medical degree course, including practical training: **4 years**
Entrance examination: **No**
Foreign students eligible: **No**

MEDICAL COLLEGE
M.S. UNIVERSITY OF BARODA
SAYIJI GUNJ
BARODA 390001
Tel.: +91 (265) 421 594
Year instruction started: **1949**
Language of instruction: **English**
Duration of basic medical degree course, including practical training: **4 years**
Entrance examination: **No**
Foreign students eligible: **No**

M.P. SHAH MEDICAL COLLEGE
SAURASHTRA UNIVERSITY
JAMNAGAR 361001
Year instruction started: **1955**

PRAMUKHSWAMI MEDICAL COLLEGE
SARDAR PATEL UNIVERSITY
KARAMSAD 388325
Year instruction started: **1987**

GOVERNMENT MEDICAL COLLEGE
SOUTH GUJARAT UNIVERSITY
SURAT 395001
Year instruction started: **1964**

■ **HARYANA**
P.T. BLAGWAT DAYAL SHARMA MEDICAL COLLEGE
MAHARISHI DAYANAND UNIVERSITY
ROHTAK 124001
Year instruction started: **1960**

■ HIMACHAL PRADESH
INDIRA GANDHI MEDICAL COLLEGE
HIMACHAL PRADESH UNIVERSITY
SHIMLA 171001
Tel.: +91 (166) 778 20
Telex: 203073 papbx in
Year instruction started: **1966**
Language of instruction: **English**
Duration of basic medical degree course, including practical training: **5–6 years**
Entrance examination: **Yes**
Foreign students eligible: **Yes**

■ JAMMU AND KASHMIR
GOVERNMENT MEDICAL COLLEGE
JAMMU UNIVERSITY
JAMMU 180001
Year instruction started: **1972**

GOVERNMENT MEDICAL COLLEGE
KASHMIR UNIVERSITY
SRINAGAR 190010
Year instruction started: **1959**

■ KARNATAKA
BANGALORE MEDICAL COLLEGE
BANGALORE UNIVERSITY
BANGALORE 560001
Year instruction started: **1955**

DR B.R. AMBEDKAR MEDICAL COLLEGE
BANGALORE UNIVERSITY
KADUGONDANAHALLI
BANGALORE 560045
Tel.: +91 (80) 547 6498/547 1784
Fax: +91 (80) 547 8904
Year instruction started: **1981**
Language of instruction: **English**
Duration of basic medical degree course, including practical training: **5 years**
Entrance examination: **Yes**
Foreign students eligible: **Yes**

KEMPEGOWDA INSTITUTE OF MEDICAL SCIENCES
BANGALORE UNIVERSITY
K.R. ROAD
V.V. PURAM
BANGALORE 560004
Tel.: +91 (80) 603 560/661 3225
Fax: +91 (80) 661 3225/660 0440
Year instruction started: **1980**
Language of instruction: **English**
Duration of basic medical degree course, including practical training: **4 years**
Entrance examination: **Yes**
Foreign students eligible: **Yes**

M.S. RAMAIAH MEDICAL COLLEGE
BANGALORE UNIVERSITY
M.S. RAMAIAH NAGAR
M.S.R.I.T POST
BANGALORE 560054
Tel.: +91 (80) 336 9852
Fax: +91 (80) 344 0441
Year instruction started: **1979**
Language of instruction: **English**
Duration of basic medical degree course, including practical training: **5 years**
Entrance examination: **Yes**
Foreign students eligible: **Yes**

ST JOHN'S MEDICAL COLLEGE
BANGALORE UNIVERSITY
SARJAPUR ROAD
BANGALORE 560034
Tel.: +91 (80) 553 0724
Fax: +91 (80) 553 1786
Year instruction started: **1963**
Language of instruction: **English**
Duration of basic medical degree course, including practical training: **4 years**
Entrance examination: **Yes**
Foreign students eligible: **Yes**

J.L.N. MEDICAL COLLEGE
KARNATAK UNIVERSITY
POONA BANGALORE ROAD
NEHRU NAGAR
BELGAUM 590010
Year instruction started: **1963**

GOVERNMENT MEDICAL COLLEGE
VIJAYNAGARA INSTITUTE OF MEDICAL SCIENCES
GULBARGA UNIVERSITY
BELLARY 583104
Tel.: +91 (8392) 721 04/725 09
Year instruction started: **1961**
Language of instruction: **English**
Duration of basic medical degree course, including practical training: **4 years**
Entrance examination: **Yes**
Foreign students eligible: **Yes**

ADICHUNCHANAGIRI INSTITUTE OF MEDICAL SCIENCES
MYSORE UNIVERSITY
BALAGANGADHARANATHA NAGARA
BELLUR 571448
Tel.: +91 (8233) 674 33
Fax: +91 (8233) 673 44
Year instruction started: **1986**
Language of instruction: **English**
Duration of basic medical degree course, including practical training: **5 years**
Entrance examination: **Yes**
Foreign students eligible: **Yes**

AL-AMEEN MEDICAL COLLEGE
KARNATAKA UNIVERSITY
BIJAPUR 586101
Year instruction started: **1984**

B.L.D.E. ASSOCIATION'S SRI B.M. PATIL MEDICAL COLLEGE AND HOSPITAL
    RESEARCH CENTRE
KARNATAKA UNIVERSITY
SMT BANGARAMMA SAJJAN CAMPUS
SHOLAPUR ROAD
BIJAPUR 586103
Tel.: +91 (8352) 220 69
Fax: +91 (8352) 226 09
Year instruction started: **1986**
Language of instruction: **English**
Duration of basic medical degree course, including practical training: **4 years**
Entrance examination: **Yes**
Foreign students eligible: **Yes**

JAGADGURU JAYADEVA MURUGARAJENDRA MEDICAL COLLEGE
KUVEMPU UNIVERSITY
PO BOX 301
DAVANGERE 577004
Tel.: +91 (8192) 313 88
Fax: +91 (8192) 312 01
Year instruction started: **1965**
Language of instruction: **English**
Duration of basic medical degree course, including practical training: **4 years**
Entrance examination: **Yes**
Foreign students eligible: **Yes**

MAHADEVAPPA RAMPURE MEDICAL COLLEGE
GULBARGA UNIVERSITY
GULBARGA 585105
Year instruction started: **1963**

KARNATAKA INSTITUTE OF MEDICAL SCIENCES
KARNATAKA UNIVERSITY
HUBLI 580020
Year instruction started: **1957**

SRI DEVARAJ URS MEDICAL COLLEGE
BANGALORE UNIVERSITY
TAMAKA
KOLAR 563101
Tel.: +91 (8152) 226 38/226 37/226 03
Fax: +91 (8152) 251 36
Year instruction started: **1986**
Language of instruction: **English**
Duration of basic medical degree course, including practical training: **5 years**
Entrance examination: **Yes**
Foreign students eligible: **Yes**

KASTURBA MEDICAL COLLEGE
MANIPAL ACADEMY OF HIGHER EDUCATION
LIGHT HOUSE HILL ROAD
PO BOX 53
MANGALORE 575001
Tel.: +91 (824) 423 452/423 654/426 482
Fax: +91 (824) 428 183

Year instruction started: **1955**
Language of instruction: **English**
Duration of basic medical degree course, including practical training: **5 years**
Entrance examination: **Yes**
Foreign students eligible: **Yes**

KASTURBA MEDICAL COLLEGE
MANIPAL ACADEMY OF HIGHER EDUCATION
PO BOX 8
MANIPAL 576119
Tel.: +91 (8252) 712 01
Fax: +91 (8252) 700 61/700 62
Telex: 833231 mahe in
E-mail: mahe@kmc.ernet.in
Year instruction started: **1953**
Language of instruction: **English**
Duration of basic medical degree course, including practical training: **4 years**
Entrance examination: **Yes**
Foreign students eligible: **Yes**

J.S.S. MEDICAL COLLEGE
MYSORE UNIVERSITY
SRI SHIVARATHREESHWARA NAGAR
MYSORE 570015
Tel.: +91 (821) 307 32
Fax: +91 (821) 563 819
Year instruction started: **1984**
Language of instruction: **English**
Duration of basic medical degree course, including practical training: **5 years**
Entrance examination: **Yes**
Foreign students eligible: **Yes**

MYSORE MEDICAL COLLEGE
MYSORE UNIVERSITY
MYSORE 570001
Year instruction started: **1924**

SRI SIDDHARTHA MEDICAL COLLEGE
BANGALORE UNIVERSITY
TUMKUR 572101
Year instruction started: **1988**

■ **KERALA**
T.D. MEDICAL COLLEGE
KERALA UNIVERSITY
ALLEPPEY 688005
Year instruction started: **1963**

MEDICAL COLLEGE
CALICUT UNIVERSITY
CALICUT 673008
Year instruction started: **1957**

KOTTAYAM MEDICAL COLLEGE
MAHATMA GANDHI UNIVERSITY
GANDHI NAGAR POST OFFICE
KOTTAYAM 686008
Tel.: +91 (481) 597 284
Fax: +91 (481) 597 284
Year instruction started: **1961**
Language of instruction: **English**
Duration of basic medical degree course, including practical training: **5 years**
Entrance examination: **Yes**
Foreign students eligible: **No**

TRICHUR MEDICAL COLLEGE
CALICUT UNIVERSITY
MULAMKUNNATHUKAVU
TRICHUR 680596
Tel.: +91 (487) 720 311/720 312/720 313
Fax: +91 (487) 721 355
Year instruction started: **1982**
Language of instruction: **English**
Duration of basic medical degree course, including practical training: **5 years**
Entrance examination: **Yes**
Foreign students eligible: **Yes**

MEDICAL COLLEGE
KERALA UNIVERSITY
PATTOM PALACE POST OFFICE
TRIVANDRUM 695011
Year instruction started: **1951**

■ **MADHYA PRADESH**
GANDHI MEDICAL COLLEGE
BARKATULLAH UNIVERSITY
BHOPAL 462021
Year instruction started: **1955**

GAJRA RAJA MEDICAL COLLEGE
JIWAJI UNIVERSITY
GWALIOR 474003
Year instruction started: **1946**

M.G.M. MEDICAL COLLEGE
DEVI AHILYA VISHWAVIDYALAYA
INDORE 452001
Year instruction started: **1948**

MEDICAL COLLEGE
RANI DURGAVATI VISHWAVIDYALAYA
JABALPUR 482001
Year instruction started: **1955**

J.L.N. MEDICAL COLLEGE
RAVI SHANKAR UNIVERSITY
RAIPUR 492001
Year instruction started: **1963**

S.S. MEDICAL COLLEGE
A.P. SINGH UNIVERSITY
REWA 486001
Year instruction started: **1963**

■ **MAHARASHTRA**
S.R.T.R. MEDICAL COLLEGE
DR BABASAHAB AMBEDKAR MARATHWADA UNIVERSITY
AMBAJOGAI 431517
Year instruction started: **1974**

DR PANJABRAO ALIAS BHAUSAHEB DESHMUKH MEMORIAL MEDICAL
    COLLEGE
AMRAVATI UNIVERSITY
SHIVAJI NAGAR
AMRAVATI 444603
Tel.: +91 (721) 662 323/662 303

Year instruction started: **1984**
Language of instruction: **English**
Duration of basic medical degree course, including practical training: **4 years**
Entrance examination: **No**
Foreign students eligible: **Yes**

GOVERNMENT MEDICAL COLLEGE
DR BABASAHAB AMBEDKAR MARATHWADA UNIVERSITY
AURANGABAD 431001
Year instruction started: **1956**

MAHATMA GANDHI MISSION'S MEDICAL COLLEGE
DR BABASAHAB AMBEDKAR MARATHWADA UNIVERSITY
AURANGABAD
Year instruction started: **1989**

GRANT MEDICAL COLLEGE
BOMBAY UNIVERSITY
BYCULLA
BOMBAY 400008
Year instruction started: **1845**

K.J. SOMAIYA MEDICAL COLLEGE AND RESEARCH CENTRE
BOMBAY UNIVERSITY
SOMAIYA AYURVIHAR COMPLEX
EASTERN HIGHWAY
SION
BOMBAY 400022
Tel.: +91 (22) 409 0933/409 0253/409 0767
Year instruction started: **1991**
Duration of basic medical degree course, including practical training: **5 years**

LOKMANYA TILAK MUNICIPAL MEDICAL COLLEGE
BOMBAY UNIVERSITY
SION
BOMBAY 400022
Year instruction started: **1964**

SETH G.S. MEDICAL COLLEGE
BOMBAY UNIVERSITY
ACHARYA DONDE MARG
PAREL
BOMBAY 400012
Tel.: +91 (22) 413 6051/413 6052/413 6053
Fax: +91 (22) 414 3435

Year instruction started: **1926**
Language of instruction: **English**
Duration of basic medical degree course, including practical training: **5–6 years**
Entrance examination: **Yes**
Foreign students eligible: **No**

TOPIWALA NATIONAL MEDICAL COLLEGE
BOMBAY UNIVERSITY
DR A.L. NAIR ROAD
BOMBAY 400008
Tel.: +91 (22) 308 1490
Year instruction started: **1921**
Language of instruction: **English**
Duration of basic medical degree course, including practical training: **4.5 years**
Entrance examination: **Yes**
Foreign students eligible: **No**

SRI BHAUSAHEB HIRE GOVERNMENT MEDICAL COLLEGE
NORTH MAHARASHTRA UNIVERSITY
DHULE
Year instruction started: **1988**

KRISHNA INSTITUTE OF MEDICAL SCIENCES
SHIVAJI UNIVERSITY
NEAR DHEBEWADI ROAD
KARAD 415110
Tel.: +91 (2164) 415 55/415 56/415 57
Fax: +91 (2164) 421 70
Year instruction started: **1984**
Language of instruction: **English**
Duration of basic medical degree course, including practical training: **5 years**
Entrance examination: **No**
Foreign students eligible: **Yes**

DR D.Y. PATIL EDUCATION SOCIETY'S MEDICAL COLLEGE
SHIVAJI UNIVERSITY
KASABA BAVADA
KOLHAPUR 416006
Tel.: +91 (231) 653 298
Fax: +91 (231) 653 426

Year instruction started: **1989**
Language of instruction: **English**
Duration of basic medical degree course, including practical training: **5 years**
Entrance examination: **No**
Foreign students eligible: **Yes**

MAHARASHTRA INSTITUTE OF MEDICAL SCIENCES AND RESEARCH
SWAMI RAMANAND TEERTH UNIVERSITY
LATUR
Year instruction started: **1990**

RURAL MEDICAL COLLEGE OF PRAVARA MEDICAL TRUST
POONA UNIVERSITY
LONI BK POST OFFICE
AHMEDNAGAR DISTRICT
LONI 413736
Tel.: +91 (2422) 536 00
Fax: +91 (2422) 534 13
Year instruction started: **1984**
Language of instruction: **English**
Duration of basic medical degree course, including practical training: **5–6 years**
Entrance examination: **No**
Foreign students eligible: **Yes**

MIRAJ MEDICAL COLLEGE
SHIVAJI UNIVERSITY
MIRAJ 416410
Year instruction started: **1962**

GOVERNMENT MEDICAL COLLEGE
NAGPUR UNIVERSITY
GENERAL HOSPITAL
NAGPUR 440001
Year instruction started: **1947**

INDIRA GANDHI MEDICAL COLLEGE
NAGPUR UNIVERSITY
CENTRAL AVENUE ROAD
NAGPUR 440018
Year instruction started: **1968**

N.K.P. SALVE INSTITUTE OF MEDICAL SCIENCES
NAGPUR UNIVERSITY
NAGPUR
Year instruction started: **1990**

GOVERNMENT MEDICAL COLLEGE
SWAMI RAMANAND TEERTH MARATHWADA UNIVERSITY
NANDED 431601
Year instruction started: **1988**
Language of instruction: **English**
Duration of basic medical degree course, including practical training: **5 years**
Entrance examination: **Yes**
Foreign students eligible: **No**

N.D.M.V.P. SAMAJ MEDICAL COLLEGE
POONA UNIVERSITY
VASANTDADA NAGAR
NASHIK 422003
Tel.: +91 (253) 303 802/573 422
Fax: +91 (253) 511 916/574 511
Year instruction started: **1990**
Language of instruction: **English**
Duration of basic medical degree course, including practical training: **5 years**
Entrance examination: **No**
Foreign students eligible: **Yes**

DR D.Y. PATIL MEDICAL COLLEGE
BOMBAY UNIVERSITY
DR D.Y. PATIL VIDYANAGAR, SECTOR 7
NEW BOMBAY 400706
Tel.: +91 (22) 767 2516/767 2517
Year instruction started: **1989**
Language of instruction: **English**
Duration of basic medical degree course, including practical training: **5 years**
Entrance examination: **No**
Foreign students eligible: **Yes**

MAHATMA GANDHI MISSION'S MEDICAL COLLEGE
BOMBAY UNIVERSITY
PUNE–MUMBAI HIGHWAY
KAMOTHE
NEW BOMBAY 410209
Tel.: +91 (22) 742 1723
Year instruction started: **1989**
Language of instruction: **English**
Duration of basic medical degree course, including practical training: **5 years**
Entrance examination: **No**
Foreign students eligible: **Yes**

BHARATI VIDYAPEETH MEDICAL COLLEGE
BHARATI VIDYAPEETH DEEMED UNIVERSITY
KATRAJ-DHANKAWADI
PUNE 411043
Tel.: +91 (212) 433 226/435 175
Fax: +91 (212) 439 121
Year instruction started: **1989**
Language of instruction: **English**
Duration of basic medical degree course, including practical training: **5–6 years**
Entrance examination: **No**
Foreign students eligible: **Yes**

ARMED FORCES MEDICAL COLLEGE
POONA UNIVERSITY
SOLAPUR ROAD
PUNE 411040
Tel.: +91 (212) 673 290
Fax: +91 (212) 674 759
Year instruction started: **1962**
Language of instruction: **English**
Duration of basic medical degree course, including practical training: **4 years**
Entrance examination: **Yes**
Foreign students eligible: **Yes**

B.J. MEDICAL COLLEGE
POONA UNIVERSITY
PUNE 411001
Year instruction started: **1946**

DR VAISHAMPAYAN MEMORIAL MEDICAL COLLEGE
SHIVAJI UNIVERSITY
GOLIBAR MAIDAN
SHOLAPUR 413003
Year instruction started: **1963**

J.N. MEDICAL COLLEGE
NAGPUR UNIVERSITY
SWANGI
WARDHA
Year instruction started: **1990**

MAHATMA GANDHI INSTITUTE OF MEDICAL SCIENCES
NAGPUR UNIVERSITY
SEVAGRAM
WARDHA 442102
Year instruction started: **1969**

SHRI VASANTRAO NAIR GOVERNMENT MEDICAL COLLEGE
AMRAVATI UNIVERSITY
YAVATMAL
Year instruction started: **1989**

■ **MANIPUR**
REGIONAL INSTITUTE OF MEDICAL SCIENCES
MANIPUR UNIVERSITY
IMPHAL 795001
Year instruction started: **1972**

■ **ORISSA**
MAHARAJA KRISHNA CHANDRA GAJAPATI MEDICAL COLLEGE
BERHAMPUR UNIVERSITY
GANJAN DISTRICT
BERHAMPUR 760004
Year instruction started: **1962**

S.C.B. MEDICAL COLLEGE
UTKAL UNIVERSITY
CUTTACK 753001
Year instruction started: **1944**

V.S.S. MEDICAL COLLEGE
SAMBALPUR UNIVERSITY
MEDICAL COLLEGE CAMPUS
BURLA
SAMBALPUR 768017
Tel.: +91 (663) 430 768
Year instruction started: **1959**
Language of instruction: **English**
Duration of basic medical degree course, including practical training: **4 years**
Entrance examination: **Yes**
Foreign students eligible: **Yes**

■ **PONDICHERRY**
JAWAHARLAL INSTITUTE OF MEDICAL EDUCATION AND RESEARCH
PONDICHERRY UNIVERSITY
PONDICHERRY 605006
Year instruction started: **1956**

■ **PUNJAB**
GOVERNMENT MEDICAL COLLEGE
GURU NANAK DEV UNIVERSITY
MAGITHA ROAD
AMRITSAR 143001
Tel.: +91 (183) 220 618
Year instruction started: **1943**
Language of instruction: **English**
Duration of basic medical degree course, including practical training: **4 years**
Entrance examination: **Yes**
Foreign students eligible: **No**

GURU GOVIND SINGH MEDICAL COLLEGE
PUNJABI UNIVERSITY
FARIDKOT 151203
Year instruction started: **1973**

CHRISTIAN MEDICAL COLLEGE
PUNJAB UNIVERSITY
BROWN ROAD
LUDHIANA 141008
Tel.: +91 (161) 665 950
Fax: +91 (161) 609 958
Telex: 386312 cmc in
Year instruction started: **1953**
Language of instruction: **English**
Duration of basic medical degree course, including practical training: **4 years**
Entrance examination: **Yes**
Foreign students eligible: **Yes**

DAYANAND MEDICAL COLLEGE AND HOSPITAL
PUNJAB UNIVERSITY
PO BOX 265
LUDHIANA 141001
Tel.: +91 (161) 405 501/404 446/471 500
Fax: +91 (161) 472 620

Year instruction started: **1934**
Language of instruction: **English**
Duration of basic medical degree course, including practical training: **4.5 years**
Entrance examination: **Yes**
Foreign students eligible: **Yes**

GOVERNMENT MEDICAL COLLEGE
PUNJABI UNIVERSITY
PATIALA 147001
Tel.: +91 (175) 212 018
Year instruction started: **1954**
Language of instruction: **English**
Duration of basic medical degree course, including practical training: **4 years**
Entrance examination: **Yes**
Foreign students eligible: **No**

■ **RAJASTHAN**
JAWAHARLAL NEHRU MEDICAL COLLEGE
RAJASTHAN UNIVERSITY
AJMER 305001
Year instruction started: **1965**

SARDAR PATEL MEDICAL COLLEGE
RAJASTHAN UNIVERSITY
NAGNECHIJI ROAD
BIKANER 334001
Tel.: +91 (151) 523 443/528 022
Year instruction started: **1959**
Language of instruction: **English**
Duration of basic medical degree course, including practical training: **4 years**
Entrance examination: **Yes**
Foreign students eligible: **No**

SAWAI MAN SINGH MEDICAL COLLEGE
RAJASTHAN UNIVERSITY
JAIPUR 302003
Year instruction started: **1947**

DR S.N. MEDICAL COLLEGE
RAJASTHAN UNIVERSITY
JODHPUR 342001
Year instruction started: **1965**

R.N.T. MEDICAL COLLEGE
RAJASTHAN UNIVERSITY
UDAIPUR 313001
Year instruction started: **1961**

■ **TAMIL NADU**
RAJAH MUTHIAH MEDICAL COLLEGE
ANNAMALAI UNIVERSITY
ANNAMALAINAGAR 608002
Tel.: +91 (4144) 220 68
Fax: +91 (4144) 230 80
Year instruction started: **1985**
Language of instruction: **English**
Duration of basic medical degree course, including practical training: **5 years**
Entrance examination: **Yes**
Foreign students eligible: **Yes**

CHENNAI MEDICAL COLLEGE
DR M.G.R. MEDICAL UNIVERSITY
CHENNAI 600032
Year instruction started: **1860**
Language of instruction: **English**
Duration of basic medical degree course, including practical training: **4 years**
Entrance examination: **Yes**
Foreign students eligible: **Yes**

CHINGLEPUT MEDICAL COLLEGE
DR M.G.R. MEDICAL UNIVERSITY
CHINGLEPUT 603001
Year instruction started: **1965**

COIMBATORE MEDICAL COLLEGE
DR M.G.R. MEDICAL UNIVERSITY
AVINAI ROAD
AERODROME POST OFFICE
COIMBATORE 641014
Tel.: +91 (422) 574 375/574 376/574 377
Year instruction started: **1967**
Language of instruction: **English**
Duration of basic medical degree course, including practical training: **5 years**
Entrance examination: **Yes**
Foreign students eligible: **No**

P.S.G. INSTITUTE OF MEDICAL SCIENCES AND RESEARCH
DR M.G.R. MEDICAL UNIVERSITY
AVANASHI ROAD
PEELAMEDU
PO BOX 1674
COIMBATORE 641004
Tel.: +91 (422) 570 170/570 171/570 172
Fax: +91 (422) 573 833
Year instruction started: **1988**
Language of instruction: **English**
Duration of basic medical degree course, including practical training: **5–6 years**
Entrance examination: **Yes**
Foreign students eligible: **Yes**

KILPAUK MEDICAL COLLEGE
DR M.G.R. MEDICAL UNIVERSITY
MADRAS 600010
Year instruction started: **1960**

SRI RAMACHANDRA MEDICAL COLLEGE
DR M.G.R. MEDICAL UNIVERSITY
RAMACHANDRA NAGAR 1
PORUR
MADRAS 600116
Tel.: +91 (44) 482 8413
Fax: +91 (44) 482 7008
Telex: 4125050 pco in
Year instruction started: **1985**
Language of instruction: **English**
Duration of basic medical degree course, including practical training: **5 years**
Entrance examination: **Yes**
Foreign students eligible: **Yes**

STANLEY MEDICAL COLLEGE
DR M.G.R. MEDICAL UNIVERSITY
MADRAS 600001
Year instruction started: **1938**

MADURAI MEDICAL COLLEGE
DR M.G.R. MEDICAL UNIVERSITY
MADURAI 625020
Year instruction started: **1954**

MOHAN KUMARAMANGALAM MEDICAL COLLEGE
DR M.G.R. MEDICAL UNIVERSITY
SALEM
Year instruction started: **1986**

THANJAVUR MEDICAL COLLEGE
DR M.G.R. MEDICAL UNIVERSITY
THANJAVUR 613001
Year instruction started: **1959**

TIRUNELVELI MEDICAL COLLEGE
DR M.G.R. MEDICAL UNIVERSITY
TIRUNELVELI 627002
Year instruction started: **1965**

CHRISTIAN MEDICAL COLLEGE
DR M.G.R. MEDICAL UNIVERSITY
NORTH ARCOT DISTRICT
THORAPADI POST OFFICE
VELLORE 632002
Tel.: +91 (416) 226 03
Fax: +91 (416) 327 88/322 68/320 35
Telex: 405202 cmch in
E-mail: abraham@cmc.ernet.in
Year instruction started: **1942**
Language of instruction: **English**
Duration of basic medical degree course, including practical training: **5–6 years**
Entrance examination: **Yes**
Foreign students eligible: **Yes**

■ UTTAR PRADESH
S.N. MEDICAL COLLEGE
AGRA UNIVERSITY
AGRA 282001
Year instruction started: **1939**

J.N. MEDICAL COLLEGE
ALIGARH MUSLIM UNIVERSITY
ALIGARH 202001
Year instruction started: **1961**

M.L.N. MEDICAL COLLEGE
ALLAHABAD UNIVERSITY
ALLAHABAD 211001
Year instruction started: **1961**

BABA RAGHAV DAS MEDICAL COLLEGE
GORAKHPUR UNIVERSITY
GORAKHPUR 273013
Year instruction started: **1972**

M.L.B. MEDICAL COLLEGE
BUNDELKHAND UNIVERSITY
KANPUR ROAD
JHANSI 284128
Tel.: +91 (0517) 440 858
Fax: +91 (0517) 440 858
Year instruction started: **1968**
Language of instruction: **English**
Duration of basic medical degree course, including practical training: **5 years**
Entrance examination: **Yes**
Foreign students eligible: **No**

G.S.V.M. MEDICAL COLLEGE
KANPUR UNIVERSITY
KANPUR 208001
Year instruction started: **1955**

K.G. MEDICAL COLLEGE
LUCKNOW UNIVERSITY
LUCKNOW 226001
Year instruction started: **1911**

L.L.R.M. MEDICAL COLLEGE
MEERUT UNIVERSITY
MEERUT 250001
Year instruction started: **1966**

INSTITUTE OF MEDICAL SCIENCES
BANARAS HINDU UNIVERSITY
VARANASI 221005
Year instruction started: **1960**

■ **WEST BENGAL**
B.S. MEDICAL COLLEGE
CALCUTTA UNIVERSITY
BANKURA 711303
Year instruction started: **1956**

BURDWAN MEDICAL COLLEGE AND HOSPITAL
BURDWAN UNIVERSITY
BABURBAG
BURDWAN 713104
Year instruction started: **1969**
Language of instruction: **English**
Duration of basic medical degree course, including practical training: **5–6 years**
Entrance examination: **Yes**
Foreign students eligible: **No**

CALCUTTA NATIONAL MEDICAL COLLEGE
CALCUTTA UNIVERSITY
CALCUTTA 700014
Year instruction started: **1948**

MEDICAL COLLEGE
CALCUTTA UNIVERSITY
CALCUTTA 700012
Year instruction started: **1838**

N.R.S. MEDICAL COLLEGE
CALCUTTA UNIVERSITY
CALCUTTA 700014
Year instruction started: **1948**

R.G. KAR MEDICAL COLLEGE
CALCUTTA UNIVERSITY
CALCUTTA 700004
Year instruction started: **1916**

MEDICAL COLLEGE
NORTH BENGAL UNIVERSITY
SILIGURI 734401
Year instruction started: **1969**

INDONESIA

Total population in 1995: **200 453 000**
Number of physicians per 100 000 population (1993): **12**
Number of medical schools: **32**
Duration of basic medical degree course, including practical training: **6–8 years**
Title of degree awarded: ***Dokter*** (**Doctor**)

Medical registration/licence to practise: **Registration is obligatory with the Ministry of Health, *Jalan H.R. Rasuna Said Kav., Jakarta 12950*. The licence to practise medicine is granted by the provincial health authorities to graduates from a recognized medical school.**
Work in government service after graduation: —
Agreements with other countries: —

FAKULTAS KEDOKTERAN
UNIVERSITAS SYIAH KUALA
KAMPUS DARUSSALAM
BANDA ACEH
D.I. ACEH
Tel.: +62 (651) 520 53
Fax: +62 (651) 520 53
Year instruction started: **1980**
Language of instruction: **Indonesian**
Duration of basic medical degree course, including practical training: **6 years**
Entrance examination: **Yes**
Foreign students eligible: **Yes**

FAKULTAS KEDOKTERAN
UNIVERSITAS KRISTEN MARANATHA
JALAN PROFESSOR DR SOERIA SOEMANTRI 65
BANDUNG
JAWA BARAT
Tel.: +62 (22) 214 463
Fax: +62 (22) 215 154
Year instruction started: **1965**
Language of instruction: **Indonesian**
Duration of basic medical degree course, including practical training: **6 years**
Entrance examination: **Yes**
Foreign students eligible: **Yes**

FAKULTAS KEDOKTERAN
UNIVERSITAS PADJADJARAN
JALAN PASIRKALIKI 190
BANDUNG 40161
JAWA BARAT
Tel.: +62 (22) 232 170
Fax: +62 (22) 230 776
Year instruction started: **1957**
Language of instruction: **Indonesian**
Duration of basic medical degree course, including practical training: **6 years**
Entrance examination: **Yes**
Foreign students eligible: **Yes**

FAKULTAS KEDOKTERAN
UNIVERSITAS LAMBUNG MANGKURAT
JALAN BRIG. JEN HASAN BASRI
BANJARMASIN
KALIMANTAN SELATAN
Year instruction started: **1995**
Language of instruction: **Indonesian**
Duration of basic medical degree course, including practical training: **6 years**
Entrance examination: **Yes**
Foreign students eligible: **Yes**

FAKULTAS KEDOKTERAN
UNIVERSITAS KRISTEN INDONESIA
JALAN MAY. JEN. SUTOYO
CAWANG 13630
JAKARTA TIMUR
Tel.: +62 (21) 801 0553/800 2144
Fax: +62 (21) 809 3133
E-mail: fkuki@jakarta.wasantara.net.id
Year instruction started: **1962**
Language of instruction: **Indonesian**
Duration of basic medical degree course, including practical training: **6 years**
Entrance examination: **Yes**
Foreign students eligible: **Yes**

FAKULTAS KEDOKTERAN
UNIVERSITAS YARSI
JALAN LET. JEN. SUPRAPTO
CEMPAKA PUTIH 10510
JAKARTA PUSAT
Tel.: +62 (21) 424 4574/420 6674
Fax: +62 (21) 424 3171
Year instruction started: **1967**
Language of instruction: **Indonesian**
Duration of basic medical degree course, including practical training: **7 years**
Entrance examination: **Yes**
Foreign students eligible: **Yes**

FAKULTAS KEDOKTERAN
UNIVERSITAS AHMAD YANI
JALAN TERUSAN JENDRAL SUDIRMAN
PO BOX 148
CIMAHI
JAWA BARAT

Tel.: +62 (22) 664 2781/664 2782/664 2783
Fax: +62 (22) 665 7187
Year instruction started: **1993**
Language of instruction: **Indonesian**
Duration of basic medical degree course, including practical training: **7 years**
Entrance examination: **Yes**
Foreign students eligible: **No**

FAKULTAS KEDOKTERAN
UNIVERSITAS UDAYANA
JALAN PANGLIMA BESAR SUDIRMAN
DENPASAR
BALI
Year instruction started: **1962**

FAKULTAS KEDOKTERAN
UNIVERSITAS INDONESIA
JALAN SALEMBA 6
PO BOX 1358
JAKARTA 10430
DKI JAKARTA
Tel.: +62 (21) 330 373
Fax: +62 (21) 330 372
Year instruction started: **1950**
Language of instruction: **Indonesian**
Duration of basic medical degree course, including practical training: **6 years**
Entrance examination: **Yes**
Foreign students eligible: **Yes**

FAKULTAS KEDOKTERAN
UNIVERSITAS UPN VETERAN
JALAN PONDOK LABU
JAKARTA
Tel.: +62 (21) 769 6904
Fax: +62 (21) 769 3275
Year instruction started: **1995**
Language of instruction: **Indonesian**
Duration of basic medical degree course, including practical training: **6 years**
Entrance examination: **Yes**
Foreign students eligible: **Yes**

FAKULTAS KEDOKTERAN
UNIVERSITAS KRISTEN KRIDA WACANA
JALAN TANJUNG DUREN RAYA 4
JAKARTA BARAT

Tel.: +62 (21) 566 6952
Fax: +62 (21) 566 6951
Year instruction started: **1967**
Language of instruction: **Indonesian**
Duration of basic medical degree course, including practical training: **6 years**
Entrance examination: **Yes**
Foreign students eligible: **Yes**

FAKULTAS KEDOKTERAN
UNIVERSITAS TARUMA NEGARA
JALAN JEN. S. PARMAN 1
JAKARTA BARAT 11440
Tel.: +62 (21) 567 0815/567 1781
Fax: +62 (21) 566 3126
Year instruction started: **1967**
Language of instruction: **Indonesian**
Duration of basic medical degree course, including practical training: **6 years**
Entrance examination: **Yes**
Foreign students eligible: **Yes**

FAKULTAS KEDOKTERAN
UNIVERSITAS TRISAKTI
JALAN KYAI TAPA 260
GROGOL
JAKARTA BARAT 11440
Tel.: +62 (21) 567 2731/565 5786
Fax: +62 (21) 566 0706
E-mail: fkusakti@rad.net.id
Year instruction started: **1965**
Language of instruction: **Indonesian**
Duration of basic medical degree course, including practical training: **7 years**
Entrance examination: **Yes**
Foreign students eligible: **Yes**

FAKULTAS KEDOKTERAN
UNIVERSITAS KATOLIK INDONESIA ARMAJAYA
KOMPLEKS RS ATAMAJAYA
JALAN PLUIT RAYA 2
JAKARTA UTARA 14440
Tel.: +62 (21) 660 6127/660 6128/660 6129
Fax: +62 (21) 660 6123

Year instruction started: **1967**
Language of instruction: **Indonesian**
Duration of basic medical degree course, including practical training: **6 years**
Entrance examination: **Yes**
Foreign students eligible: **No**

FAKULTAS KEDOKTERAN
UNIVERSITAS BRAWIJAYA
JALAN MAYOR JENDRAL HARJONO 171
MALANG 65145
JAWA TIMUR
Tel.: +62 (341) 564 755
Fax: +62 (341) 564 755
Year instruction started: **1963**
Language of instruction: **Indonesian**
Duration of basic medical degree course, including practical training: **6 years**
Entrance examination: **Yes**
Foreign students eligible: **Yes**

FAKULTAS KEDOKTERAN
UNIVERSITAS ISLAM SUMATRA UTARA
JALAN SISINGAMANGARAJA 2A
MEDAN
SUMATRA UTARA
Tel.: +62 (61) 372 733
Fax: +62 (61) 542 495
Year instruction started: **1965**
Language of instruction: **Indonesian**
Duration of basic medical degree course, including practical training: **6 years**
Entrance examination: **Yes**
Foreign students eligible: **Yes**

FAKULTAS KEDOKTERAN
UNIVERSITAS METHODIST INDONESIA
JALAN SETIABUDI PASAR II
TANJUNG SARI
MEDAN 20132
SUMATRA UTARA
Tel.: +62 (61) 812 160
Fax: +62 (61) 812 161
Year instruction started: **1968**
Language of instruction: **Indonesian**
Duration of basic medical degree course, including practical training: **7 years**
Entrance examination: **Yes**
Foreign students eligible: **Yes**

FAKULTAS KEDOKTERAN
UNIVERSITAS SUMATERA UTARA
JALAN DR T. MANSUR 5
MEDAN 20155
SUMATRA UTERA
Tel.: +62 (61) 811 045
Fax: +62 (61) 816 264
E-mail: fkusu@karet.usu.ac.id
Year instruction started: **1952**
Language of instruction: **Indonesian**
Duration of basic medical degree course, including practical training: **6 years**
Entrance examination: **Yes**
Foreign students eligible: **Yes**

FAKULTAS KEDOKTERAN
UNIVERSITAS SAM RATULANGI
JALAN GUNUNG WENANG
MENADO
SULAWESI UTARA
Year instruction started: **1961**

FAKULTAS KEDOKTERAN
UNIVERSITAS ANDALAS
KAMPUS KEDOKTERAN
JALAN PERINTIS
PO BOX 49
PADANG 25127
SUMATRA BARAT
Tel.: +62 (751) 317 46
Fax: +62 (751) 317 46
Year instruction started: **1956**
Language of instruction: **Indonesian**
Duration of basic medical degree course, including practical training: **6 years**
Entrance examination: **Yes**
Foreign students eligible: **Yes**

FAKULTAS KEDOKTERAN
UNIVERSITAS BAITTURACHMAN
PADANG
SUMATRA BARAT
Tel.: +62 (751) 291 34/280 53

Year instruction started: **1995**
Language of instruction: **Indonesian**
Duration of basic medical degree course, including practical training: **6 years**
Entrance examination: **Yes**
Foreign students eligible: **Yes**

FAKULTAS KEDOKTERAN
UNIVERSITAS SRIWIJAYA
KOMPLEKS RSUP
JALAN MAYOR MAHIDIN
PALEMBANG 30126
SUMATRA SELATAN
Tel.: +62 (711) 352 342
Fax: +62 (711) 352 342
Year instruction started: **1962**
Language of instruction: **Indonesian**
Duration of basic medical degree course, including practical training: **6 years**
Entrance examination: **Yes**
Foreign students eligible: **Yes**

FAKULTAS KEDOKTERAN
UNIVERSITAS DIPONEGORO
JALAN DR SUTOMO 18
SEMARANG
JAWA TENGAH
Tel.: +62 (24) 311 480
Fax: +62 (24) 311 480
Year instruction started: **1961**
Language of instruction: **Indonesian**
Duration of basic medical degree course, including practical training: **6 years**
Entrance examination: **Yes**
Foreign students eligible: **Yes**

FAKULTAS KEDOKTERAN
UNIVERSITAS ISLAM SULTAN AGUNG
JALAN DEMAK RAYA
SEMARANG
JAWA TENGAH
Tel.: +62 (24) 583 588
Fax: +62 (24) 582 455
Year instruction started: **1964**
Language of instruction: **Indonesian**
Duration of basic medical degree course, including practical training: **6 years**
Entrance examination: **Yes**
Foreign students eligible: **Yes**

FAKULTAS KEDOKTERAN
UNIVERSITAS AIRLANGGA
JALAN MAYOR JENDRAL PROFESSOR DR MOESTOPO 47
SURABAYA 60131
JAWA TIMUR
Tel.: +62 (31) 534 2051/534 2052/534 2053
Fax: +62 (31) 532 2472
Year instruction started: **1954**
Language of instruction: **Indonesian**
Duration of basic medical degree course, including practical training: **6 years**
Entrance examination: **Yes**
Foreign students eligible: **Yes**

FAKULTAS KEDOKTERAN
UNIVERSITAS HAND TUAH
KOMPLEKS TIMUR RSAL
JALAN GADUNG 1
SURABAYA
JAWA TIMUR
Tel.: +62 (31) 843 3626
Fax: +62 (31) 843 3646
Year instruction started: **1985**
Language of instruction: **Indonesian**
Duration of basic medical degree course, including practical training: **8 years**
Entrance examination: **Yes**
Foreign students eligible: **No**

FAKULTAS KEDOKTERAN
UNIVERSITAS WIJAYAKUSUMA
JALAN DUKUH KUPANG XXV
SURABAYA 60225
JAWA TIMUR
Tel.: +62 (31) 568 6531
Fax: +62 (31) 568 6531
Year instruction started: **1987**
Language of instruction: **Indonesian**
Duration of basic medical degree course, including practical training: **7 years**
Entrance examination: **Yes**
Foreign students eligible: **Yes**

FAKULTAS KEDOKTERAN
UNIVERSITAS SEBELAS MARET
JALAN IR SUTAMI 36A
KENTINGAN
SURAKARTA
JAWA TENGAH
Year instruction started: **1976**

FAKULTAS KEDOKTERAN
UNIVERSITAS HASANUDDIN
JALAN PERINTIS DEMERDEKAAN KM 11
UJUNG PANDANG
SULAWESI SELATAN
Tel.: +62 (411) 512 010
Fax: +62 (411) 512 010
Year instruction started: **1956**
Language of instruction: **Indonesian**
Duration of basic medical degree course, including practical training: **6 years**
Entrance examination: **Yes**
Foreign students eligible: **Yes**

FAKULTAS KEDOKTERAN
UNIVERSITAS MUSLIM INDONESIA
JALAN URIP SUMOHARDJO KM 5 2A
UJUNG PANDANG
SULAWESI SELATAN
Tel.: +62 (411) 873 018
Fax: +62 (411) 327 009
Year instruction started: **1992**
Language of instruction: **Indonesian**
Duration of basic medical degree course, including practical training: **6 years**
Entrance examination: **Yes**
Foreign students eligible: **Yes**

FAKULTAS KEDOKTERAN
UNIVERSITAS GADJAH MADA
JALAN FARMAKO SEKIP
YOGYAKARTA 55281
Year instruction started: **1946**

FAKULTAS KEDOKTERAN
UNIVERSITAS MUHAMADIYAH
JALAN HQS TJOKROAMINOTO
YOGYAKARTA

Tel.: +62 (274) 514 753/517 011
Fax: +62 (274) 565 444
Year instruction started: **1993**
Language of instruction: **Indonesian**
Duration of basic medical degree course, including practical training: **6 years**
Entrance examination: **Yes**
Foreign students eligible: **Yes**

IRAN (ISLAMIC REPUBLIC OF)

Total population in 1995: **69 975 000**
Number of physicians per 100 000 population (1993): —
Number of medical schools: **46**
Duration of basic medical degree course, including practical training: **7 years (a further 2 years must be spent in government service before the degree is awarded)**
Title of degree awarded: **Doctor of Medicine**
Medical registration/licence to practise: **Registration is obligatory with the Medical Council of Iran, Academy of Medical Sciences of the Islamic Republic of Iran, Pasdaran Avenue, PO Box 4655, Teheran 19395.**
Work in government service after graduation: **Obligatory (2 years)**
Agreements with other countries: —

AHVAZ MEDICAL SCHOOL
AHVAZ UNIVERSITY OF MEDICAL SCIENCES AND HEALTH SERVICES
SHAHER DANSHGAH-GOLOSTAN STREET
PO BOX 159
AHVAZ 61355
Tel.: +98 (61) 335 024/339 092
Fax: +98 (61) 335 200
Year instruction started: **1955**
Language of instruction: **Farsi**
Duration of basic medical degree course, including practical training: **7 years**
Entrance examination: **Yes**
Foreign students eligible: **Yes**

SCHOOL OF MEDICINE
ARAK UNIVERSITY OF MEDICAL SCIENCES AND HEALTH SERVICES
AALAMOLHODA
PO BOX 646
ARAK
Tel.: +98 (861) 360 55/360 56/360 57
Fax: +98 (861) 300 21/337 05

Year instruction started: **1989**
Language of instruction: **Farsi**
Duration of basic medical degree course, including practical training: **7 years**
Entrance examination: **Yes**

MEDICAL SCHOOL
ARDABIL ISLAMIC AZAD UNIVERSITY
PO BOX 467
ARDABIL 55135
Tel.: +98 (451) 319 61
Fax: +98 (451) 310 99
Year instruction started: **1985**
Language of instruction: **Farsi**
Duration of basic medical degree course, including practical training: **7 years**
Entrance examination: **Yes**
Foreign students eligible: **No**

FACULTY OF MEDICINE
ARDABIL UNIVERSITY OF MEDICAL SCIENCES
SHOHADA SQUARE
ARDABIL 55136
Tel.: +98 (451) 213 00/280 02
Fax: +98 (451) 213 00
Year instruction started: **1992**
Language of instruction: **Farsi**
Duration of basic medical degree course, including practical training: **7 years**
Entrance examination: **Yes**
Foreign students eligible: **No**

MEDICAL SCHOOL
BABOL UNIVERSITY OF MEDICAL SCIENCES AND HEALTH SERVICES
BABOL
Year instruction started: **1985**

SCHOOL OF MEDICINE
BANDAR ABBAS UNIVERSITY OF MEDICAL SCIENCES AND HEALTH SERVICES
SHAHID MOTAHARI
PO BOX 4188
BANDAR ABBAS 79145
Tel.: +98 (761) 336 89
Year instruction started: **1987**
Language of instruction: **Farsi, English**
Duration of basic medical degree course, including practical training: **7 years**
Entrance examination: **Yes**
Foreign students eligible: **No**

BIRJAND UNIVERSITY OF MEDICAL SCIENCES AND HEALTH SERVICES
MOALLEM STREET
BIRJAND 97178
Tel.: +98 (6324) 300 75/300 81/300 82
Fax: +98 (6324) 300 76
Year instruction started: **1986**
Language of instruction: **Farsi**
Duration of basic medical degree course, including practical training: **7 years**
Entrance examination: **Yes**
Foreign students eligible: **No**

BUSHEHR UNIVERSITY OF MEDICAL SCIENCES AND HEALTH SERVICES
MOALEM STREET
PO BOX 3631
BUSHEHR
Tel.: +98 (771) 220 75/263 17
Fax: +98 (771) 261 54
Year instruction started: **1995**
Language of instruction: **Farsi**
Duration of basic medical degree course, including practical training: **7 years**
Entrance examination: **Yes**
Foreign students eligible: **No**

FASA FACULTY OF MEDICAL SCIENCES AND HEALTH SERVICES
DANESHKADEH BOULEVARD
FASA 74615
Tel.: +98 (731) 909 94/909 95/909 96
Year instruction started: **1978**
Language of instruction: **Farsi, English**
Duration of basic medical degree course, including practical training: **7 years**
Entrance examination: **Yes**
Foreign students eligible: **No**

GHAZVIN MEDICAL SCHOOL
GHAZVIN UNIVERSITY OF MEDICAL SCIENCES AND HEALTH SERVICES
SHAHID BAHONAR BOULEVARD
GHAZVIN
Tel.: +98 (281) 360 01/360 02/360 03
Fax: +98 (281) 360 07
Year instruction started: **1985**
Language of instruction: **Farsi**
Duration of basic medical degree course, including practical training: **7 years**
Entrance examination: **Yes**
Foreign students eligible: **Yes**

GONABAD FACULTY OF MEDICAL SCIENCES AND HEALTH SERVICES
IMAM KHOMEINI AVENUE
PO BOX 47
GONABAD 96916
Tel.: +98 (5326) 2328
Fax: +98 (5326) 3815
Year instruction started: **1993**
Language of instruction: **Farsi, English**
Duration of basic medical degree course, including practical training: **7 years**
Entrance examination: **Yes**
Foreign students eligible: **Yes**

GORGAN UNIVERSITY OF MEDICAL SCIENCES AND HEALTH SERVICES
SARY-GORGAN AVENUE 2ND KM
GORGAN
Tel.: +98 (271) 318 00/318 01/318 02
Fax: +98 (271) 318 00
Year instruction started: **1991**
Language of instruction: **Farsi, English**
Duration of basic medical degree course, including practical training: **7 years**
Entrance examination: **Yes**
Foreign students eligible: **Yes**

HAMADAN UNIVERSITY OF MEDICAL SCIENCES AND HEALTH SERVICES
KHAJEH RASHID CROSSROADS
PO BOX 518
HAMADAN 65176
Tel.: +98 (81) 220 683/220 684
Fax: +98 (81) 220 273
Year instruction started: **1976**
Language of instruction: **Farsi**
Duration of basic medical degree course, including practical training: **7 years**
Entrance examination: **Yes**
Foreign students eligible: **Yes**

ILAM UNIVERSITY OF MEDICAL SCIENCES AND HEALTH SERVICES
KESHVARI SQUARE
PO BOX 364
ILAM 69315
Tel.: +98 (841) 375 38/375 39/375 40
Fax: +98 (841) 340 60

Year instruction started: **1989**
Language of instruction: **Farsi**
Duration of basic medical degree course, including practical training: **7 years**
Entrance examination: **Yes**
Foreign students eligible: **Yes**

FACULTY OF MEDICINE
ISFAHAN UNIVERSITY OF MEDICAL SCIENCES AND HEALTH SERVICES
HEZAR JERIB STREET
PO BOX 319
ISFAHAN 81745
Tel.: +98 (31) 222 550/222 199
Fax: +98 (31) 264 50
Year instruction started: **1946**
Language of instruction: **Farsi**
Duration of basic medical degree course, including practical training: **7 years**
Entrance examination: **Yes**
Foreign students eligible: **Yes**

JAHROM FACULTY OF MEDICAL SCIENCES AND HEALTH SERVICES
JAHROM
Tel.: +98 (791) 315 20/315 21/315 22
Fax: +98 (791) 315 20
Year instruction started: **1986**
Language of instruction: **Farsi**
Duration of basic medical degree course, including practical training: **7 years**
Entrance examination: **Yes**
Foreign students eligible: **Yes**

KASHAN UNIVERSITY OF MEDICAL SCIENCES AND HEALTH SERVICES
KHYABAN ABAZAR
PO BOX 87137-111
KASHAN 87134
Tel.: +98 (361) 430 22/430 23/430 24
Fax: +98 (361) 556 112
Year instruction started: **1986**
Language of instruction: **Farsi, English**
Duration of basic medical degree course, including practical training: **7 years**
Entrance examination: **Yes**
Foreign students eligible: **Yes**

AFZALE-POUR MEDICAL SCHOOL
KERMAN UNIVERSITY OF MEDICAL SCIENCES AND HEALTH SERVICES
22 BAHMAN BOULEVARD
PO BOX 444
KERMAN
Tel.: +98 (341) 231 640
Fax: +98 (341) 231 585
Year instruction started: **1976**
Language of instruction: **Farsi**
Duration of basic medical degree course, including practical training: **7 years**
Entrance examination: **Yes**
Foreign students eligible: **Yes**

KERMANSHAH UNIVERSITY OF MEDICAL SCIENCES AND HEALTH SERVICES
BOLVAR-E-SHAHID BEHESHTI
KERMANSHAH 67147
Tel.: +98 (831) 597 95/501 77/500 97
Fax: +98 (831) 500 13
Year instruction started: **1985**
Language of instruction: **Farsi**
Duration of basic medical degree course, including practical training: **7 years**
Entrance examination: **Yes**
Foreign students eligible: **Yes**

LORESTAN UNIVERSITY OF MEDICAL SCIENCES AND HEALTH SERVICES
SHAFA STREET
KHORAMABAD
Tel.: +98 (661) 350 13
Fax: +98 (661) 307 71
Year instruction started: **1991**
Language of instruction: **Farsi, English**
Duration of basic medical degree course, including practical training: **7 years**
Entrance examination: **Yes**
Foreign students eligible: **No**

ISLAMIC AZAD UNIVERSITY SCHOOL OF MEDICINE
MALEK ABAD BOULEVARD
FARHAD STREET
MASHHAD 91857
Tel.: +98 (51) 783 979
Language of instruction: **Farsi, English**
Duration of basic medical degree course, including practical training: **7 years**
Entrance examination: **Yes**
Foreign students eligible: **Yes**

MEDICAL SCHOOL
MASHHAD UNIVERSITY OF MEDICAL SCIENCES AND HEALTH SERVICES
DANESHGAH STREET
PO BOX 91735-588
MASHHAD 91376
Tel.: +98 (51) 440 81/440 82/440 83
Fax: +98 (51) 919 22
Year instruction started: **1949**
Language of instruction: **Farsi**
Duration of basic medical degree course, including practical training: **7 years**
Entrance examination: **Yes**
Foreign students eligible: **Yes**

NAJAF ABAD MEDICAL FACULTY
ISLAMIC AZAD UNIVERSITY
UNIVERSITY BOULEVARD
NAJEF ABAD 85135
Tel.: +98 (331) 512 75
Fax: +98 (331) 513 72
Language of instruction: **Farsi, English**
Duration of basic medical degree course, including practical training: **7 years**
Entrance examination: **Yes**
Foreign students eligible: **Yes**

FACULTY OF MEDICINE
WEST AZERBAIJAN UNIVERSITY OF MEDICAL SCIENCES AND HEALTH
    SERVICES
DJAHAD AVENUE
PO BOX 1138
OROUMIEH 57147
Tel.: +98 (441) 322 96
Fax: +98 (441) 218 41
Year instruction started: **1977**
Language of instruction: **Farsi**
Duration of basic medical degree course, including practical training: **7 years**
Entrance examination: **Yes**
Foreign students eligible: **No**

QOM UNIVERSITY OF MEDICAL SCIENCES
SHAHID LAVASANI AVENUE
PO BOX 3534
QOM 37185
Year instruction started: **1997**

Language of instruction: **Farsi, English**
Duration of basic medical degree course, including practical training: **7 years**
Entrance examination: **Yes**
Foreign students eligible: **No**

RAFSANJAN UNIVERSITY OF MEDICAL SCIENCES AND HEALTH SERVICES
IMAM KHOMAINI
RAFSANJAN
Tel.: +98 (3431) 6962
Fax: +98 (3431) 6310
Year instruction started: **1986**
Language of instruction: **Farsi**
Duration of basic medical degree course, including practical training: **7 years**
Entrance examination: **Yes**
Foreign students eligible: **No**

MEDICAL SCHOOL
GILAN UNIVERSITY OF MEDICAL SCIENCES AND HEALTH SERVICES
NAMJOO AVENUE
RASHT 41335
Tel.: +98 (131) 394 29/312 82
Fax: +98 (131) 370 70
Year instruction started: **1984**
Language of instruction: **Farsi**
Duration of basic medical degree course, including practical training: **7 years**
Entrance examination: **Yes**
Foreign students eligible: **Yes**

SABZEVAR FACULTY OF MEDICAL SCIENCES AND HEALTH SERVICES
TEHRAN ROAD
SABZEVAR 96135
Tel.: +98 (5221) 419 91/419 92/419 93
Fax: +98 (5221) 419 91
Year instruction started: **1992**
Language of instruction: **Farsi**
Duration of basic medical degree course, including practical training: **7 years**
Entrance examination: **Yes**
Foreign students eligible: **No**

KURDISTAN UNIVERSITY OF MEDICAL SCIENCES AND HEALTH SERVICES
PASDARAN BOULEVARD
SANANDAJ
Tel.: +98 (871) 311 05
Fax: +98 (871) 328 00

Year instruction started: **1985**
Language of instruction: **Farsi, English**
Duration of basic medical degree course, including practical training: **7 years**
Entrance examination: **Yes**
Foreign students eligible: **Yes**

MAZANDARAN UNIVERSITY OF MEDICAL SCIENCES AND HEALTH SERVICES
JOYBAR THREEWAY
SARI 48154
Tel.: +98 (151) 216 21
Fax: +98 (151) 256 69
Year instruction started: **1988**
Language of instruction: **Farsi**
Duration of basic medical degree course, including practical training: **7 years**
Entrance examination: **Yes**

SEMNAN UNIVERSITY OF MEDICAL SCIENCES AND HEALTH SERVICES
BOLVAR BACIJE
PO BOX 193
SEMNAN 35195
Fax: +98 (2231) 311 2379
Year instruction started: **1986**
Language of instruction: **Farsi**
Duration of basic medical degree course, including practical training: **7 years**

MEDICAL FACULTY
SHAHR-E-KORD UNIVERSITY OF MEDICAL SCIENCES AND HEALTH
    SERVICES
SHAHID BEHESHTI AVENUE
PO BOX 618
SHAHR-E-KORD 88155
Tel.: +98 (381) 272 20/272 21
Fax: +98 (381) 243 84
Year instruction started: **1986**
Language of instruction: **Farsi**
Duration of basic medical degree course, including practical training: **7 years**
Entrance examination: **Yes**
Foreign students eligible: **No**

SHAHROOD FACULTY OF MEDICAL SCIENCES AND HEALTH SERVICES
SHOHADA AVENUE
SHAHROOD 36184
Fax: +98 (2731) 340 90
Year instruction started: **1992**
Language of instruction: **English**

MEDICAL SCHOOL
SHIRAZ UNIVERSITY OF MEDICAL SCIENCES AND HEALTH SERVICES
SHIRAZ
Year instruction started: **1949**

FACULTY OF MEDICINE, TABRIZ MEDICAL UNIT
ISLAMIC AZAD UNIVERSITY
SHESHGELAN AVENUE
TABRIZ 51386
Tel.: +98 (41) 299 73
Fax: +98 (41) 318 687
Year instruction started: **1985**
Language of instruction: **Farsi**
Duration of basic medical degree course, including practical training: **7 years**
Entrance examination: **Yes**
Foreign students eligible: **Yes**

FACULTY OF MEDICINE
TABRIZ UNIVERSITY OF MEDICAL SCIENCES AND HEALTH SERVICES
TABRIZ
Year instruction started: **1947**
Duration of basic medical degree course, including practical training: **7 years**

SCHOOL OF MEDICINE
IRAN UNIVERSITY OF MEDICAL SCIENCES AND HEALTH SERVICES
SATTARKHAN AVENUE
NIAYESH STREET
TEHERAN 14456
Tel.: +98 (21) 979 024/978 591
Fax: +98 (21) 989 947
Year instruction started: **1975**
Language of instruction: **Farsi**
Duration of basic medical degree course, including practical training: **7 years**
Entrance examination: **Yes**
Foreign students eligible: **No**

TEHERAN SCHOOL OF MEDICINE
ISLAMIC AZAD UNIVERSITY
PO BOX 19395-1495
TEHERAN 19168
Tel.: +98 (21) 200 6660/200 6661/200 6662
Fax: +98 (21) 260 714

E-mail: ghods@neda.net
Year instruction started: **1985**
Language of instruction: **Farsi**
Duration of basic medical degree course, including practical training: **7 years**
Entrance examination: **Yes**

MEDICAL SCHOOL
SHAHID BEHESHTI UNIVERSITY OF MEDICAL SCIENCES AND HEALTH
　　SERVICES
EVEEN AVENUE
TEHERAN 19395-4719
Tel.: +98 (21) 240 0511/214 1420
Fax: +98 (21) 240 0681
Year instruction started: **1986**
Language of instruction: **Farsi, English**
Duration of basic medical degree course, including practical training: **7 years**
Entrance examination: **Yes**
Foreign students eligible: **Yes**

TEHERAN SCHOOL OF MEDICAL SCIENCES AND HEALTH SERVICES
TAJRISH SQUARE
TEHERAN
Year instruction started: **1934**

TEHERAN MEDICAL SCHOOL
TEHERAN UNIVERSITY OF MEDICAL SCIENCES AND HEALTH SERVICES
KESHAVARZ BOULEVARD
POURSINA AVENUE
PO BOX 5799
TEHERAN 14155
Tel.: +98 (21) 640 5373
Fax: +98 (21) 640 9641
Year instruction started: **1932**
Language of instruction: **Farsi, English**
Duration of basic medical degree course, including practical training: **7 years**
Entrance examination: **Yes**
Foreign students eligible: **Yes**

YASUJ UNIVERSITY OF MEDICAL SCIENCES AND HEALTH SERVICES
MOTAHARI BOULEVARD
YASUJ 75914
Tel.: +98 (741) 902 13
Fax: +98 (741) 5305

Year instruction started: **1990**
Language of instruction: **Farsi**
Duration of basic medical degree course, including practical training: **7 years**
Entrance examination: **Yes**
Foreign students eligible: **Yes**

ALI BEN ABITALIB MEDICAL COLLEGE
ISLAMIC AZAD UNIVERSITY
SAFA-EIYEH
PO BOX 89195
YAZD
Tel.: +98 (351) 840 697
Fax: +98 (351) 845 775
Year instruction started: **1986**
Language of instruction: **Farsi**
Duration of basic medical degree course, including practical training: **7 years**
Entrance examination: **Yes**
Foreign students eligible: **No**

YAZD SHAHID SADOUGHI UNIVERSITY OF MEDICAL SCIENCES AND
    HEALTH SERVICES
BOU ALI STREET SAFAIEH
PO BOX 734
YAZD
Tel.: +98 (351) 454 45
Fax: +98 (351) 454 46
Year instruction started: **1983**
Language of instruction: **Farsi**
Duration of basic medical degree course, including practical training: **7 years**
Entrance examination: **Yes**
Foreign students eligible: **No**

ZAHEDAN UNIVERSITY OF MEDICAL SCIENCES AND HEALTH SERVICES
MIDANE MASHAHIR
PO BOX 936
ZAHEDAN 98135
Tel.: +98 (541) 448 584
Fax: +98 (541) 442 481
Year instruction started: **1976**
Language of instruction: **Farsi, English**
Duration of basic medical degree course, including practical training: **7 years**
Entrance examination: **Yes**
Foreign students eligible: **Yes**

ZANJAN MEDICAL SCHOOL
ZANJAN UNIVERSITY OF MEDICAL SCIENCES AND HEALTH SERVICES
AZADI BOULEVARD
ZANJAN 45154
Tel.: +98 (2821) 247 77
Fax: +98 (2821) 396 24
Year instruction started: **1987**
Language of instruction: **Farsi**
Duration of basic medical degree course, including practical training: **7 years**
Entrance examination: **No**
Foreign students eligible: **Yes**

IRAQ

Total population in 1995: **20 607 000**
Number of physicians per 100 000 population (1993): **51**
Number of medical schools: **10**
Duration of basic medical degree course, including practical training: **6 years**
Title of degree awarded: **Bachelor of Medicine and Bachelor of Surgery (MB, ChB); Bachelor of Science in Medicine and General Surgery (BSc)**
Medical registration/licence to practise: **Registration is obligatory with the Iraqi Medical Association, Al Maarri Street, PO Box 6282, Al Mansour City, Baghdad. The licence to practise medicine is granted to holders of a Bachelor of Science in Medicine and General Surgery from a recognized medical school in the country. Graduates must have completed a 2-year internship, 1 year of rural service and national service. Those who have qualified abroad must have their degree validated by the Ministry of Higher Education and Scientific Research. Foreigners may practise if they hold a contract with a government agency or if a reciprocal agreement exists between their country and Iraq.**
Work in government service after graduation: **Obligatory for nationals (25 years)**
Agreements with other countries: —

COLLEGE OF MEDICINE
AL-ANBAR UNIVERSITY
PO BOX 55
AL-ANBAR
Tel.: +964 (8) 864 856

COLLEGE OF MEDICINE
BABEL UNIVERSITY
PO BOX 4
BABEL
Tel.: +964 (30) 249 672

SADDAM COLLEGE OF MEDICINE
SADDAM UNIVERSITY
KADHIMIA MAHALLAH 427
PO BOX 14222
BAGHDAD 11427
Tel.: +964 (1) 522 6452
Telex: 213068 samed ik
Year instruction started: **1987**
Language of instruction: **English**
Duration of basic medical degree course, including practical training: **6 years**
Entrance examination: **Yes**
Foreign students eligible: **No**

COLLEGE OF MEDICINE
UNIVERSITY OF AL-MUSTANSIRIYAH
PO BOX 14022
BAGHDAD
Tel.: +964 (1) 541 3392/541 2419
Telex: 213252 medco ik
Year instruction started: **1975**
Language of instruction: **English**
Duration of basic medical degree course, including practical training: **6 years**
Entrance examination: **No**
Foreign students eligible: **Yes**

COLLEGE OF MEDICINE
UNIVERSITY OF BAGHDAD
BAB AL-MUADHAM
PO BOX 61023
BAGHDAD 12114
Tel.: +964 (1) 886 1514
Year instruction started: **1927**
Language of instruction: **English**
Duration of basic medical degree course, including practical training: **6 years**
Entrance examination: **No**
Foreign students eligible: **Yes**

FACULTY OF MEDICINE
UNIVERSITY OF BASRAH
PO BOX 939
BASRAH
Tel.: +964 (40) 211 671/311 890

Year instruction started: **1967**
Language of instruction: **English**
Duration of basic medical degree course, including practical training: **6 years**
Entrance examination: **Yes**
Foreign students eligible: **Yes**

SALAHADIN MEDICAL SCHOOL
UNIVERSITY OF SALAHADIN
ERBIL
Year instruction started: **1978**

COLLEGE OF MEDICINE
KUFA UNIVERSITY
PO BOX 18
KUFA
Tel.: +964 (33) 342 822
Year instruction started: **1977**
Language of instruction: **English**
Duration of basic medical degree course, including practical training: **6 years**
Entrance examination: **No**
Foreign students eligible: **Yes**

COLLEGE OF MEDICINE
UNIVERSITY OF MOSUL
AL-SHEFAA
MOSUL
Tel.: +964 (60) 777 340
Year instruction started: **1959**
Language of instruction: **English**
Duration of basic medical degree course, including practical training: **6 years**
Entrance examination: **No**
Foreign students eligible: **Yes**

FACULTY OF MEDICINE
UNIVERSITY OF TIKRIT
YARMOOK STREET
PO BOX 45
TIKRIT 28001
Tel.: +964 (21) 825 293
Telex: 216700 untik ik
Year instruction started: **1989**
Language of instruction: **English**
Duration of basic medical degree course, including practical training: **6 years**
Entrance examination: **Yes**
Foreign students eligible: **Yes**

IRELAND

Total population in 1995: **3 554 000**
Number of physicians per 100 000 population (1993): **167**
Number of medical schools: **5**
Duration of basic medical degree course, including practical training: **5 or 6 years**
Title of degree awarded: **Bachelor of Medicine and Bachelor of Surgery (MB, BCh)**
Medical registration/licence to practise: **Registration is obligatory with the Medical Council, Porto Bello Court, Lower Rathmines Road, Dublin 6. Graduates must have completed a 1-year internship (6 months of medicine and 6 months of surgery) and received a certificate of experience signed by the Dean of the medical school. Those who have qualified abroad must provide the original degree certificate and a certificate from the authority with which they are currently registered.**
Work in government service after graduation: **Not obligatory**
Agreements with other countries: **Agreements exist with other countries of the European Union (Directive 93/16/EEC governing the employment of doctors) and with certain universities in Australia, New Zealand and South Africa.**

FACULTY OF MEDICINE
NATIONAL UNIVERSITY OF IRELAND
UNIVERSITY COLLEGE
CORK
Year instruction started: **1841**

MEDICAL SCHOOL
ROYAL COLLEGE OF SURGEONS IN IRELAND
123 ST STEPHEN'S GREEN
DUBLIN 2
Tel.: +353 (1) 402 2281
Fax: +353 (1) 402 2460
Telex: 30795 rcsi ei
E-mail: registrar@rcsi.ie
Year instruction started: **1784**
Language of instruction: **English**
Duration of basic medical degree course, including practical training: **6 years**
Entrance examination: **No**
Foreign students eligible: **Yes**

FACULTY OF MEDICINE
NATIONAL UNIVERSITY OF IRELAND
UNIVERSITY COLLEGE OF DUBLIN
EARLSFORT TERRACE
DUBLIN 2
Year instruction started: **1854**

FACULTY OF HEALTH SCIENCES
UNIVERSITY OF DUBLIN
TRINITY COLLEGE
DUBLIN 2
Tel.: +353 (1) 608 1727/608 1075
Fax: +353 (1) 671 3956
E-mail: maslevin@mail.tcd.ie
Year instruction started: **1711**
Language of instruction: **English**
Duration of basic medical degree course, including practical training: **5 or 6 years**
Entrance examination: **No**
Foreign students eligible: **Yes**

FACULTY OF MEDICINE
NATIONAL UNIVERSITY OF IRELAND
UNIVERSITY COLLEGE
GALWAY
Year instruction started: **1849**

ISRAEL

Total population in 1995: **5 664 000**
Number of physicians per 100 000 population (1993): **459**
Number of medical schools: **4**
Duration of basic medical degree course, including practical training: **6 or 7 years**
Title of degree awarded: **Doctor of Medicine**
Medical registration/licence to practise: —
Work in government service after graduation: —
Agreements with other countries: —

IRVING AND JOYCE GOLDMAN SCHOOL OF MEDICINE
BEN GURION UNIVERSITY OF THE NEGEV
BEN-GURION DRIVE
PO BOX 653
BEER-SHEVA 84105
Tel.: +972 (7) 623 9068
Fax: +972 (7) 627 7342

Year instruction started: **1974**
Language of instruction: **Hebrew**
Duration of basic medical degree course, including practical training: **6 years**
Entrance examination: **Yes**
Foreign students eligible: **No**

THE BRUCE RAPPAPORT FACULTY OF MEDICINE
TECHNION–ISRAEL INSTITUTE OF TECHNOLOGY
EFRON STREET
BAT GALIM
PO BOX 9649
HAIFA 31096
Tel.: +972 (4) 829 5308
Fax: +972 (4) 851 7008
E-mail: rosalieb@tx.technion.ac.il
Year instruction started: **1969**
Language of instruction: **Hebrew**
Duration of basic medical degree course, including practical training: **6 years**
Entrance examination: **No**
Foreign students eligible: **Yes**

HADASSAH MEDICAL SCHOOL
THE HEBREW UNIVERSITY
PO BOX 12272
JERUSALEM 91120
Tel.: +972 (2) 675 8011
Fax: +972 (2) 678 4010
Year instruction started: **1949**
Language of instruction: **Hebrew, English**
Duration of basic medical degree course, including practical training: **7 years**
Foreign students eligible: **Yes**

SACKLER SCHOOL OF MEDICINE
TEL AVIV UNIVERSITY
RAMAT AVIV
TEL AVIV-YAFO 69978
Year instruction started: **1964**

ITALY

Total population in 1995: **57 226 000**
Number of physicians per 100 000 population (1993): —
Number of medical schools: **31**
Duration of basic medical degree course, including practical training: **6 or 7 years**

Title of degree awarded: *Laurea in Medicina e Chirurgia* (Diploma in Medicine and Surgery)
Medical registration/licence to practise: —
Work in government service after graduation: —
Agreements with other countries: **An agreement exists with other countries of the European Union (Directive 93/16/EEC governing the employment of doctors).**

FACOLTA DI MEDICINA E CHIRURGIA
UNIVERSITA DI ANCONA
PIAZZA ROMA 22
I-60100 ANCONA
Year instruction started: **1970**

FACOLTA DI MEDICINA E CHIRURGIA
UNIVERSITA DELL'AQUILA
VIA VETOIO COPPITO II
I-67100 AQUILA
Tel.: +39 (862) 433 301
Fax: +39 (862) 433 306
Year instruction started: **1969**
Language of instruction: **Italian**
Duration of basic medical degree course, including practical training: **6 years**
Entrance examination: **Yes**
Foreign students eligible: **Yes**

FACOLTA DI MEDICINA E CHIRURGIA
UNIVERSITA DI BARI
PIAZZA GIULIO CESARE 11
I-70124 BARI
Tel.: +39 (80) 547 8701
Fax: +39 (80) 547 8701
Year instruction started: **1925**
Language of instruction: **Italian**
Duration of basic medical degree course, including practical training: **6 years**
Entrance examination: **Yes**
Foreign students eligible: **Yes**

FACOLTA DI MEDICINA E CHIRURGIA
UNIVERSITA DI BOLOGNA
VIA SAN VITALE 59
I-40138 BOLOGNA
Year instruction started: **13th century**

FACOLTA DI MEDICINA E CHIRURGIA
UNIVERSITA DEGLI STUDI DI BRESCIA
VIA VALSABBINA 19
I-25100 BRESCIA
Year instruction started: **1982**

FACOLTA DI MEDICINA E CHIRURGIA
UNIVERSITA DEGLI STUDI DI CAGLIARI
VIALE DELL'UNIVERSITA 40
I-09100 CAGLIARI
Year instruction started: **1626**

FACOLTA DI MEDICINA E CHIRURGIA
UNIVERSITA DI CATANIA
VIALE PLEBISCITO 628
I-95124 CATANIA
Year instruction started: **1434**

FACOLTA DI MEDICINA E CHIRURGIA
UNIVERSITA DI REGGIO CALABRIA
VIALE PIO X 162
PRESSO OSPEDALE
I-88100 CATANZARO
Year instruction started: **1982**

FACOLTA DI MEDICINA E CHIRURGIA
LIBERA UNIVERSITA DEGLI STUDI "G. D'ANNUNZIO"
VIA DEI VESTINI
I-66100 CHIETI
Year instruction started: **1965**

FACOLTA DI MEDICINA E CHIRURGIA
UNIVERSITA DI FERRARA
CORSO GIOVECCA 203
I-44100 FERRARA
Year instruction started: **1391**

FACOLTA DI MEDICINA E CHIRURGIA
UNIVERSITA DI FIRENZE
VIALE MORGAGNI 85
I-50134 FIRENZE
Tel.: +39 (55) 417 928
Fax: +39 (55) 437 9384

Year instruction started: **14th century**
Language of instruction: **Italian**
Duration of basic medical degree course, including practical training: **6 years**
Entrance examination: **Yes**
Foreign students eligible: **Yes**

FACOLTA DI MEDICINA E CHIRURGIA
UNIVERSITA DI GENOVA
VIA DE TONI
I-16132 GENOVA
Tel.: +39 (10) 353 7235
Fax: +39 (10) 353 7352
Year instruction started: **1471**
Language of instruction: **Italian**
Duration of basic medical degree course, including practical training: **7 years**
Entrance examination: **Yes**
Foreign students eligible: **Yes**

FACOLTA DI MEDICINA E CHIRURGIA
UNIVERSITA DI MESSINA
VIA UGO BASSI
I-98100 MESSINA
Year instruction started: **1548**

FACOLTA DI MEDICINA E CHIRURGIA
UNIVERSITA DI MILANO
VIA FESTO DEL PERDONO 7
I-20122 MILANO
Year instruction started: **1924**

FACOLTA DI MEDICINA E CHIRURGIA
UNIVERSITA DI MODENA
VIA DEL POZZO 71
I-41100 MODENA
Year instruction started: **18th century**

FACOLTA DI MEDICINA E CHIRURGIA I
UNIVERSITA DI NAPOLI
VIA MEZZOCANNONE 16
I-80134 NAPOLI
Year instruction started: **1224**

FACOLTA DI MEDICINA E CHIRURGIA II
UNIVERSITA DI NAPOLI
VIA SERGIO PANSINI 5
I-80131 NAPOLI
Year instruction started: **1972**

FACOLTA DI MEDICINA E CHIRURGIA
UNIVERSITA DI PADOVA
VIA FACCIOLATI 71
I-35127 PADOVA
Year instruction started: **1222**

FACOLTA DI MEDICINA E CHIRURGIA
UNIVERSITA DI PALERMO
VIA DEL VESPRO 129
I-90127 PALERMO
Year instruction started: **1841**

FACOLTA DI MEDICINA E CHIRURGIA
UNIVERSITA DI PARMA
VIA GRAMSCI 14
I-43100 PARMA
Year instruction started: **1347**

FACOLTA DI MEDICINA E CHIRURGIA
UNIVERSITA DI PAVIA
PIAZZALE GOLGI 25
I-27100 PAVIA
Year instruction started: **1361**

FACOLTA DI MEDICINA E CHIRURGIA
UNIVERSITA DI PERUGIA
POLICLINICO MONTELUCE
I-06100 PERUGIA

FACOLTA DI MEDICINA E CHIRURGIA
UNIVERSITA DI PISA
VIA ROMA 55
I-56100 PISA
Year instruction started: **1343**

FACOLTA DI MEDICINA E CHIRURGIA "AGOSTINO GEMELLI"
UNIVERSITA CATTOLICA DEL SACRO CUORE
LARGO FRANCESCO VITO 1
I-00168 ROMA
Tel.: +39 (6) 301 51
Fax: +39 (6) 305 1343
Telex: 611330 ucatro i
Year instruction started: **1961**
Language of instruction: **Italian**
Duration of basic medical degree course, including practical training: **6 years**
Entrance examination: **Yes**
Foreign students eligible: **Yes**

FACOLTA DI MEDICINA E CHIRURGIA
UNIVERSITA DI ROMA—LA SAPIENZA
CITTA UNIVERSITARIA
PIAZZALE ALDO MORO 5
I-00185 ROMA
Year instruction started: **1303**

FACOLTA DI MEDICINA E CHIRURGIA
UNIVERSITA DI ROMA—TOR VERGATA
VIA DI TOR VERGATA 135
I-00133 ROMA
Tel.: +39 (6) 725 969 83
Fax: +39 (6) 202 5485
E-mail: guerrieri@utovrm.it
Year instruction started: **1982**
Language of instruction: **Italian**
Duration of basic medical degree course, including practical training: **6 years**
Entrance examination: **Yes**
Foreign students eligible: **Yes**

FACOLTA DI MEDICINA E CHIRURGIA
UNIVERSITA DI SASSARI
PIAZZALE UNIVERSITA
I-07100 SASSARI
Year instruction started: **1632**

FACOLTA DI MEDICINA E CHIRURGIA
UNIVERSITA DI SIENA
VIA DEL PORRIONE 80
I-53100 SIENA
Year instruction started: **1859**

FACOLTA DI MEDICINA E CHIRURGIA
UNIVERSITA DI TORINO
CORSO RAFFAELLO 30
I-10125 TORINO
Year instruction started: **1404**

FACOLTA DI MEDICINA E CHIRURGIA
UNIVERSITA DI TRIESTE
VIA MANZONI 16
I-34134 TRIESTE
Year instruction started: **1965**

CORSA DI LAUREA IN MEDICINA E CHIRURGIA
UNIVERSITA DEGLI STUDI DI VERONA
MENEGONE—BORGO ROMA
I-37134 VERONA
Tel.: +39 (45) 807 4466
Fax: +39 (45) 820 2222
E-mail: vettore@borgoroma.univr.it
Year instruction started: **1988**
Language of instruction: **Italian**
Duration of basic medical degree course, including practical training: **6 years**
Entrance examination: **Yes**
Foreign students eligible: **Yes**

JAMAICA

Total population in 1995: **2 491 000**
Number of physicians per 100 000 population (1993): **57**
Number of medical schools: **1**
Duration of basic medical degree course, including practical training: **5 years**
Title of degree awarded: **Bachelor of Medicine and Bachelor of Surgery (MB, BS)**
Medical registration/licence to practise: —
Work in government service after graduation: —
Agreements with other countries: —

FACULTY OF MEDICAL SCIENCES
UNIVERSITY OF THE WEST INDIES
MONA
KINGSTON
Tel.: +1876 (927) 2556
Fax: +1876 (927) 2556

Year instruction started: **1948**
Language of instruction: **English**
Duration of basic medical degree course, including practical training: **5 years**
Entrance examination: **No**
Foreign students eligible: **Yes**

JAPAN

Total population in 1995: **125 351 000**
Number of physicians per 100 000 population (1993): **177**
Number of medical schools: **80**
Duration of basic medical degree course, including practical training: **6 years**
Title of degree awarded: *Igakushi* **(Bachelor of Medicine)**
Medical registration/licence to practise: **Registration is obligatory with the Ministry of Health and Welfare, 1-2-2 Kasumigaseki, Chiyoda-ku, Tokyo. The licence to practise medicine is granted to graduates of a recognized medical school who have successfully completed a national medical practitioners' examination. Graduates of foreign medical schools must have their degree validated.**
Work in government service after graduation: **Not obligatory**
Agreements with other countries: **None**

■ AICHI
AICHI MEDICAL UNIVERSITY
21 KARIMATA IWASAKU
NAGAKUTE-CHO
AICHI-GUN 480-11
Tel.: +81 (52) 264 4811
Fax: +81 (56) 162 4866
Year instruction started: **1972**
Language of instruction: **Japanese**
Duration of basic medical degree course, including practical training: **6 years**
Entrance examination: **Yes**
Foreign students eligible: **Yes**

MEDICAL SCHOOL
NAGOYA CITY UNIVERSITY
1 KAWASUMI MIZUO-CHO
MIZUO-KU
NAGOYA 467
Tel.: +81 (52) 853 8077/851 5511
Fax: +81 (52) 842 0863

Year instruction started: **1943**
Language of instruction: **Japanese, English**
Duration of basic medical degree course, including practical training: **6 years**
Entrance examination: **Yes**
Foreign students eligible: **Yes**

SCHOOL OF MEDICINE
NAGOYA UNIVERSITY
65 TSURUMAI-CHO
SHOWA-KU
NAGOYA 466
Tel.: +81 (52) 741 2111
Fax: +81 (52) 744 2428
Year instruction started: **1871**
Language of instruction: **Japanese**
Duration of basic medical degree course, including practical training: **6 years**
Entrance examination: **Yes**
Foreign students eligible: **Yes**

SCHOOL OF MEDICINE
FUJITA HEALTH UNIVERSITY
1-98 DENGAKUGAKUBO
KUTSUKAKE-MACHI
TOYOAKE 470-11
Tel.: +81 (562) 932 600
Fax: +81 (562) 934 593
Year instruction started: **1972**
Language of instruction: **Japanese**
Duration of basic medical degree course, including practical training: **6 years**
Entrance examination: **Yes**
Foreign students eligible: **Yes**

■ **AKITA**
SCHOOL OF MEDICINE
AKITA UNIVERSITY
1-1 HONDO 1-CHOME
AKITA 010
Tel.: +81 (188) 331 166
Year instruction started: **1970**

■ **AOMORI**
SCHOOL OF MEDICINE
HIROSAKI UNIVERSITY
5 ZAIFU-CHO
HIROSAKI 036
Tel.: +81 (172) 335 111
Year instruction started: **1944**

■ **CHIBA**
SCHOOL OF MEDICINE
CHIBA UNIVERSITY
8-1 INOHANA 1-CHOME
CHUO-KU
CHIBA 260
Tel.: +81 (43) 222 7171
Fax: +81 (43) 227 1798
Year instruction started: **1874**
Language of instruction: **Japanese**
Duration of basic medical degree course, including practical training: **6 years**
Entrance examination: **Yes**
Foreign students eligible: **Yes**

■ **EHIME**
SCHOOL OF MEDICINE
EHIME UNIVERSITY
SHIZUKAWA SHIGENOBU-CHO
ONSEN-GUN 791-0295
Tel.: +81 (89) 944 1111
Fax: +81 (89) 960 5131
Year instruction started: **1973**
Language of instruction: **Japanese**
Duration of basic medical degree course, including practical training: **6 years**
Entrance examination: **Yes**
Foreign students eligible: **Yes**

■ **FUKUI**
FUKUI MEDICAL UNIVERSITY
23-3 SIMOAIZUKI
MATSUOKA-CHO
YOSIDA-GUN 910-11
Tel.: +81 (776) 613 111
Fax: +81 (776) 618 153

Year instruction started: **1980**
Language of instruction: **Japanese**
Duration of basic medical degree course, including practical training: **6 years**
Entrance examination: **Yes**
Foreign students eligible: **Yes**

■ **FUKUOKA**
SCHOOL OF MEDICINE
FUKUOKA UNIVERSITY
45-1 NANAKUMA 7-CHOME
JONAN-KU
FUKUOKA 814-80
Tel.: +81 (92) 801 1011
Fax: +81 (92) 865 6032
Year instruction started: **1972**
Language of instruction: **Japanese**
Duration of basic medical degree course, including practical training: **6 years**
Entrance examination: **Yes**
Foreign students eligible: **Yes**

FACULTY OF MEDICINE
KYUSHU UNIVERSITY
1-1 MAIDASHI 3-CHOME
HIGASHI-KU
FUKUOKA 812
Tel.: +81 (92) 641 1151
Fax: +81 (92) 631 2794
Year instruction started: **1903**
Language of instruction: **Japanese, English**
Duration of basic medical degree course, including practical training: **6 years**
Entrance examination: **Yes**
Foreign students eligible: **Yes**

SANGYO UNIVERSITY OF OCCUPATIONAL AND ENVIRONMENTAL HEALTH
1-1 ISEIGAOKA
YAHATANISHI-KU
KITAKYUSHU 807
Tel.: +81 (93) 691 7207
Fax: +81 (93) 602 5432
Year instruction started: **1978**
Language of instruction: **Japanese**
Duration of basic medical degree course, including practical training: **6 years**
Entrance examination: **Yes**
Foreign students eligible: **Yes**

SCHOOL OF MEDICINE
KURUME UNIVERSITY
67 ASAHI-MACHI
KURUME 830
Tel.: +81 (942) 353 311
Fax: +81 (942) 314 374
Year instruction started: **1928**
Language of instruction: **Japanese**
Duration of basic medical degree course, including practical training: **6 years**
Entrance examination: **Yes**
Foreign students eligible: **Yes**

■ **FUKUSHIMA**
FUKUSHIMA MEDICAL COLLEGE
1 HIKARIGAOKA
FUKUSHIMA 960-12
Tel.: +81 (245) 482 111
Year instruction started: **1944**

■ **GIFU**
SCHOOL OF MEDICINE
GIFU UNIVERSITY
40 TSUKASA-MACHI
GIFU 500
Tel.: +81 (582) 651 241
Year instruction started: **1943**

■ **GUNMA**
SCHOOL OF MEDICINE
GUNMA UNIVERSITY
39-22 SHOWA-MACHI 3-CHOME
MAEBASHI 371
Tel.: +81 (272) 207 111
Year instruction started: **1943**

■ **HIROSHIMA**
SCHOOL OF MEDICINE
HIROSHIMA UNIVERSITY
2-3 KASUMI 1-CHOME
MINAMI-KU
HIROSHIMA 734
Tel.: +81 (82) 257 5555
Fax: +81 (82) 257 5087
E-mail: kchoshi@mcai.med.hiroshima-u.ac.jp

Year instruction started: **1945**
Language of instruction: **Japanese**
Duration of basic medical degree course, including practical training: **6 years**
Entrance examination: **Yes**
Foreign students eligible: **Yes**

■ **HOKKAIDO**
ASAHIKAWA MEDICAL COLLEGE
3-11 NISHIKAGURA-4-SEN 5-CHOME
ASAHIKAWA 078
Tel.: +81 (16) 665 2111
Fax: +81 (16) 665 8275
Year instruction started: **1973**
Language of instruction: **Japanese**
Duration of basic medical degree course, including practical training: **6 years**
Entrance examination: **Yes**
Foreign students eligible: **Yes**

SCHOOL OF MEDICINE
HOKKAIDO UNIVERSITY
NISHI 7-CHOME KITA 15-JO
KITA-KU
SAPPORO 060
Tel.: +81 (11) 716 2111
Year instruction started: **1919**

SAPPORO MEDICAL COLLEGE
NISHI 17-CHOME MINAMI 1-JO
CHUO-KU
SAPPORO 060
Tel.: +81 (11) 611 2111
Year instruction started: **1944**

■ **HYOGO**
FACULTY OF MEDICINE
KOBE UNIVERSITY
5-1 KUSUNOKI-CHO 7-CHOME
CHUO-KU
KOBE 650
Tel.: +81 (78) 341 7451
Fax: +81 (78) 351 5197

Year instruction started: **1944**
Language of instruction: **Japanese**
Duration of basic medical degree course, including practical training: **6 years**
Entrance examination: **Yes**
Foreign students eligible: **Yes**

HYOGO MEDICAL UNIVERSITY
1-1 MUKOGAWA-CHO
NISHINOMIYA 663
Tel.: +81 (798) 456 111
Year instruction started: **1972**

■ **IBARAKI**
SCHOOL OF MEDICINE
UNIVERSITY OF TSUKUBA
1-1 TENNODAI 1-CHOME
TSUKUBA 305
Tel.: +81 (298) 533 000
Fax: +81 (298) 533 037
Year instruction started: **1974**
Language of instruction: **Japanese**
Duration of basic medical degree course, including practical training: **6 years**
Entrance examination: **Yes**
Foreign students eligible: **Yes**

■ **ISHIKAWA**
KANAZAWA MEDICAL UNIVERSITY
1-1 DAIGAKU
UCHINADA-MACHI
KAHOKU-GUN 920-02
Tel.: +81 (762) 862 211
Fax: +81 (762) 862 373
Year instruction started: **1972**
Language of instruction: **Japanese**
Duration of basic medical degree course, including practical training: **6 years**
Entrance examination: **Yes**
Foreign students eligible: **Yes**

FACULTY OF MEDICINE
KANAZAWA UNIVERSITY
13-1 TAKARA-MACHI
KANAZAWA 920
Tel.: +81 (762) 628 151
Fax: +81 (762) 624 202

Year instruction started: **1945**
Language of instruction: **Japanese**
Duration of basic medical degree course, including practical training: **6 years**
Entrance examination: **Yes**
Foreign students eligible: **Yes**

■ IWATE

SCHOOL OF MEDICINE
IWATE MEDICAL UNIVERSITY
19-1 UCHIMARU
MORIOKA 020
Tel.: +81 (19) 651 5111
Fax: +81 (19) 624 1231
Year instruction started: **1928**
Language of instruction: **Japanese**
Duration of basic medical degree course, including practical training: **6 years**
Entrance examination: **Yes**
Foreign students eligible: **Yes**

■ KAGAWA

KAGAWA MEDICAL UNIVERSITY
1750-1 IKENOBE
MIKI-CHO
KITA-GUN 761-07
Tel.: +81 (878) 985 111
Year instruction started: **1980**

■ KAGOSHIMA

FACULTY OF MEDICINE
KAGOSHIMA UNIVERSITY
35-1 SAKURAGAOKA 8-CHOME
KAGOSHIMA 890
Tel.: +81 (992) 755 111
Fax: +81 (992) 755 014
Year instruction started: **1942**
Language of instruction: **Japanese**
Duration of basic medical degree course, including practical training: **6 years**
Entrance examination: **Yes**
Foreign students eligible: **Yes**

■ KANAGAWA

SCHOOL OF MEDICINE
TOKAI UNIVERSITY
BOSEIDAI
ISEHARA 259-11
Tel.: +81 (463) 931 121
Fax: +81 (463) 931 130
E-mail: nakamura@is.icc.u-tokai.ac.jp
Year instruction started: **1974**
Language of instruction: **Japanese, English**
Duration of basic medical degree course, including practical training: **6 years**
Entrance examination: **Yes**
Foreign students eligible: **Yes**

SCHOOL OF MEDICINE
ST MARIANNA UNIVERSITY
16-1 SUGAO 2-CHOME
MIYAMAE-KU
KAWASAKI 216
Tel.: +81 (44) 977 8111
Fax: +81 (44) 977 8133
Year instruction started: **1971**
Language of instruction: **Japanese**
Entrance examination: **Yes**
Foreign students eligible: **No**

SCHOOL OF MEDICINE
KITASATO UNIVERSITY
15-1 KITASATO 1-CHOME
SAGAMIHARA 228
Tel.: +81 (427) 789 339/788 111
Fax: +81 (427) 789 262
Year instruction started: **1970**
Language of instruction: **Japanese**
Duration of basic medical degree course, including practical training: **6 years**
Entrance examination: **Yes**
Foreign students eligible: **Yes**

YOKOHAMA CITY UNIVERSITY
3-9 FUKUURA
KANAZAWA-KU
YOKOHAMA 236
Tel.: +81 (45) 787 2511
Year instruction started: **1944**

■ KOCHI
KOCHI MEDICAL SCHOOL
OKOH-CHO
NANGOKU 783
Tel.: +81 (888) 665 811
Fax: +81 (888) 802 264
Year instruction started: **1978**
Language of instruction: **Japanese**
Duration of basic medical degree course, including practical training: **6 years**
Entrance examination: **Yes**
Foreign students eligible: **Yes**

■ KUMAMOTO
SCHOOL OF MEDICINE
KUMAMOTO UNIVERSITY
2-1 HONJO 2-CHOME
KUMAMOTO 860
Tel.: +81 (96) 344 2111
Year instruction started: **1904**

■ KYOTO
KYOTO PREFECTURAL UNIVERSITY OF MEDICINE
HIROKOJI, KAMARAMACHI-DORI
KAMIGYO-KU
KYOTO 602
Tel.: +81 (75) 251 5111
Year instruction started: **1903**

FACULTY OF MEDICINE
KYOTO UNIVERSITY
YOSHIDA-KONO-CHO
SAKYO-KU
KYOTO 606-01
Tel.: +81 (75) 753 7531
Year instruction started: **1899**

■ MIE
SCHOOL OF MEDICINE
MIE UNIVERSITY
2-174 EDOBASHI
TSU 514
Tel.: +81 (592) 321 111
Fax: +81 (592) 327 498
Year instruction started: **1943**

■ MIYAGI

FACULTY OF MEDICINE
TOHOKU UNIVERSITY
2-1 SEIRYO-MACHI
AOBA-KU
SENDAI 980
Tel.: +81 (22) 274 1111
Year instruction started: **1887**

■ MIYAZAKI

MIYAZAKI MEDICAL COLLEGE
5200 KIHARA
KIYOTAKE-CHO
MIYAZAKI-GUN 889-16
Tel.: +81 (985) 851 510
Year instruction started: **1974**

■ NAGANO

FACULTY OF MEDICINE
SHINSHU UNIVERSITY
1-1 ASAHI 3-CHOME
MATSUMOTO 390
Tel.: +81 (263) 354 600
Fax: +81 (263) 336 458
Year instruction started: **1944**
Language of instruction: **Japanese**
Duration of basic medical degree course, including practical training: **6 years**
Entrance examination: **Yes**
Foreign students eligible: **Yes**

■ NAGASAKI

SCHOOL OF MEDICINE
NAGASAKI UNIVERSITY
12-4 SAKAMOTO-MACHI 1-CHOME
NAGASAKI 852
Tel.: +81 (958) 497 000/472 111
Fax: +81 (958) 497 012
Year instruction started: **1868**
Language of instruction: **Japanese**
Duration of basic medical degree course, including practical training: **6 years**
Entrance examination: **Yes**
Foreign students eligible: **Yes**

■ NARA

NARA MEDICAL UNIVERSITY
840 SHIJO-CHO
KASHIHARA 634
Tel.: +81 (744) 223 051
Year instruction started: **1945**
Language of instruction: **Japanese**
Duration of basic medical degree course, including practical training: **6 years**
Entrance examination: **Yes**
Foreign students eligible: **Yes**

■ NIIGATA

SCHOOL OF MEDICINE
NIIGATA UNIVERSITY
757 ICHIBAN-CHO
ASAHIMACHI-DORI
NIIGATA 951
Tel.: +81 (25) 223 6161
Fax: +81 (25) 225 5885
Year instruction started: **1937**
Language of instruction: **Japanese**
Duration of basic medical degree course, including practical training: **6 years**
Entrance examination: **Yes**
Foreign students eligible: **Yes**

■ OITA

MEDICAL UNIVERSITY OF OITA
1-1 IDAIGAOKA
HAZAMA-CHO
OITA-GUN 879-55
Tel.: +81 (975) 865 170
Fax: +81 (975) 865 119
Year instruction started: **1976**
Language of instruction: **Japanese**
Duration of basic medical degree course, including practical training: **6 years**
Entrance examination: **Yes**
Foreign students eligible: **Yes**

■ OKAYAMA

KAWASAKI MEDICAL SCHOOL
577 MATSUSHIMA
KURASHIKI 701-01
Tel.: +81 (86) 462 1111
Fax: +81 (86) 464 1019

E-mail: dean@cc.kawasaki-m.ac.jp
Year instruction started: **1970**
Language of instruction: **Japanese**
Duration of basic medical degree course, including practical training: **6 years**
Entrance examination: **Yes**
Foreign students eligible: **Yes**

SCHOOL OF MEDICINE
OKAYAMA UNIVERSITY
5-1 SHIKATA-CHO 2-CHOME
OKAYAMA 700
Tel.: +81 (86) 223 7151
Fax: +81 (86) 233 3559
Year instruction started: **1870**
Language of instruction: **Japanese**
Duration of basic medical degree course, including practical training: **6 years**
Entrance examination: **Yes**
Foreign students eligible: **Yes**

■ **OKINAWA**
FACULTY OF MEDICINE
RYUKYUS UNIVERSITY
207 UEHARA
NISHIHARA-MACHI
NAKAGAMI-GUN 903-01
Tel.: +81 (98) 895 3331
Fax: +81 (98) 895 2779
Year instruction started: **1981**
Language of instruction: **Japanese**
Duration of basic medical degree course, including practical training: **6 years**
Entrance examination: **Yes**
Foreign students eligible: **Yes**

■ **OSAKA**
KANSAI MEDICAL SCHOOL
1 FUMIZONO-CHO
MORIGUCHI 570
Tel.: +81 (6) 992 1001
Year instruction started: **1928**

SCHOOL OF MEDICINE
OSAKA CITY UNIVERSITY
4-54 ASACHI-MACHI 1-CHOME
ABENO-KU
OSAKA 545
Tel.: +81 (6) 645 2121
Year instruction started: **1944**

SCHOOL OF MEDICINE
KINKI UNIVERSITY
377-2 OHNO-HIGASHI
OSAKA-SAYAMA 589
Tel.: +81 (723) 660 221
Year instruction started: **1974**

FACULTY OF MEDICINE
OSAKA UNIVERSITY
2-2 YAMADAOKA
SUITA 565
Tel.: +81 (6) 879 5111
Year instruction started: **1903**

OSAKA MEDICAL COLLEGE
2-7 DAIGAKU-MACHI
TAKATSUKI 569
Tel.: +81 (726) 831 221
Year instruction started: **1927**

■ **SAGA**
SAGA MEDICAL SCHOOL
1-1 NABESHIMA 5-CHOME
SAGA 849
Tel.: +81 (952) 316 511
Fax: +81 (952) 326 254
E-mail: president@post.saga-med.ac.jp
Year instruction started: **1978**
Language of instruction: **Japanese**
Duration of basic medical degree course, including practical training: **6 years**
Entrance examination: **Yes**
Foreign students eligible: **Yes**

■ SAITAMA

SAITAMA MEDICAL SCHOOL
38 MOROHONGO
MOROYAMA-MACHI
IRUMA-GUN 350-4
Tel.: +81 (492) 761 111
Year instruction started: **1972**

NATIONAL DEFENCE MEDICAL COLLEGE
3-2 NAMIKI
TOKOROZAWA 359
Tel.: +81 (429) 951 511/951 211
Fax: +81 (429) 951 283
Year instruction started: **1974**
Language of instruction: **Japanese**
Duration of basic medical degree course, including practical training: **6 years**
Entrance examination: **Yes**
Foreign students eligible: **No**

■ SHIGA

SHIGA MEDICAL UNIVERSITY
SETATSUKINOWA-CHO
OTSU 520-21
Tel.: +81 (775) 482 111
Year instruction started: **1975**

■ SHIMANE

SHIMANE MEDICAL UNIVERSITY
89-1 ENYA-CHO
IZUMO 693
Tel.: +81 (853) 232 111
Fax: +81 (853) 241 799
Year instruction started: **1976**
Language of instruction: **Japanese**
Duration of basic medical degree course, including practical training: **6 years**
Entrance examination: **Yes**
Foreign students eligible: **No**

■ SHIZUOKA

HAMAMATSU MEDICAL UNIVERSITY
3600 HANDA-CHO
HAMAMATSU 431-31
Tel.: +81 (53) 435 2111
Year instruction started: **1974**

■ TOCHIGI

JICHI MEDICAL UNIVERSITY
3311 YAKUSHIJI
MINAMI-KAWAUCHI-CHO
KAWAUCHI-GUN 329-04
Tel.: +81 (285) 442 111
Year instruction started: **1972**
Language of instruction: **Japanese**
Duration of basic medical degree course, including practical training: **6 years**
Entrance examination: **Yes**
Foreign students eligible: **No**

SCHOOL OF MEDICINE
DOKKYO UNIVERSITY
880 KITAKOBAYASHI
MIBU-MACHI
SHIMO-TSUGA-GUN 321-02
Tel.: +81 (282) 861 111
Year instruction started: **1973**

■ TOKUSHIMA

SCHOOL OF MEDICINE
UNIVERSITY OF TOKUSHIMA
18-15 KURAMOTO-CHO 3-CHOME
TOKUSHIMA 770
Tel.: +81 (886) 313 111
Fax: +81 (886) 337 009
Year instruction started: **1943**
Language of instruction: **Japanese**
Duration of basic medical degree course, including practical training: **6 years**
Entrance examination: **Yes**
Foreign students eligible: **Yes**

■ TOKYO

SCHOOL OF MEDICINE
JUNTENDO UNIVERSITY
1-1 HONGO 2-CHOME
BUNKYO-KU 113
Tel.: +81 (3) 381 331 11
Year instruction started: **1943**

NIPPON MEDICAL UNIVERSITY
1-5 SENDAGI 1-CHOME
BUNKYO-KU 113
Tel.: +81 (3) 382 221 31
Fax: +81 (3) 382 477 12
E-mail: admin@ams.ac.jp
Year instruction started: **1904**
Language of instruction: **Japanese, English**
Duration of basic medical degree course, including practical training: **6 years**
Entrance examination: **Yes**
Foreign students eligible: **Yes**

SCHOOL OF MEDICINE
TOKYO MEDICAL AND DENTAL UNIVERSITY
5-45 YUSHIMA 1-CHOME
BUNKYO-KU 113
Tel.: +81 (3) 381 361 11
Year instruction started: **1944**

FACULTY OF MEDICINE
UNIVERSITY OF TOKYO
3-1 HONGO 7-CHOME
BUNKYO-KU 113
Tel.: +81 (3) 381 221 11
Fax: +81 (3) 381 590 97
E-mail: fukuhara@m.u-tokyo.ac.jp
Year instruction started: **1868**
Language of instruction: **Japanese**
Duration of basic medical degree course, including practical training: **6 years**
Entrance examination: **Yes**
Foreign students eligible: **Yes**

SCHOOL OF MEDICINE
NIHON UNIVERSITY
30-1 OHYAGUCHI-KAMI-MACHI
ITABASHI-KU 173
Tel.: +81 (3) 397 281 11
Fax: +81 (3) 397 200 15
Year instruction started: **1944**

SCHOOL OF MEDICINE
TEIKYO UNIVERSITY
11-1 KAGA 2-CHOME
ITABASHI-KU 173
Tel.: +81 (3) 396 412 11

Year instruction started: **1971**
Language of instruction: **Japanese**
Duration of basic medical degree course, including practical training: **6 years**
Entrance examination: **Yes**
Foreign students eligible: **Yes**

SCHOOL OF MEDICINE
TOKYO JIKEI UNIVERSITY
25-8 NISHI-SHINBASHI 3-CHOME
MINATO-KU 105
Tel.: +81 (3) 343 311 11
Fax: +81 (3) 343 519 22
Year instruction started: **1881**
Language of instruction: **Japanese**
Duration of basic medical degree course, including practical training: **6 years**
Entrance examination: **Yes**
Foreign students eligible: **Yes**

SCHOOL OF MEDICINE
KYORIN UNIVERSITY
20-2 SHINKAWA 6-CHOME
MITAKA 181
Tel.: +81 (422) 475 511
Fax: +81 (422) 440 892
Year instruction started: **1970**
Language of instruction: **Japanese**
Duration of basic medical degree course, including practical training: **6 years**
Entrance examination: **Yes**
Foreign students eligible: **Yes**

SCHOOL OF MEDICINE
TOHO UNIVERSITY
21-16 OMORI-NISHI 5-CHOME
OTA-KU 143
Tel.: +81 (3) 376 241 51
Fax: +81 (3) 376 105 46
Year instruction started: **1925**
Language of instruction: **Japanese**
Duration of basic medical degree course, including practical training: **6 years**
Entrance examination: **Yes**
Foreign students eligible: **Yes**

SCHOOL OF MEDICINE
SHOWA UNIVERSITY
5-8 HATANODAI 1-CHOME
SHINAGAWA-KU 142
Tel.: +81 (3) 378 480 00
Fax: +81 (3) 378 600 72
Year instruction started: **1928**

SCHOOL OF MEDICINE
KEIO UNIVERSITY
35 SHINANO-MACHI
SHINJUKU-KU 160
Tel.: +81 (3) 335 312 11
Year instruction started: **1917**
Language of instruction: **Japanese**
Duration of basic medical degree course, including practical training: **6 years**
Entrance examination: **Yes**
Foreign students eligible: **Yes**

TOKYO MEDICAL COLLEGE
1-1 SHINJUKU 6-CHOME
SHINJUKU-KU 160
Tel.: +81 (3) 335 161 41
Fax: +81 (3) 322 670 30
Year instruction started: **1916**
Language of instruction: **Japanese**
Duration of basic medical degree course, including practical training: **6 years**
Entrance examination: **Yes**
Foreign students eligible: **Yes**

TOKYO WOMEN'S MEDICAL COLLEGE
8-1 KAWADA-CHO
SHINJUKU-KU 162
Tel.: +81 (3) 335 381 11
Fax: +81 (3) 335 367 93
Year instruction started: **1912**

■ **TOTTORI**
FACULTY OF MEDICINE
TOTTORI UNIVERSITY
86 NISHI-MACHI
YONAGO 683
Tel.: +81 (859) 331 111
Fax: +81 (859) 348 207

Year instruction started: **1945**
Language of instruction: **Japanese**
Duration of basic medical degree course, including practical training: **6 years**
Entrance examination: **Yes**
Foreign students eligible: **Yes**

■ TOYAMA
FACULTY OF MEDICINE
TOYAMA MEDICAL AND PHARMACEUTICAL UNIVERSITY
2630 SUGITANI
TOYAMA 930-01
Tel.: +81 (764) 342 281
Fax: +81 (764) 341 463
Year instruction started: **1976**
Language of instruction: **Japanese**
Duration of basic medical degree course, including practical training: **6 years**
Entrance examination: **Yes**
Foreign students eligible: **Yes**

■ WAKAYAMA
WAKAYAMA MEDICAL COLLEGE
27 KYUBAN-CHO
WAKAYAMA 640
Tel.: +81 (734) 312 151
Fax: +81 (734) 237 794
Year instruction started: **1945**

■ YAMAGATA
SCHOOL OF MEDICINE
YAMAGATA UNIVERSITY
2-2 IIDA-NISHI 2-CHOME
YAMAGATA 990-23
Tel.: +81 (236) 331 122
Fax: +81 (236) 322 019
Year instruction started: **1973**

■ YAMAGUCHI
SCHOOL OF MEDICINE
YAMAGUCHI UNIVERSITY
1144 KOGUSHI
UBE 755
Tel.: +81 (836) 222 111
Year instruction started: **1944**

■ **YAMANASHI**
YAMANASHI MEDICAL COLLEGE
1110 SHIMOKATO
TAMAHO-CHO
NAKAKOMA-GUN 409-38
Tel.: +81 (552) 731 111
Fax: +81 (552) 736 742/737 108
Year instruction started: **1980**
Language of instruction: **Japanese**
Duration of basic medical degree course, including practical training: **6 years**
Entrance examination: **Yes**
Foreign students eligible: **No**

JORDAN

Total population in 1995: **5 581 000**
Number of physicians per 100 000 population (1993): **158**
Number of medical schools: **2**
Duration of basic medical degree course, including practical training: **6 years**
Title of degree awarded: **Bachelor of Medicine and Surgery**
Medical registration/licence to practise: **Registration is obligatory with the Jordan Medical Association. The licence to practise medicine is granted by the Ministry of Health, PO Box 915, Amman 11118, to graduates on completion of an 11-month internship in the four main departments of a teaching hospital. Graduates of foreign medical schools must have their degree validated. Foreigners must hold a residence permit.**
Work in government service after graduation: **Not obligatory**
Agreements with other countries: **An agreement exists with the Arab Board of Medical Specialities which provides for mutual recognition of Jordanian and Arab degrees in medicine and surgery.**

FACULTY OF MEDICINE
UNIVERSITY OF JORDAN
UNIVERSITY STREET
AMMAN
Tel.: +962 (6) 843 555
Fax: +962 (6) 832 318
Telex: 21629 unvj jo
Year instruction started: **1971**
Language of instruction: **English**
Duration of basic medical degree course, including practical training: **6 years**
Entrance examination: **No**
Foreign students eligible: **Yes**

FACULTY OF MEDICINE
JORDAN UNIVERSITY OF SCIENCE AND TECHNOLOGY
PO BOX 3030
IRBID
Tel.: +962 (2) 295 111
Fax: +962 (2) 295 123
Telex: 55545 just jo
Year instruction started: **1984**
Language of instruction: **English**
Duration of basic medical degree course, including practical training: **6 years**
Entrance examination: **No**
Foreign students eligible: **Yes**

KAZAKHSTAN

Total population in 1995: **16 820 000**
Number of physicians per 100 000 population (1993): **360**
Number of medical schools: **6**
Duration of basic medical degree course, including practical training: **5–7 years (a
  further 2 or 3 years of supervised practice are required before the degree is
  awarded)**
Title of degree awarded: ***Kandidat* (Candidate), *Doktor Medicinskih Nauk*
  (Doctor of Medical Science)**
Medical registration/licence to practise: **Registration is obligatory with the
  Oblastnye i Gorodskie Departamenty Zdravoomranenija (Oblast and Munici-
  pal Health Departments). The licence to practise medicine is granted by
  the Ministry of Health, *pr. Ablajhana 63, 480003 Almaty*, and the Ministry
  of Education to graduates of a recognized medical school who hold a
  certificate of specialization.**
Work in government service after graduation: —
Agreements with other countries: —

AKMOLA MEDICAL INSTITUTE
95 DELEGATSKAJA
AKMOLA 473029
Year instruction started: **1964**

MEDICAL INSTITUTE OF AKTJUBINSK
ULICA LENINA 52
AKTJUBINSK 463022
Tel.: +7 (327) 221 273
Year instruction started: **1957**
Language of instruction: **Kazakh, Russian**

ALMA ATINSKIJ STATE MEDICAL INSTITUTE
88 TOLEBI STREET
ALMATY 480012
Year instruction started: **1931**

KARAGANDA STATE MEDICAL INSTITUTE
ULICA GOGOLJA 40
KARAGANDA 470061
Tel.: +7 (321) 254 6891
Fax: +7 (321) 258 2486
Year instruction started: **1950**
Language of instruction: **Kazakh, Russian, English**
Entrance examination: **No**
Foreign students eligible: **Yes**

SEMIPALATINSK STATE MEDICAL INSTITUTE
ABAJ STREET 103
SEMIPALATINSK 490019
Tel.: +7 (322) 623 965/622 251
Fax: +7 (322) 663 401
Year instruction started: **1953**
Language of instruction: **Kazakh, Russian**
Duration of basic medical degree course, including practical training: **7 years**
Entrance examination: **Yes**
Foreign students eligible: **Yes**

SHYMKENT MEDICAL INSTITUTE
1 LENIN STREET
SHYMKENT 486018

KENYA

Total population in 1995: **27 799 000**
Number of physicians per 100 000 population (1993): **15**
Number of medical schools: **2**
Duration of basic medical degree course, including practical training: **6 years**
Title of degree awarded: **Bachelor of Medicine and Bachelor of Surgery (MB, ChB)**
Medical registration/licence to practise: —
Work in government service after graduation: —
Agreements with other countries: —

FACULTY OF HEALTH SCIENCES
MOI UNIVERSITY
LUMUMBA AVENUE
PO BOX 4606
ELDORET
Tel.: +254 (321) 615 62
Fax: +254 (321) 330 41
Telex: 35047 moivarsity ke
E-mail: medlibmoi@ken.healthnet.org
Year instruction started: **1990**
Language of instruction: **English**
Duration of basic medical degree course, including practical training: **6 years**
Entrance examination: **No**
Foreign students eligible: **Yes**

COLLEGE OF HEALTH SCIENCES
UNIVERSITY OF NAIROBI
PO BOX 19676
NAIROBI
Year instruction started: **1967**

KUWAIT

Total population in 1995: **1 687 000**
Number of physicians per 100 000 population (1993): **178**
Number of medical schools: **1**
Duration of basic medical degree course, including practical training: **7 years**
Title of degree awarded: **Bachelor of Medical Science, Bachelor of Medicine and Bachelor of Surgery (BMedSc, BM, BCh)**
Medical registration/licence to practise: —
Work in government service after graduation: —
Agreements with other countries: —

FACULTY OF MEDICINE
KUWAIT UNIVERSITY
HEALTH SCIENCES CENTRE
PO BOX 24923
SAFAT
JABRIYA DISTRICT 13110
Tel.: +965 531 9491/531 2300
Fax: +965 531 8454
Telex: 44595 alrazi kt
E-mail: accountname@hsccwww.kuniv.edu.kw

Year instruction started: **1973**
Language of instruction: **English**
Duration of basic medical degree course, including practical training: **7 years**
Entrance examination: **Yes**
Foreign students eligible: **Yes**

KYRGYZSTAN

Total population in 1995: **4 469 000**
Number of physicians per 100 000 population (1993): **310**
Number of medical schools: **1**
Duration of basic medical degree course, including practical training: **5 years**
Title of degree awarded: —
Medical registration/licence to practise: —
Work in government service after graduation: —
Agreements with other countries: —

KYRGYZ STATE MEDICAL ACADEMY
AHUNBAEV STREET 92
BISHKEK 720061
Tel.: +996 (3312) 445 051
Fax: +996 (3312) 425 352
E-mail: kgma@imfiko.bishkek.su
Year instruction started: **1939**
Language of instruction: **Russian**
Duration of basic medical degree course, including practical training: **5 years**
Entrance examination: **Yes**
Foreign students eligible: **Yes**

LAO PEOPLE'S DEMOCRATIC REPUBLIC

Total population in 1995: **5 035 000**
Number of physicians per 100 000 population (1993): —
Number of medical schools: **1**
Duration of basic medical degree course, including practical training: **6 years**
Title of degree awarded: **Doctor of Medicine**
Medical registration/licence to practise: **Registration is obligatory with the Ministry of Public Health, Vientiane. The licence to practise medicine is awarded to graduates of a recognized medical school. Foreigners may only practise if they have graduated from the Faculty of Medicine, Vientiane.**
Work in government service after graduation: **Obligatory**
Agreements with other countries: —

FACULTE DES SCIENCES MEDICALES
RUE SAM SENE THAI
BP 7444
SISATTANAK
VIENTIANE
Tel.: +856 (21) 4055/4033/4034
Fax: +856 (21) 4055
Year instruction started: **1968**
Language of instruction: **Lao**
Duration of basic medical degree course, including practical training: **6 years**
Entrance examination: **Yes**

LATVIA

Total population in 1995: **2 504 000**
Number of physicians per 100 000 population (1993): **303**
Number of medical schools: **2**
Duration of basic medical degree course, including practical training: —
Title of degree awarded: —
Medical registration/licence to practise: —
Work in government service after graduation: —
Agreements with other countries: —

LATVIJAS MEDICINAS AKADEMIJA
DZIRCIEMA IELA 16
RIGA LV 1007
Tel.: +371 (2) 450 708
Fax: +371 (2) 828 155
Year instruction started: **1919**
Language of instruction: **Latvian, Russian, English**
Duration of basic medical degree course, including practical training: **5–6 years**
Entrance examination: **Yes**
Foreign students eligible: **Yes**

LATVIJAS UNIVERSITATE
MEDICINAS FAKULTATE
RAINA BULV. 19
RIGA LV 1059
Tel.: +371 (2) 722 8701
Fax: +371 (2) 782 0113
Year instruction started: **1998**

LEBANON

Total population in 1995: **3 084 000**
Number of physicians per 100 000 population (1993): **191**
Number of medical schools: **4**
Duration of basic medical degree course, including practical training: **4–7 years**
Title of degree awarded: **Doctor of Medicine (MD)**
Medical registration/licence to practise: —
Work in government service after graduation: —
Agreements with other countries: —

FACULTY OF MEDICINE
AMERICAN UNIVERSITY OF BEIRUT
BLISS STREET
BEIRUT
Fax: +1 (212) 444 5817
Year instruction started: **1868**
Language of instruction: **English**
Duration of basic medical degree course, including practical training: **4 years**
Entrance examination: **Yes**
Foreign students eligible: **Yes**

FACULTY OF MEDICINE
BEIRUT ARAB UNIVERSITY
PO BOX 11-5020
BEIRUT
Tel.: +961 (1) 300 110
Fax: +961 (1) 818 402
E-mail: bau@inco.com.lb
Year instruction started: **1995**
Language of instruction: **English**
Duration of basic medical degree course, including practical training: **6 years**

SCHOOL OF MEDICINE
FACULTY OF MEDICAL SCIENCES
LEBANESE UNIVERSITY
MUSEUM PLACE
BEIRUT
Year instruction started: **1983**

FACULTE DE MEDECINE
UNIVERSITE SAINT-JOSEPH
RUE DE DAMAS
BP 11-5076
BEYROUTH

Tel.: +961 (1) 392 644
Fax: +961 (1) 386 796
Year instruction started: **1883**
Language of instruction: **French, English**
Duration of basic medical degree course, including practical training: **7 years**
Entrance examination: **Yes**
Foreign students eligible: **Yes**

LIBERIA

Total population in 1995: **2 245 000**
Number of physicians per 100 000 population (1993): —
Number of medical schools: **1**
Duration of basic medical degree course, including practical training: **5 years**
Title of degree awarded: **Doctor of Medicine**
Medical registration/licence to practise: **The licence to practise medicine is granted by the Liberian Medical Board, c/o Ministry of Health and Social Welfare, PO Box 9009, Monrovia, to graduates of a recognized medical school who have worked for 1 year as an intern and for 1 year in a rural area.**
Work in government service after graduation: **Obligatory (1 year in a rural area)**
Agreements with other countries: —

A.M. DOGLIOTTI COLLEGE OF MEDICINE
UNIVERSITY OF LIBERIA
PO BOX 1018
MONROVIA
Year instruction started: **1968**
Language of instruction: **English**
Duration of basic medical degree course, including practical training: **5 years**
Entrance examination: **No**
Foreign students eligible: **Yes**

LIBYAN ARAB JAMAHIRIYA

Total population in 1995: **5 593 000**
Number of physicians per 100 000 population (1993): **137**
Number of medical schools: **4**
Duration of basic medical degree course, including practical training: **6 years (a further year of supervised clinical practice is required before the degree is awarded)**
Title of degree awarded: **Bachelor of Medicine and Bachelor of Surgery (MB, BS)**

Medical registration/licence to practise: **Registration is obligatory with the General Medical Syndicate, Great Libyan Arab Jamahiriya, Jarabi Street, PO Box 7768, Ain Zaro, Tripoli. The licence to practise medicine is granted by the General Directorate for Health Affairs, Ministry of Health and Social Security, Tripoli, to graduates of a recognized medical school on completion of a 1-year internship. Those with foreign medical qualifications require special authorization to practise.**
Work in government service after graduation: **Obligatory**
Agreements with other countries: **Agreements exist with universities in other Arab countries and in eastern and western Europe.**

FACULTY OF MEDICINE
AL ARAB MEDICAL UNIVERSITY
PO BOX 1451
BENGHAZI
Tel.: +218 (61) 222 2195
Fax: +218 (61) 222 1152
Year instruction started: **1970**

SEBHA MEDICAL UNIVERSITY
PO BOX 19838
SEBHA
Tel.: +218 (71) 629 293
Fax: +218 (71) 629 201

FACULTY OF MEDICINE
ALTAHDI UNIVERSITY
PO BOX 633
SIRTE
Tel.: +218 (54) 653 25
Fax: +218 (54) 625 05
Year instruction started: **1991**
Language of instruction: **English**
Duration of basic medical degree course, including practical training: **6 years**
Entrance examination: **Yes**
Foreign students eligible: **Yes**

FACULTY OF MEDICINE
UNIVERSITY OF AL FATEH
PO BOX 13628
TRIPOLI
Tel.: +218 (21) 360 2971
Fax: +218 (21) 360 2971
Year instruction started: **1974**

LITHUANIA

Total population in 1995: **3 728 000**
Number of physicians per 100 000 population (1993): **399**
Number of medical schools: **2**
Duration of basic medical degree course, including practical training: **6 years**
Title of degree awarded: —
Medical registration/licence to practise: —
Work in government service after graduation: —
Agreements with other countries: —

KAUNO MEDICINOS UNIVERSITETO
MICKEVICIAUS 9
KAUNAS 3000
Tel.: +370 (7) 226 110
Fax: +370 (7) 220 733
E-mail: vilgra@kma.lt
Year instruction started: **1919**
Language of instruction: **Lithuanian, English**
Duration of basic medical degree course, including practical training: **6 years**
Entrance examination: **Yes**
Foreign students eligible: **Yes**

MEDICINOS FAKULTETAS
VILNIAUS UNIVERSITETO
CIURLIONIO 21
VILNIUS 2009
Tel.: +370 (2) 630 243
Fax: +370 (2) 263 167
Year instruction started: **1781**
Language of instruction: **Lithuanian**
Duration of basic medical degree course, including practical training: **6 years**
Entrance examination: **Yes**
Foreign students eligible: **Yes**

MADAGASCAR

Total population in 1995: **15 353 000**
Number of physicians per 100 000 population (1993): **24**
Number of medical schools: **2**
Duration of basic medical degree course, including practical training: **7 or 8 years**
Title of degree awarded: ***Docteur en Médecine (Diplôme d'État)* (Doctor of Medicine (State Diploma))**

Medical registration/licence to practise: **Registration is obligatory with the** *Ministère de la Santé et de la Population, BP 88, 101 Antananarivo.* **The licence to practise medicine is granted by the** *Ordre des Médecins, place Charles Renel, Antaninandro, Antananarivo 101,* **to graduates of a recognized medical school who have completed a 2-year internship. Foreigners require authorization from the Ministry of Health to practise.**
Work in government service after graduation: **Not obligatory**
Agreements with other countries: —

FACULTE DE MEDECINE D'ANTANANARIVO
UNIVERSITE DE MADAGASCAR
BP 375
ANTANANARIVO 101
Tel.: +261 (20) 297 71/212 60/207 23
Fax: +261 (20) 277 04
Year instruction started: **1962**
Language of instruction: **French**
Duration of basic medical degree course, including practical training: **8 years**
Entrance examination: **No**
Foreign students eligible: **Yes**

FACULTE DE MEDECINE
ETABLISSEMENT D'ENSEIGNEMENT SUPERIEUR DES SCIENCES DE LA SANTE
UNIVERSITE DE MADAGASCAR
BP 652
MAHAJANGA 401
Year instruction started: **1984**
Language of instruction: **French**
Duration of basic medical degree course, including practical training: **7 years**
Entrance examination: **No**
Foreign students eligible: **Yes**

MALAWI

Total population in 1995: **9 845 000**
Number of physicians per 100 000 population (1993): **2**
Number of medical schools: **1**
Duration of basic medical degree course, including practical training: **5 years**
Title of degree awarded: **Bachelor of Medicine and Bachelor of Surgery (MB, BS)**
Medical registration/licence to practise: —
Work in government service after graduation: —
Agreements with other countries: —

COLLEGE OF MEDICINE
UNIVERSITY OF MALAWI
PRIVATE BAG 360
CHICHIRI
BLANTYRE 3
Tel.: +265 677 291
Fax: +265 674 700
Year instruction started: **1991**
Language of instruction: **English**
Duration of basic medical degree course, including practical training: **5 years**
Entrance examination: **No**
Foreign students eligible: **Yes**

MALAYSIA

Total population in 1995: **20 581 000**
Number of physicians per 100 000 population (1993): **43**
Number of medical schools: **5**
Duration of basic medical degree course, including practical training: **5–6 years**
Title of degree awarded: ***Doktor Perubatan* (Doctor of Medicine)**
Medical registration/licence to practise: **Registration is obligatory with the Malaysian Medical Council, Ministry of Health, 50590 Kuala Lumpur. The licence to practise medicine is granted to graduates of a recognized medical school who have successfully completed an internship of at least 1 year. Those with foreign medical qualifications must provide evidence of adequate experience. Foreigners may receive a licence to practise for a limited period under special conditions and must be registered in their own country.**
Work in government service after graduation: **Obligatory (3 years)**
Agreements with other countries: **None**

FAKULTI PERUBATAN
UNIVERSITI KEBANGSAAN MALAYSIA
JALAN TENTERAM
BANDAR TUN RAZAK
CHERAS 56000
KUALA LUMPUR
Tel.: +60 (3) 973 3333
Fax: +60 (3) 291 2659
Year instruction started: **1973**
Language of instruction: **Malay, English**
Duration of basic medical degree course, including practical training: **5 years**
Entrance examination: **No**
Foreign students eligible: **No**

PUSAT PENGAJAIN SAINS PERUBATAN
UNIVERSITI SAINS MALAYSIA
KUBANG KERIAN
KOTA BHARU 16150
KELANTAN
Tel.: +60 (9) 765 1711
Fax: +60 (9) 765 3370
E-mail: ppsp@kb.usm.my
Year instruction started: **1979**
Language of instruction: **Malay, English**
Duration of basic medical degree course, including practical training: **5 years**
Entrance examination: **No**
Foreign students eligible: **No**

FAKULTI PERUBATAN DAN SAINS KESIHATAN
UNIVERSITI MALAYSIA SARAWAK
KOTA SAMARAHAN 94300
SARAWAK
Tel.: +60 (82) 428 110
Fax: +60 (82) 427 716
E-mail: medical@fhs.unimas.my
Year instruction started: **1994**
Language of instruction: **Malay, English**
Duration of basic medical degree course, including practical training: **5 years**
Entrance examination: **No**
Foreign students eligible: **No**

FAKULTI PERUBATAN
UNIVERSITI MALAYA
LEMBAH PANTAI
KUALA LUMPUR
Tel.: +60 (3) 750 2429
Fax: +60 (3) 755 7740
Year instruction started: **1964**
Language of instruction: **Malay, English**
Duration of basic medical degree course, including practical training: **5 years**
Entrance examination: **No**
Foreign students eligible: **Yes**

INTERNATIONAL MEDICAL UNIVERSITY
21 JALAN SELANGOR
PETALING JAYA 46050
SELANGOR DARUL EHSAN

Tel.: +60 (3) 758 4249
Fax: +60 (3) 758 4239
E-mail: imu@imu.edu.my
Year instruction started: **1993**
Language of instruction: **English**
Duration of basic medical degree course, including practical training: **5–6 years**
Entrance examination: **No**
Foreign students eligible: **Yes**

MALI

Total population in 1995: **11 134 000**
Number of physicians per 100 000 population (1993): **4**
Number of medical schools: **1**
Duration of basic medical degree course, including practical training: **7 years**
Title of degree awarded: ***Docteur en Médecine*** **(Doctor of Medicine)**
Medical registration/licence to practise: **—**
Work in government service after graduation: **Not obligatory**
Agreements with other countries: **An agreement exists among French-speaking African countries.**

ECOLE NATIONALE DE MEDECINE, DE PHARMACIE ET
    D'ODONTOSTOMATOLOGIE DU MALI
BP 1805
BAMAKO 223
Tel.: +223 225 277
Fax: +223 229 658
Year instruction started: **1969**
Language of instruction: **French**
Duration of basic medical degree course, including practical training: **7 years**
Entrance examination: **Yes**
Foreign students eligible: **Yes**

MALTA

Total population in 1995: **369 000**
Number of physicians per 100 000 population (1993): **250**
Number of medical schools: **1**
Duration of basic medical degree course, including practical training: **5 years**
Title of degree awarded: ***Dottorat fil-Medicina u l-Kirurgija*** **(Doctor of Medicine and Surgery)**
Medical registration/licence to practise: **Registration is obligatory with the Medical Council, Castellania Palace, 15 Merchants Street, Valletta CMRO02. The licence to practise medicine is granted by the President of**

Malta to graduates of a recognized medical school who have worked for 2 years as an intern on a rotating basis in a teaching hospital. Those with foreign medical degrees must pass a statutory examination. Foreigners must obtain a work permit and are eligible for a temporary licence only.

Work in government service after graduation: **Obligatory (2 years)**

Agreements with other countries: **Agreements exist with Ireland and the United Kingdom.**

MEDICAL SCHOOL
UNIVERSITY OF MALTA
GUARDAMANGIA
Tel.: +356 239 783/221 019
Fax: +356 235 638
Year instruction started: **1676**
Language of instruction: **English**
Duration of basic medical degree course, including practical training: **5 years**
Entrance examination: **No**
Foreign students eligible: **Yes**

MARSHALL ISLANDS

Total population in 1995: —
Number of physicians per 100 000 population (1993): —
Number of medical schools: **None**
Medical registration/licence to practise: **Registration is obligatory with the Ministry of Health and Environment, PO Box 16, Majuro, Marshall Islands 96960. The licence to practise medicine is granted by the Marshall Islands Medical Licensing Board, PO Box 16, Majuro, to graduates of a recognized medical school provided they have a current licence to practise elsewhere and have no criminal record.**

Work in government service after graduation: **Obligatory (prior to receipt of a full licence to practise)**

Agreements with other countries: **None**

MAURITIUS

Total population in 1995: **1 129 000**
Number of physicians per 100 000 population (1993): **85**
Number of medical schools: **None**
Medical registration/licence to practise: **Registration is obligatory with the Medical and Dental Councils of Mauritius, 6 Avenue des Jacinthes, Morc.**

St Jean, Quatre Bornes. The licence to practise medicine is granted to graduates of a recognized medical school on completion of a 1-year internship either in Mauritius or in the country of graduation. Foreigners must hold a work permit.

Work in government service after graduation: **Not obligatory**
Agreements with other countries: **None**

MEXICO

Total population in 1995: **92 718 000**
Number of physicians per 100 000 population (1993): **107**
Number of medical schools: **55**
Duration of basic medical degree course, including practical training: **4–7 years (a further year of supervised practice is required before the degree is awarded)**
Title of degree awarded: ***Médico Cirujano* (Physician and Surgeon)**
Medical registration/licence to practise: **The licence to practise medicine is granted by the *Secretaria de Educación Pública* (SEP), *Dirección General de Profesiones, Insurgentes Sur 2387, San Angel, 01000 México, DF*, and is regulated by Article 5 of the Constitution.**
Work in government service after graduation: **Not obligatory**
Agreements with other countries: —

■ AGUASCALIENTES
ESCUELA DE MEDICINA
CENTRO BIOMEDICO
UNIVERSIDAD AUTONOMA DE AGUASCALIENTES
AVENIDA UNIVERSIDAD 940
AGUASCALIENTES 20100
Tel.: +52 (491) 123 345
Fax: +52 (491) 143 222
Year instruction started: **1972**
Language of instruction: **Spanish**
Duration of basic medical degree course, including practical training: **5 years**
Entrance examination: **Yes**
Foreign students eligible: **Yes**

■ BAJA CALIFORNIA
ESCUELA DE MEDICINA
CENTRO DE ESTUDIOS UNIVERSITARIOS XOCHICALCO
SAN FRANCISCO 1139
FRACC. MISION
APDO 1377
ENSENADA 22830

Tel.: +52 (617) 743 980/743 981
Fax: +52 (617) 743 980/743 981
Year instruction started: **1974**
Language of instruction: **Spanish**
Duration of basic medical degree course, including practical training: **6 years**
Entrance examination: **No**
Foreign students eligible: **Yes**

ESCUELA DE MEDICINA DE MEXICALI
UNIVERSIDAD AUTONOMA DE BAJA CALIFORNIA
CENTRO CIVICO COMERCIAL DE MEXICALI
CALLE DE LOS MISIONEROS S/N
MEXICALI 21000
Tel.: +52 (65) 575 356/575 998
Fax: +52 (65) 572 658
Year instruction started: **1972**
Language of instruction: **Spanish, English**
Duration of basic medical degree course, including practical training: **7 years**
Entrance examination: **Yes**
Foreign students eligible: **No**

ESCUELA DE MEDICINA DE TIJUANA
UNIVERSIDAD AUTONOMA DE BAJA CALIFORNIA
EX-EJIDO TAMPICO
APDO 13-A
TIJUANA 22350
Tel.: +52 (66) 821 033
Fax: +52 (66) 821 233
Year instruction started: **1974**

■ **CAMPECHE**
FACULTAD DE MEDICINA
UNIVERSIDAD DEL SUDESTE
AVENIDA PATRICIO TRUEBA Y REGIL
CAMPECHE 24090
Tel.: +52 (981) 315 68
Fax: +52 (981) 315 34
E-mail: venus@uacam.mx
Language of instruction: **Spanish**
Duration of basic medical degree course, including practical training: **6 years**
Entrance examination: **Yes**
Foreign students eligible: **Yes**

■ **CHIAPAS**
FACULTAD DE MEDICINA HUMANA
UNIVERSIDAD AUTONOMA DE CHIAPAS
CAMPUS II
10/A AVENIDA SUR Y CALLE CENTRAL S/N
APDO 575
TUXTLA GUTIERREZ 29000
Tel.: +52 (961) 375 35/249 24
Fax: +52 (961) 222 92
E-mail: jlaquino@montebello.unach.mx
Year instruction started: **1975**
Language of instruction: **Spanish**
Duration of basic medical degree course, including practical training: **7 years**
Entrance examination: **Yes**
Foreign students eligible: **Yes**

■ **CHIHUAHUA**
FACULTAD DE MEDICINA
UNIVERSIDAD AUTONOMA DE CHIHUAHUA
AVENIDA COLON Y ROSALES S/N
APDO 1090
CHIHUAHUA
Tel.: +52 (14) 152 059
Fax: +52 (14) 152 543
Year instruction started: **1954**

ESCUELA DE MEDICINA
INSTITUTO DE CIENCIAS BIOMEDICAS
UNIVERSIDAD AUTONOMA DE CIUDAD JUAREZ
ANILLO ENVOLVENTE Y ESTOCOLMO
APDO 1729-D
CIUDAD JUAREZ 32310
Tel.: +52 (16) 167 075
Fax: +52 (16) 162 111
Year instruction started: **1973**
Language of instruction: **Spanish**
Duration of basic medical degree course, including practical training: **7 years**
Entrance examination: **Yes**
Foreign students eligible: **Yes**

■ COAHUILA

ESCUELA DE MEDICINA DE SALTILLO
UNIVERSIDAD AUTONOMA DE COAHUILA
FRANCISCO MURGUIA SUR 205
SALTILLO 25000
Tel.: +52 (84) 128 095
Fax: +52 (84) 128 095
Year instruction started: **1974**

ESCUELA DE MEDICINA DE TORREON
UNIVERSIDAD AUTONOMA DE COAHUILA
AVENIDA MORELOS ORIENTE 900
TORREON 27000
Tel.: +52 (17) 137 044
Fax: +52 (17) 136 783
Year instruction started: **1957**

■ COLIMA

FACULTAD DE MEDICINA
UNIVERSIDAD DE COLIMA
AVENIDA UNIVERSIDAD 333
LAS VIBORAS
COLIMA 28040
Tel.: +52 (331) 432 54
Fax: +52 (331) 202 12
E-mail: solorioj@volcan.ucol.mx, rcedillo@volcan.ucol.mx
Year instruction started: **1977**
Language of instruction: **Spanish**
Duration of basic medical degree course, including practical training: **6 years**
Entrance examination: **Yes**
Foreign students eligible: **Yes**

■ DISTRITO FEDERAL

CENTRO INTERDISCIPLINARIO DE CIENCIAS DE LA SALUD
INSTITUTO POLITECNICO NACIONAL
KM 39.5, CARRETERA XOCHIMILCO OAXTEPEC
APDO 5
MILPA ALTA
MEXICO 12000

Tel.: +52 (5) 729 5000
Year instruction started: **1975**
Language of instruction: **Spanish**
Duration of basic medical degree course, including practical training: **5 years**
Entrance examination: **Yes**
Foreign students eligible: **Yes**

ESCUELA NACIONAL DE MEDICINA Y HOMEOPATIA
INSTITUTO POLITECNICO NACIONAL
GUILLERMO MASSIEU HELGUERA 239
FRACCIONAMIENTO "LA ESCALERA"
TICOMAN
MEXICO 07320
Tel.: +52 (5) 729 6000
Fax: +52 (5) 754 3258
E-mail: enmyh@vmredipn.ipn.mx
Year instruction started: **1896**
Language of instruction: **Spanish, English**
Duration of basic medical degree course, including practical training: **5 years**
Entrance examination: **Yes**
Foreign students eligible: **Yes**

ESCUELA SUPERIOR DE MEDICINA
INSTITUTO POLITECNICO NACIONAL
PLAN DE SAN LUIS Y DIAZ MIRON
MEXICO 11340
Tel.: +52 (5) 341 3789
Fax: +52 (5) 729 6000
E-mail: esm@vmredipn.ipn.mx
Year instruction started: **1938**
Language of instruction: **Spanish**
Duration of basic medical degree course, including practical training: **7 years**
Entrance examination: **Yes**
Foreign students eligible: **Yes**

DIVISION DE CIENCIAS BIOLOGICAS Y DE LA SALUD
UNIVERSIDAD AUTONOMA METROPOLITANA
UNIDAD XOCHIMILCO
DELEGACION COYOACAN
CALZADA DEL HUESO 1100
MEXICO 04960
Tel.: +52 (5) 724 5200
Fax: +52 (5) 724 5218
Year instruction started: **1974**

ESCUELA MEDICO MILITAR
UNIVERSIDAD DEL EJERCITO Y FUERZA AEREA
CERRADA DE PALOMAS Y PERIFERICO
DELEGACION MIGUEL HGO
MEXICO 11200
Tel.: +52 (5) 407 726
Fax: +52 (5) 202 121
Year instruction started: **1917**
Language of instruction: **Spanish**
Duration of basic medical degree course, including practical training: **6 years**
Entrance examination: **Yes**
Foreign students eligible: **Yes**

FACULTAD MEXICANA DE MEDICINA
UNIVERSIDAD DE SALLE
FUENTES 31
TLALPAN
APDO 22271
MEXICO 14000
Tel.: +52 (5) 606 3157
Fax: +52 (5) 606 2690
Year instruction started: **1970**
Language of instruction: **Spanish**
Duration of basic medical degree course, including practical training: **5 years**
Entrance examination: **Yes**
Foreign students eligible: **Yes**

FACULTAD DE ESTUDIOS SUPERIORES ZARAGOZA
UNIVERSIDAD NACIONAL AUTONOMA DE MEXICO
JOSE C. BONILLA 66
APDO 9020
COLONIA EJERCITO DE ORIENTE IZTAPALAPA
MEXICO 09230
Tel.: +52 (5) 623 0540/744 1076
Fax: +52 (5) 744 1217
Year instruction started: **1976**
Language of instruction: **Spanish, English**
Duration of basic medical degree course, including practical training: **6 years**
Entrance examination: **Yes**
Foreign students eligible: **Yes**

FACULTAD DE MEDICINA
UNIVERSIDAD NACIONAL AUTONOMA DE MEXICO
CIUDAD UNIVERSITARIA
MEXICO 04510

Tel.: +52 (5) 623 2403
Fax: +52 (5) 623 2155
Year instruction started: **1578**
Language of instruction: **Spanish**
Duration of basic medical degree course, including practical training: **6 years**
Entrance examination: **No**
Foreign students eligible: **Yes**

■ DURANGO
FACULTAD DE MEDICINA DE DURANGO
UNIVERSIDAD JUAREZ DEL ESTADO DE DURANGO
AVENIDA UNIVERSIDAD Y FANNY ANITUA
APDO 229
DURANGO 34000
Tel.: +52 (81) 121 779
Fax: +52 (81) 136 902
Year instruction started: **1957**

FACULTAD DE MEDICINA DE GOMEZ PALACIO
UNIVERSIDAD JUAREZ DEL ESTADO DE DURANGO
SIXTO UGALDE Y CALZADA LA SALLE I
GOMEZ PALACIO 35050
Tel.: +52 (17) 145 122
Fax: +52 (17) 146 476
Year instruction started: **1976**
Language of instruction: **Spanish, English**
Duration of basic medical degree course, including practical training: **7 years**
Entrance examination: **Yes**
Foreign students eligible: **Yes**

■ ESTADO DE MEXICO
ESCUELA DE MEDICINA UNIVERSIDAD ANAHUAC
AVENIDA LOMAS ANAHUAC S/N
HUIXQUILUCAN 52760
Tel.: +52 (728) 627 0210
Fax: +52 (728) 589 9796
Year instruction started: **1975**
Language of instruction: **Spanish, English**
Duration of basic medical degree course, including practical training: **6 years**
Entrance examination: **Yes**
Foreign students eligible: **Yes**

ESCUELA NACIONAL DE ESTUDIOS PROFESIONALES IZTACALA
UNIVERSIDAD NACIONAL AUTONOMA DE MEXICO
AVENIDA DE LOS BARRIOS S/N
LOS REYES
APDO 314
TLALNEPANTLA 54090
Tel.: +52 (5) 623 1148
Fax: +52 (5) 623 1218
Year instruction started: **1975**
Language of instruction: **Spanish, English**
Duration of basic medical degree course, including practical training: **5 years**
Entrance examination: **Yes**
Foreign students eligible: **Yes**

FACULTAD DE MEDICINA
UNIVERSIDAD AUTONOMA DEL ESTADO DE MEXICO
PASEO TOLLOCAN ESQUINA JESUS CARRANZA S/N
TOLUCA 50180
Tel.: +52 (72) 173 552
Fax: +52 (72) 174 142
Year instruction started: **1955**
Language of instruction: **Spanish**
Duration of basic medical degree course, including practical training: **7 years**
Entrance examination: **Yes**
Foreign students eligible: **Yes**

■ **GUANAJUATO**
FACULTAD DE MEDICINA DE LEON
UNIVERSIDAD DE GUANAJUATO
20 DE ENERO 929
COLONIA OBREGON
APDO 623
LEON 37320
Tel.: +52 (47) 161 197/145 859
Fax: +52 (47) 131 834
E-mail: angel@infosel.net.mx
Year instruction started: **1945**
Language of instruction: **Spanish**
Duration of basic medical degree course, including practical training: **6.5 years**
Entrance examination: **Yes**
Foreign students eligible: **Yes**

■ **HIDALGO**
ESCUELA DE MEDICINA
UNIVERSIDAD AUTONOMA DE HIDALGO
DR ELISEO RAMIREZ ULLOA 400
PACHUCA
Tel.: +52 (771) 720 00
Fax: +52 (771) 721 23
Year instruction started: **1945**

■ **JALISCO**
FACULTAD DE MEDICINA
UNIVERSIDAD AUTONOMA DE GUADALAJARA
AVENIDA PATRIA 1201
LOMAS DEL VALLE 3A
APDO 1-440
GUADALAJARA
Tel.: +52 (3) 641 7051/641 5051
Fax: +52 (3) 834 0520
Year instruction started: **1935**
Language of instruction: **Spanish, English**
Duration of basic medical degree course, including practical training: **6 years**
Entrance examination: **No**
Foreign students eligible: **Yes**

CARRERA DE MEDICINA
CENTRO UNIVERSITARIO DE CIENCIAS DE LA SALUD
UNIVERSIDAD DE GUADALAJARA
SIERRA MOJADA 950
COLONIA INDEPENDENCIA
APDO 1-433
GUADALAJARA 44340
Tel.: +52 (3) 175 022
Fax: +52 (3) 175 506
Year instruction started: **1792**
Language of instruction: **Spanish**
Duration of basic medical degree course, including practical training: **6 years**
Entrance examination: **Yes**
Foreign students eligible: **Yes**

■ **MICHOACAN**
FACULTAD DE MEDICINA "DR IGNACIO CHAVEZ"
UNIVERSIDAD MICHOACAN DE SAN NICOLAS DE HIDALGO
SALVADOR GONZALEZ HERREJON
MORELIA 58000

Tel.: +52 (43) 120 510
Fax: +52 (43) 128 239
Year instruction started: **1830**
Language of instruction: **Spanish, English**
Duration of basic medical degree course, including practical training: **7 years**
Entrance examination: **Yes**
Foreign students eligible: **No**

■ MORELOS
FACULTAD DE MEDICINA
UNIVERSIDAD AUTONOMA DE ESTADO DE MORELOS
AVENIDA UNIVERSIDAD 1001
COLONIA CHAMILPA
CUERNAVACA 62210
Tel.: +52 (73) 297 048
Fax: +52 (73) 297 048
E-mail: montesj@buzon.uaem.mx
Year instruction started: **1976**
Language of instruction: **Spanish**
Duration of basic medical degree course, including practical training: **6 years**
Entrance examination: **Yes**
Foreign students eligible: **Yes**

■ NAYARIT
ESCUELA DE MEDICINA
UNIVERSIDAD AUTONOMA DE NAYARIT
AVENIDA DE LA CULTURA S/N
APDO 536
TEPIC 63175
Tel.: +52 (321) 142 160
Fax: +52 (321) 142 160
Year instruction started: **1975**
Language of instruction: **Spanish**
Duration of basic medical degree course, including practical training: **6 years**
Entrance examination: **Yes**
Foreign students eligible: **Yes**

■ NUEVO LEON
FACULTAD DE MEDICINA
CARRERA DE MEDICINA
UNIVERSIDAD DE MONTEMORELOS
AVENIDA LIBERTAD PONIENTE 1300
APDO 16-10
MONTEMORELOS 67530

Tel.: +52 (826) 335 10
Fax: +52 (826) 334 19
Year instruction started: **1975**
Language of instruction: **Spanish**
Duration of basic medical degree course, including practical training: **7 years**
Entrance examination: **Yes**
Foreign students eligible: **Yes**

ESCUELA DE MEDICINA "IGNACIO A. SANTOS"
INSTITUTO TECNOLOGICO Y DE ESTUDIOS SUPERIORES DE MONTERREY
AVENIDA I. MORONES PRIETO 3000 PONIENTE
MONTERREY 64710
Tel.: +52 (83) 480 426
Fax: +52 (83) 475 413
E-mail: cdiaz@campus.mty.itesm.mx
Year instruction started: **1978**
Language of instruction: **Spanish**
Duration of basic medical degree course, including practical training: **7 years**
Entrance examination: **Yes**
Foreign students eligible: **Yes**

FACULTAD DE MEDICINA
UNIVERSIDAD AUTONOMA DE NUEVO LEON
AVENIDA FRANCISCO I MADERO AL PONIENTE Y DR
APDO 1563
MONTERREY 64460
Tel.: +52 (83) 294 153/483 373
Fax: +52 (83) 485 477
E-mail: meduanl@ccr.dsi.uani.mx
Year instruction started: **1859**
Language of instruction: **Spanish, English**
Duration of basic medical degree course, including practical training: **7 years**
Entrance examination: **Yes**
Foreign students eligible: **Yes**

FACULTAD DE MEDICINA
DIVISION DE CIENCIAS DE LA SALUD
UNIVERSIDAD DE MONTERREY
AVENIDA I. MORONES PRIETO 4500 PONIENTE
APDO 321
SAN PEDRO GARZA GARCIA 66238
Tel.: +52 (83) 383 388
Fax: +52 (83) 384 452

E-mail: ztriana@ummac01.mty.udem.mx
Year instruction started: **1969**
Language of instruction: **Spanish**
Duration of basic medical degree course, including practical training: **6 years**
Entrance examination: **Yes**
Foreign students eligible: **Yes**

■ OAXACA
ESCUELA DE MEDICINA Y CIRUGIA
UNIVERSIDAD AUTONOMA "BENITO JUAREZ" DE OAXACA
EX-HACIENDA DE AQUILERA
OAXACA DE JUAREZ 68020
Tel.: +52 (951) 530 58
Fax: +52 (951) 530 58
Year instruction started: **1827**

ESCUELA DE MEDICINA Y CIRUGIA
UNIVERSIDAD REGIONAL DEL SURESTE
PROLONGACION 20 DE NOVIEMBRE S/N
APDO 483
OAXACA DE JUAREZ 68120
Tel.: +52 (951) 414 10/463 18/619 46
Fax: +52 (951) 414 10/414 88/463 18
Year instruction started: **1977**
Language of instruction: **Spanish**
Duration of basic medical degree course, including practical training: **7 years**
Entrance examination: **Yes**
Foreign students eligible: **Yes**

■ PUEBLA
ESCUELA DE MEDICINA
UNIVERSIDAD AUTONOMA DE PUEBLA
CALLE 13 SUR 2702 PRIVADA DE LA 29 PONIENTE
APDO 28
PUEBLA 72000
Tel.: +52 (22) 431 447
Fax: +52 (22) 431 444
Year instruction started: **1831**

FACULTAD DE MEDICINA
UNIVERSIDAD POPULAR AUTONOMA DEL ESTADO DE PUEBLA
CALLE 21 SUR 1103
COLONIA SANTIAGO
PUEBLA 72160

Tel.: +52 (22) 320 266
Fax: +52 (22) 466 855
Year instruction started: **1973**
Language of instruction: **Spanish**
Duration of basic medical degree course, including practical training: **6 years**
Entrance examination: **Yes**
Foreign students eligible: **Yes**

■ QUERETARO
FACULTAD DE MEDICINA
UNIVERSIDAD AUTONOMA DE QUERETARO
CLAVEL 200
PRADOS DE LA CAPILLA
QUERETARO 76170
Tel.: +52 (42) 161 414
Fax: +52 (42) 161 087
Year instruction started: **1978**
Language of instruction: **Spanish**
Duration of basic medical degree course, including practical training: **7 years**
Entrance examination: **Yes**
Foreign students eligible: **Yes**

■ SAN LUIS POTOSI
FACULTAD DE MEDICINA
UNIVERSIDAD AUTONOMA DE SAN LUIS POTOSI
AVENIDA VENUSTIANO
CARRANZA 2405
APDO 142
SAN LUIS POTOSI 78210
Tel.: +52 (48) 130 500
Fax: +52 (48) 176 976
Year instruction started: **1877**

■ SINALOA
ESCUELA DE MEDICINA
UNIVERSIDAD AUTONOMA DE SINALOA
EUSTAQUIO BUELNA Y JOSEFA ORTIZ
CULIACAN 80030
Tel.: +52 (67) 150 338
Fax: +52 (67) 150 338

Year instruction started: **1977**
Language of instruction: **Spanish**
Duration of basic medical degree course, including practical training: **7 years**
Entrance examination: **Yes**
Foreign students eligible: **Yes**

■ TABASCO

ESCUELA DE MEDICINA HUMANA
UNIVERSIDAD "JUAREZ" AUTONOMA DE TABASCO
GREGORIO MENDEZ 2838
COLONIA TAMULTE
VILLAHERMOSA 86150
Tel.: +52 (931) 511 132
Fax: +52 (931) 511 105
Year instruction started: **1959**

■ TAMAULIPAS

ESCUELA DE CIENCIAS DE LA SALUD
UNIVERSIDAD MEXICO AMERICANA DEL NORTE
VICENTE GUERRERO 1317
COLONIA DEL PRADO
CIUDAD REYNOSA 88560
Tel.: +52 (89) 222 568
Fax: +52 (89) 228 568
E-mail: uman@infosel.net.mx
Year instruction started: **1983**
Language of instruction: **Spanish**
Duration of basic medical degree course, including practical training: **4 years**

ESCUELA DE MEDICINA
UNIVERSIDAD VALLE DEL BRAVO
CALLE SEPTIMA Y RIO MANTE S/N
COLONIA PROLONGACION
APDO 331
CIUDAD REYNOSA 88660
Tel.: +52 (89) 234 722
Fax: +52 (89) 234 422
Year instruction started: **1979**
Language of instruction: **Spanish**
Duration of basic medical degree course, including practical training: **6 years**
Entrance examination: **No**
Foreign students eligible: **Yes**

FACULTAD DE MEDICINA HUMANA DE MATAMOROS
UNIVERSIDAD AUTONOMA DE TAMAULIPAS
SENDERO NACIONAL KM 3
APDO 2005
MATAMOROS 87300
Tel.: +52 (88) 135 257/160 223
Fax: +52 (88) 125 062
E-mail: cadlg62m@voyager.uat.mx
Year instruction started: **1970**
Language of instruction: **Spanish**
Duration of basic medical degree course, including practical training: **6.5 years**
Entrance examination: **Yes**
Foreign students eligible: **Yes**

FACULTAD DE MEDICINA DE TAMPICO
UNIVERSIDAD AUTONOMA DE TAMAULIPAS
CENTRO UNIVERSITARIO TAMPICO–MADERO
APDO C-33
TAMPICO 89339
Tel.: +52 (12) 270 576/270 586
Year instruction started: **1950**
Language of instruction: **Spanish**
Duration of basic medical degree course, including practical training: **7 years**
Entrance examination: **Yes**
Foreign students eligible: **Yes**

ESCUELA DE MEDICINA
UNIVERSIDAD DEL NORESTE
PROLONGACION AVENIDA HIDALGO S/N, KM 137
CARRETERA TAMPICO–MANTE
APDO 469
TAMPICO 89339
Tel.: +52 (12) 281 156
Fax: +52 (12) 281 237
Year instruction started: **1970**
Language of instruction: **Spanish**
Duration of basic medical degree course, including practical training: **6 years**
Entrance examination: **Yes**
Foreign students eligible: **Yes**

■ VERACRUZ

FACULTAD DE MEDICINA CAMERINO Z. MENDOZA
UNIVERSIDAD VERACRUZANA
AVENIDA HIDALGO Y CARRILLO PUERTO
CIUDAD MENDOZA 94740
Tel.: +52 (272) 712 09/724 02
Fax: +52 (272) 712 09
Year instruction started: **1974**
Language of instruction: **Spanish**
Duration of basic medical degree course, including practical training: **5 years**
Entrance examination: **Yes**
Foreign students eligible: **Yes**

FACULTAD DE MEDICINA DE JALPA
UNIVERSIDAD VERACRUZANA
ZONA JALAPA
AVENIDA 20 DE NOVIEMBRE S/N
JALAPA 91010
Tel.: +52 (28) 153 443
Fax: +52 (28) 153 443
Year instruction started: **1974**

FACULTAD DE MEDICINA DE MINATITLAN
UNIVERSIDAD VERACRUZANA
ATENAS Y MANAGUA
MINATITLAN 96760
Tel.: +52 (922) 340 55
Fax: +52 (922) 340 55
Year instruction started: **1976**

ESCUELA DE MEDICINA DE POZA RICA
UNIVERSIDAD VERACRUZANA
BOULEVARD LAZARO CARDENAS 801
COLONIA MORELOS
POZA RICA 93340
Tel.: +52 (782) 256 14
Fax: +52 (782) 212 41
Year instruction started: **1972**

FACULTAD DE MEDICINA LIC. MIGUEL ALEMAN VALDES
UNIVERSIDAD VERACRUZANA
ITURBIDE Y CARMEN SERDAN S/N
VERACRUZ 91900
Tel.: +52 (29) 325 534
Fax: +52 (29) 325 534
Year instruction started: **1952**
Language of instruction: **Spanish**
Duration of basic medical degree course, including practical training: **6 years**
Entrance examination: **Yes**
Foreign students eligible: **Yes**

■ **YUCATAN**
FACULTAD DE MEDICINA
UNIVERSIDAD AUTONOMA DE YUCATAN
AVENIDA ITZAEZ 498
APDO 1225-A
MERIDA 97000
Tel.: +52 (99) 240 554
Fax: +52 (99) 233 297
E-mail: pecampos@tunku.uady.mx
Year instruction started: **1833**
Language of instruction: **Spanish**
Duration of basic medical degree course, including practical training: **7 years**
Entrance examination: **Yes**
Foreign students eligible: **No**

■ **ZACATECAS**
FACULTAD DE MEDICINA HUMANA Y CIENCIAS DE LA SALUD
UNIVERSIDAD AUTONOMA DE ZACATECAS
CARRETERA A LA BUFA S/N
APDO 554
ZACATECAS 98060
Tel.: +52 (492) 210 56
Fax: +52 (492) 246 10
E-mail: fmhuaz@gauss.logicnet.com.mx
Year instruction started: **1968**
Language of instruction: **Spanish**
Duration of basic medical degree course, including practical training: **7 years**
Entrance examination: **Yes**
Foreign students eligible: **Yes**

MICRONESIA (FEDERATED STATES OF)

Total population in 1995: —
Number of physicians per 100 000 population (1993): **46**
Number of medical schools: **None**
Medical registration/licence to practise: **Registration is obligatory with the Micronesian Medical Council, PO Box 1298, Kolonia, Pohnpei. The licence to practise medicine is granted by the Micronesian Medical Licensure Board to graduates of a recognized medical school who have completed a 1- or 2-year internship.**
Work in government service after graduation: **Not obligatory**
Agreements with other countries: **None**

MONGOLIA

Total population in 1995: **2 515 000**
Number of physicians per 100 000 population (1993): **452**
Number of medical schools: **2**
Duration of basic medical degree course, including practical training: **5 or 6 years**
Title of degree awarded: **Physician**
Medical registration/licence to practise: **Registration is obligatory with the Ministry of Health and Social Welfare of Mongolia, Olympic Street 2, *Ulaanbaatar 48* and the Ministry of Science, Technology, Education and Culture, Government building 3, *Baga toiruu 44, Ulaanbaatar 11*. The licence to practise medicine is granted to graduates of a Mongolian medical school who have successfully completed a national examination set by the Ministry of Health. Graduates of foreign medical schools are not entitled to practise.**
Work in government service after graduation: **Obligatory**
Agreements with other countries: —

SAINSHAND MEDICAL COLLEGE
DORNOGOBI ANIMAG
SAINSHAND 060000
Tel.: +976 (63) 2754
Fax: +976 (63) 2754
Year instruction started: **1992**
Language of instruction: **Mongolian, Russian, English**
Duration of basic medical degree course, including practical training: **5 years**
Entrance examination: **Yes**
Foreign students eligible: **Yes**

NATIONAL MEDICAL UNIVERSITY OF MONGOLIA
CHOIDOG STREET 4
ULAANBAATAR 48
Tel.: +976 (1) 321 249
Fax: +976 (1) 328 670
Year instruction started: **1942**
Language of instruction: **Mongolian, Russian, English**
Duration of basic medical degree course, including practical training: **6 years**
Entrance examination: **Yes**
Foreign students eligible: **Yes**

MONTSERRAT[1]

Total population in 1995: —
Number of physicians per 100 000 population (1993): —
Number of medical schools: **1**
Duration of basic medical degree course, including practical training: **4 years**
Title of degree awarded: **Doctor of Medicine (MD)**
Medical registration/licence to practise: —
Work in government service after graduation: —
Agreements with other countries: —

SCHOOL OF MEDICINE[2]
AMERICAN UNIVERSITY OF THE CARIBBEAN
PO BOX 400
PLYMOUTH
Tel.: +1809 (491) 2213
Year instruction started: **1978**
Language of instruction: **English**
Duration of basic medical degree course, including practical training: **4 years**
Entrance examination: **Yes**
Foreign students eligible: **Yes**

---

[1] Based on information received from the Government of the United Kingdom.
[2] The American University of the Caribbean has been relocated temporarily to the Netherlands Antilles since 1995 because of volcanic activity on Monserrat.

MOROCCO

Total population in 1995: **27 021 000**
Number of physicians per 100 000 population (1993): **34**
Number of medical schools: **2**
Duration of basic medical degree course, including practical training: **7 years (a
  further 1-year internship is required before the degree is awarded)**
Title of degree awarded: ***Docteur en Médecine* (Doctor of Medicine)**
Medical registration/licence to practise: **Registration is obligatory with the
  *Conseil national de l'Ordre des Médecins, Nouvelle Maternité Souissi, BP
  6555, Rabat.* The licence to practise medicine is granted by the *Secrétariat
  général du Gouvernement, Rabat*, to graduates of a recognized medical
  school.**
Work in government service after graduation: **Not obligatory**
Agreements with other countries: **Agreements exist with France and Spain.**

FACULTE DE MEDECINE ET DE PHARMACIE DE CASABLANCA
UNIVERSITE HASSAN II
19 RUE TARIK BNOU ZIAD
BP 9154
CASABLANCA 20150
Tel.: +212 (2) 271 630
Fax: +212 (2) 261 453
Year instruction started: **1975**
Language of instruction: **French**
Duration of basic medical degree course, including practical training: **7 years**
Entrance examination: **No**
Foreign students eligible: **Yes**

FACULTE DE MEDECINE ET DE PHARMACIE DE RABAT
UNIVERSITE MOHAMMED V
RABAT INSTITUTS
BP 6203
RABAT
Tel.: +212 (7) 770 421/770 431/770 433
Fax: +212 (7) 773 701
Year instruction started: **1962**
Language of instruction: **French**
Duration of basic medical degree course, including practical training: **7 years**
Entrance examination: **Yes**
Foreign students eligible: **Yes**

MOZAMBIQUE

Total population in 1995: **17 796 000**
Number of physicians per 100 000 population (1993): —
Number of medical schools: **1**
Duration of basic medical degree course, including practical training: **7 years**
Title of degree awarded: *Licenciatura em Medicina* (**Licence in Medicine**)
Medical registration/licence to practise: —
Work in government service after graduation: —
Agreements with other countries: —

FACULDADE DE MEDICINA
UNIVERSIDADE EDUARDO MONDLANE
AVENIDA DR SALVADOR ALLENDE
CP 257
MAPUTO
Tel.: +258 (1) 424 910
Fax: +258 (1) 425 855/427 133
E-mail: facmed@health.uem.mz
Year instruction started: **1963**
Language of instruction: **Portuguese**
Duration of basic medical degree course including practical training: **7 years**
Entrance examination: **Yes**
Foreign students eligible: **Yes**

MYANMAR

Total population in 1995: **45 922 000**
Number of physicians per 100 000 population (1993): **28**
Number of medical schools: **3**
Duration of basic medical degree course, including practical training: **6.5 years**
Title of degree awarded: **Bachelor of Medicine and Bachelor of Surgery (MB, BS)**
Medical registration/licence to practise: **Registration is obligatory with the Myanmar Medical Council. The licence to practise medicine is granted to graduates of a recognized medical school who have completed a 1-year internship. Foreigners are not eligible to practise.**
Work in government service after graduation: **Obligatory (3 years)**
Agreements with other countries: **None**

MANDALAY INSTITUTE OF MEDICINE
30TH STREET BETWEEN 73RD AND 74TH STREET
MANDALAY
Year instruction started: **1954**

INSTITUTE OF MEDICINE I
LANMADAW POST OFFICE
245 MYOMA KYAUNG STREET
YANGON
Year instruction started: **1923**

INSTITUTE OF MEDICINE II
MINGALADON
13TH MILE
PYAY ROAD
YANGON
Year instruction started: **1962**

NEPAL

Total population in 1995: **22 021 000**
Number of physicians per 100 000 population (1993): **5**
Number of medical schools: **4**
Duration of basic medical degree course, including practical training: **5.5 years**
Title of degree awarded: **Bachelor of Medicine and Bachelor of Surgery (MB, BS)**
Medical registration/licence to practise: **Registration is obligatory with the Nepal Medical Council, Bansbari, Kathmandu. The licence to practise medicine is granted to graduates of a recognized medical school who have completed a 1-year internship.**
Work in government service after graduation: **Not obligatory**
Agreements with other countries: **Agreements exist with Bangladesh, India, Pakistan and Sri Lanka.**

B.P. KOIRALA INSTITUTE OF HEALTH SCIENCES
PO BOX 7053 (KATHMANDU)
GHOPA CAMP
DHARAN
SUNSARI DISTRICT
Tel.: +977 (25) 210 17
Fax: +977 (25) 202 51
E-mail: bpkihs@npl.healthnet.org
Year instruction started: **1993**
Language of instruction: **English**
Duration of basic medical degree course, including practical training: **5.5 years**
Entrance examination: **Yes**
Foreign students eligible: **Yes**

NEPAL MEDICAL COLLEGE
JORPATI
PO BOX 13344
KATHMANDU
Tel.: +977 (1) 471 875/473 113
Fax: +977 (1) 473 118
Year instruction started: **1997**

INSTITUTE OF MEDICINE
TRIBHUVAN UNIVERSITY
KENDRIYA CAMPUS
MAHARAJGUNJ
PO BOX 1524
KATHMANDU
Tel.: +977 (1) 412 798/412 040/422 973
Fax: +977 (1) 418 186
Year instruction started: **1978**
Language of instruction: **English**
Duration of basic medical degree course, including practical training: **5.5 years**
Entrance examination: **Yes**
Foreign students eligible: **Yes**

MANIPAL COLLEGE OF MEDICAL SCIENCES
PO BOX 155
DEEP HEIGHTS
POKHARA 16
KASKI DISTRICT
Tel.: +977 (6) 121 387
Fax: +977 (6) 122 160
E-mail: mcoms@mos.com.np
Year instruction started: **1994**
Language of instruction: **English**
Duration of basic medical degree course, including practical training: **5.5 years**
Entrance examination: **Yes**
Foreign students eligible: **Yes**

NETHERLANDS

Total population in 1995: **15 575 000**
Number of physicians per 100 000 population (1993): —
Number of medical schools: **8**
Duration of basic medical degree course, including practical training: **6 years**
Title of degree awarded: *Arts* **(Physician)**
Medical registration/licence to practise: **Registration is obligatory with the Chief**

Inspector of Health Care, *Postbus 5850, 2280 HW, Rijswijk*. The licence to practise medicine is granted by the Ministry of Health, Welfare and Sport, PO Box 20350, 2500 EJ, The Hague, to graduates of a recognized medical school in the Netherlands or a country of the European Union. Those with qualifications obtained outside the European Union are granted a licence to practise at the discretion of the Minister of Health.

Work in government service after graduation: **Not obligatory**

Agreements with other countries: **An agreement exists with other countries of the European Union (Directive 93/16/EEC governing the employment of doctors).**

FACULTEIT DER GENEESKUNDE
UNIVERSITEIT VAN AMSTERDAM
MEIBERGDREEF 15
NL-1105 AZ AMSTERDAM
Year instruction started: **1632**

FACULTEIT DER GENEESKUNDE
VRIJE UNIVERSITEIT
VAN DER BOECHORSTSTRAAT 7
NL-1081 BT AMSTERDAM
Tel.: +31 (20) 444 8010
Fax: +31 (20) 444 8262
E-mail: med.educ.dept@med.vu.nl
Year instruction started: **1950**
Language of instruction: **Dutch**
Duration of basic medical degree course, including practical training: **6 years**
Entrance examination: **No**
Foreign students eligible: **Yes**

FACULTEIT DER GENEESKUNDE
RIJKSUNIVERSITEIT GRONINGEN
BLOEMSINGEL 10
NL-9712 KZ GRONINGEN
Year instruction started: **1614**

FACULTEIT DER GENEESKUNDE
RIJKSUNIVERSITEIT TE LEIDEN
WASSENAARSEWEG 62
NL-2333 AL LEIDEN
Year instruction started: **1575**

FACULTEIT DER GENEESKUNDE
RIJKSUNIVERSITEIT LIMBURG
TONGERSESTRAAT 53
POSTBUS 616
NL-6200 MD MAASTRICHT
Year instruction started: **1974**

FACULTEIT DER MEDISCHE WETENSCHAPPEN
KATHOLIEKE UNIVERSITEIT NIJMEGEN
GEERT GROOTEPLEIN NOORD 9
POSTBUS 9101
NL-6500 HB NIJMEGEN
Tel.: +31 (24) 361 9203/361 8937
Fax: +31 (24) 354 0529
Year instruction started: **1951**
Language of instruction: **Dutch**
Duration of basic medical degree course, including practical training: **6 years**
Entrance examination: **No**
Foreign students eligible: **Yes**

FACULTEIT DER GENEESKUNDE
ERASMUS UNIVERSITEIT
DR MOLEWATERPLEIN 50
POSTBUS 1738
NL-3000 DR ROTTERDAM
Tel.: +31 (10) 408 1111
Fax: +31 (10) 436 2841
E-mail: groeneveld@facb.fgg.eur.nl
Year instruction started: **1966**
Language of instruction: **Dutch**
Duration of basic medical degree course, including practical training: **6 years**
Entrance examination: **No**
Foreign students eligible: **Yes**

FACULTEIT DER GENEESKUNDE
UNIVERSITEIT UTRECHT
UNIVERSITEITSWEG 100
POSTBUS 80030
NL-3508 TA UTRECHT
Tel.: +31 (30) 253 8888
Fax: +31 (30) 253 9025

E-mail: bureau@med.ruu.nl
Year instruction started: **1636**
Language of instruction: **Dutch**
Duration of basic medical degree course, including practical training: **6 years**
Entrance examination: **No**
Foreign students eligible: **Yes**

NETHERLANDS ANTILLES

Total population in 1995: —
Number of physicians per 100 000 population (1993): —
Number of medical schools: **1**
Duration of basic medical degree course, including practical training: —
Title of degree awarded: —
Medical registration/licence to practise: —
Work in government service after graduation: —
Agreements with other countries: —

SABA SCHOOL OF MEDICINE
PO BOX 1000
SABA
NETHERLANDS ANTILLES
Tel.: +599 (4) 634 56
Fax: +599 (4) 634 58
Year instruction started: **1993**

NEW ZEALAND

Total population in 1995: **3 602 000**
Number of physicians per 100 000 population (1993): **210**
Number of medical schools: **2**
Duration of basic medical degree course, including practical training: **6 years**
Title of degree awarded: **Bachelor of Medicine and Bachelor of Surgery**
Medical registration/licence to practise: **The licence to practise medicine is granted by the Medical Council of New Zealand, 139–143 Willis Street, PO Box 11 649, Wellington. Graduates of medical schools in Australia can register without fulfilling any further requirements. The applications of graduates from other countries are considered individually.**
Work in government service after graduation: **Not obligatory**
Agreements with other countries: **An agreement exists with Australia.**

FACULTY OF MEDICINE AND HEALTH SCIENCE
UNIVERSITY OF AUCKLAND
PRIVATE BAG 92 019
AUCKLAND
Tel.: +64 (9) 373 7599
Fax: +64 (9) 373 7481
E-mail: medschool@auckland.ac.nz
Year instruction started: **1968**
Language of instruction: **English**
Duration of basic medical degree course, including practical training: **6 years**
Entrance examination: **No**
Foreign students eligible: **No**

OTAGO MEDICAL SCHOOL
UNIVERSITY OF OTAGO
GREAT KING STREET
PO BOX 913
DUNEDIN
Tel.: +64 (3) 479 5057
Fax: +64 (3) 479 0401
E-mail: medical.faculty@stonebow.otago.ac.nz
Year instruction started: **1875**
Language of instruction: **English**
Duration of basic medical degree course, including practical training: **6 years**
Entrance examination: **Yes**
Foreign students eligible: **Yes**

NICARAGUA

Total population in 1995: **4 238 000**
Number of physicians per 100 000 population (1993): **82**
Number of medical schools: **3**
Duration of basic medical degree course, including practical training: **6–7 years**
Title of degree awarded: ***Doctor en Medicina y Cirugia*** (**Doctor of Medicine and Surgery**)
Medical registration/licence to practise: —
Work in government service after graduation: —
Agreements with other countries: —

FACULTAD DE CIENCIAS MEDICAS
UNIVERSIDAD NACIONAL AUTONOMA DE NICARAGUA
LEON
Year instruction started: **1893**

FACULTAD DE CIENCIAS MEDICAS
UNIVERSIDAD AMERICANA (UAM)
MANAGUA
Tel.: +505 (2) 783 800
Fax: +505 (2) 787 558
Year instruction started: **1994**
Duration of basic medical degree course, including practical training: **6 years**

FACULTAD DE CIENCIAS MEDICAS
UNIVERSIDAD NACIONAL AUTONOMA DE NICARAGUA
CALLE DE ENEL CENTRAL 3 KM AL SUR
APDO 663
MANAGUA
Tel.: +505 (2) 277 1850
Fax: +505 (2) 278 6782
E-mail: cdocunan@ops.org.ni
Year instruction started: **1980**
Language of instruction: **Spanish**
Duration of basic medical degree course, including practical training: **7 years**
Entrance examination: **Yes**
Foreign students eligible: **Yes**

NIGER

Total population in 1995: **9 465 000**
Number of physicians per 100 000 population (1993): **3**
Number of medical schools: **1**
Duration of basic medical degree course, including practical training: **7 years**
Title of degree awarded: ***Docteur en Médecine* (*Diplôme d'État*) (Doctor of Medicine (State Diploma))**
Medical registration/licence to practise: —
Work in government service after graduation: —
Agreements with other countries: —

FACULTE DES SCIENCES DE LA SANTE
UNIVERSITE DE NIAMEY
BP 237
NIAMEY
Year instruction started: **1974**

NIGERIA

Total population in 1995: **115 020 000**
Number of physicians per 100 000 population (1993): **21**
Number of medical schools: **15**
Duration of basic medical degree course, including practical training: **5–6 years**
Title of degree awarded: **Bachelor of Medicine and Bachelor of Surgery**
Medical registration/licence to practise: **Registration is obligatory with the Medical and Dental Council of Nigeria, 25 Ahmed Onibudo Street, Victoria Island, Private Mail Bag 12611, Lagos. The licence to practise medicine is granted to graduates of a recognized medical school who have worked as an intern for 12 months on a rotating basis in an accredited hospital. Those with foreign qualifications must pass the Nigeria Medical Council Assessment Examination and serve for 1 year as an intern in Nigeria.**
Work in government service after graduation: **Obligatory (Nigerians must serve for 1 year in the National Youth Service)**
Agreements with other countries: **None**

OBAFEMI AWOLOWO COLLEGE OF HEALTH SCIENCES
OGUN STATE UNIVERSITY
PRIVATE MAIL BAG 2002
AGO-IWOYE
OGUN STATE
Year instruction started: **1983**

FACULTY OF MEDICINE
UNIVERSITY OF BENIN
PRIVATE MAIL BAG 1154
BENIN CITY
EDO STATE
Tel.: +234 (52) 600 547/600 549/600 567
Fax: +234 (52) 600 273
Telex: 41365 uniben ng
Year instruction started: **1971**
Language of instruction: **English**
Duration of basic medical degree course, including practical training: **6 years**
Entrance examination: **Yes**
Foreign students eligible: **Yes**

COLLEGE OF MEDICAL SCIENCES
UNIVERSITY OF CALABAR
PRIVATE MAIL BAG 1115
CALABAR
CROSS RIVER STATE

Tel.: +234 (87) 222 855/225 547
Fax: +234 (87) 221 766
Telex: 65103 unical ng
Year instruction started: **1978**
Language of instruction: **English**
Duration of basic medical degree course, including practical training: **5 or 6 years**
Entrance examination: **Yes**
Foreign students eligible: **Yes**

FACULTY OF MEDICINE
UNIVERSITY OF NIGERIA
ENUGU CAMPUS
PRIVATE MAIL BAG 01229
ENUGU
ENUGU STATE
Year instruction started: **1969**

COLLEGE OF MEDICINE
UNIVERSITY OF IBADAN
UNIVERSITY COLLEGE HOSPITAL
QUEEN ELIZABETH ROAD
PRIVATE MAIL BAG 5017
IBADAN
OYO STATE
Tel.: +234 (2) 241 3922
Fax: +234 (2) 241 1768
E-mail: provost.sysop@nga.healthnet.org
Year instruction started: **1948**
Language of instruction: **English**
Duration of basic medical degree course, including practical training: **5 or 6 years**
Entrance examination: **Yes**
Foreign students eligible: **Yes**

COLLEGE OF HEALTH SCIENCES
OBAFEMI AWOLOWO UNIVERSITY
PRIVATE MAIL BAG 2002
ILE-IFE
OYO STATE
Tel.: +234 (36) 233 134
Fax: +234 (36) 233 134
Year instruction started: **1972**
Language of instruction: **English**
Duration of basic medical degree course, including practical training: **6 years**
Entrance examination: **Yes**
Foreign students eligible: **Yes**

FACULTY OF HEALTH SCIENCES
UNIVERSITY OF ILORIN
PRIVATE MAIL BAG 1515
ILORIN
KWARA STATE
Tel.: +234 (31) 221 844
Telex: 33144 unilon ng
E-mail: fhs@unilorin.edu.ng
Year instruction started: **1977**
Language of instruction: **English**
Duration of basic medical degree course, including practical training: **6 years**
Entrance examination: **Yes**
Foreign students eligible: **Yes**

FACULTY OF MEDICAL SCIENCES
UNIVERSITY OF JOS
PRIVATE MAIL BAG 2084
JOS
PLATEAU STATE
Year instruction started: **1976**

COLLEGE OF MEDICINE
UNIVERSITY OF LAGOS
IDI-ARABA
PRIVATE MAIL BAG 12003
LAGOS
LAGOS STATE
Tel.: +234 (1) 832 049/801 500
Fax: +234 (1) 837 630
Telex: 27636 ng
Year instruction started: **1962**
Language of instruction: **English**
Duration of basic medical degree course, including practical training: **5 years**
Entrance examination: **Yes**
Foreign students eligible: **Yes**

COLLEGE OF MEDICAL SCIENCES
UNIVERSITY OF MAIDUGURI
PRIVATE MAIL BAG 1069
MAIDUGURI
BORNO STATE

Year instruction started: **1978**
Language of instruction: **English**
Duration of basic medical degree course, including practical training: **5 years**
Entrance examination: **No**
Foreign students eligible: **Yes**

COLLEGE OF HEALTH SCIENCES
NNAMDI AZIKIWE UNIVERSITY
NNEWI CAMPUS
PRIVATE MAIL BAG 5001
NNEWI
ANAMBRA STATE
Tel.: +234 (46) 463 663
Fax: +234 (46) 460 124
Year instruction started: **1987**
Language of instruction: **English**
Duration of basic medical degree course, including practical training: **5–6 years**
Entrance examination: **Yes**
Foreign students eligible: **Yes**

COLLEGE OF HEALTH SCIENCES
UNIVERSITY OF PORT HARCOURT
EAST-WEST ROAD
PRIVATE MAIL BAG 1
CHOBA
PORT HARCOURT
RIVERS STATE
Telex: 61183 phuni ng
Year instruction started: **1979**
Language of instruction: **English**
Duration of basic medical degree course, including practical training: **6 years**
Entrance examination: **Yes**
Foreign students eligible: **Yes**

COLLEGE OF HEALTH SCIENCES
DANFODIYO UNIVERSITY
SULTAN ABUBAKAR ROAD
PRIVATE MAIL BAG 2370
SOKOTO 02254
SOKOTO STATE

Tel.: +234 (60) 233 012
Fax: +234 (60) 230 709
Year instruction started: **1979**
Language of instruction: **English**
Duration of basic medical degree course, including practical training: **6 years**
Entrance examination: **Yes**
Foreign students eligible: **Yes**

COLLEGE OF MEDICINE AND HEALTH SCIENCES
ABIA STATE UNIVERSITY
PRIVATE MAIL BAG 2000
UTURU
ABIA STATE

FACULTY OF MEDICINE
AHMADU BELLO UNIVERSITY
ZARIA
KADUNA STATE
Year instruction started: **1967**

NORWAY

Total population in 1995: **4 348 000**
Number of physicians per 100 000 population (1993): —
Number of medical schools: **4**
Duration of basic medical degree course, including practical training: **6–6.5 years**
Title of degree awarded: ***Candidatus medicinae* (cand. med.)**
Medical registration/licence to practise: **Registration is obligatory with the Norwegian Board of Health, PO Box 8126 Dep., 0032 Oslo. The licence to practise medicine is granted to graduates who have successfully completed 1.5 years of medical practice. Those with foreign medical qualifications must have their degree approved and pass complementary tests on certain medical subjects. Foreigners must also pass a language examination.**
Work in government service after graduation: **Obligatory (1.5 years)**
Agreements with other countries: **Agreements exist with other countries of the European Union (Directive 93/16/EEC governing the employment of doctors) and Denmark, Finland, Iceland and Sweden.**

DET MEDISINSKE FAKULTET
UNIVERSITETET I BERGEN
HARALD HARFAGRESGT. 1
N-5020 BERGEN

Year instruction started: **1946**
Language of instruction: **Norwegian**
Duration of basic medical degree course, including practical training: **6–6.5 years**
Entrance examination: **No**
Foreign students eligible: **Yes**

DET MEDISINSKE FAKULTET
UNIVERSITETET I OSLO
SOSTERHJEMMET 2 ETG.
ULLEVAL SYKEHUS
POST BOKS 1078 BLINDERN
N-0316 OSLO
Year instruction started: **1814**

FAGOMRADET MEDISIN UNIVERSITETET I TROMSO
N-9037 TROMSO
Tel.: +47 (776) 446 10
Fax: +47 (776) 453 00
Year instruction started: **1972**
Language of instruction: **Norwegian**
Duration of basic medical degree course, including practical training: **6 years**
Entrance examination: **No**
Foreign students eligible: **Yes**

DET MEDISINSKE FAKULTET
UNIVERSITETET I TRONDHEIM
EIRIK JARLS GT. 10
N-7000 TRONDHEIM
Year instruction started: **1975**

OMAN

Total population in 1995: **2 302 000**
Number of physicians per 100 000 population (1993): **120**
Number of medical schools: **1**
Duration of basic medical degree course, including practical training: **7 years (a further year of supervised practice is required before the degree is awarded)**
Title of degree awarded: **Doctor of Medicine (MD)**
Medical registration/licence to practise: **Registration is obligatory with the Ministry of Health, PO Box 393, Muscat. The licence to practise medicine is granted to graduates of a recognized medical school who have completed**

a 2-year internship. Graduates of foreign medical schools must sit a local qualifying examination.

Work in government service after graduation: **Not obligatory**

Agreements with other countries: **An agreement for limited registration exists with the General Medical Council of the United Kingdom.**

COLLEGE OF MEDICINE
SULTAN QABOOS UNIVERSITY
AL KHOD
PO BOX 35
MUSCAT 123
Tel.: +968 515 102
Fax: +968 513 419
Year instruction started: **1986**
Language of instruction: **English**
Duration of basic medical degree course, including practical training: **7 years**
Entrance examination: **No**
Foreign students eligible: **No**

PAKISTAN

Total population in 1995: **139 973 000**
Number of physicians per 100 000 population (1993): **52**
Number of medical schools: **19**
Duration of basic medical degree course, including practical training: **5 years**
Title of degree awarded: **Bachelor of Medicine and Bachelor of Surgery (MB, BS)**
Medical registration/licence to practise: **Registration is obligatory with the Pakistan Medical and Dental Council, G-10/4 Mauve Area, Islamabad. The licence to practise medicine is granted to graduates of a recognized medical school. Graduates of foreign medical schools must pass a qualifying registration examination of the National Examination Board of the Pakistan Medical and Dental Council. Foreigners are only eligible for conditional registration and a licence to practise on a year-to-year basis for institutional service.**
Work in government service after graduation: **Obligatory (1 year)**
Agreements with other countries: **—**

AYUB MEDICAL COLLEGE
UNIVERSITY OF PESHAWAR
ABBOTTABAD
Year instruction started: **1979**

QUAID-E-AZAM MEDICAL COLLEGE
ISLAMIA UNIVERSITY
CIRCULAR ROAD
PO BOX 4
BAHAWALPUR
Tel.: +92 (621) 884 289
Fax: +92 (621) 875 677
Year instruction started: **1971**
Language of instruction: **English**
Duration of basic medical degree course, including practical training: **5 years**
Entrance examination: **Yes**
Foreign students eligible: **Yes**

PUNJAB MEDICAL COLLEGE
UNIVERSITY OF PUNJAB
SARDOGHA ROAD
FAISALABAD
Tel.: +92 (41) 760 470
Fax: +92 (41) 762 846
Year instruction started: **1973**
Language of instruction: **English**
Duration of basic medical degree course, including practical training: **5 years**
Entrance examination: **No**
Foreign students eligible: **Yes**

LIAQUAT MEDICAL COLLEGE
UNIVERSITY OF SIND
JAMSHORO
Tel.: +92 (221) 771 239
Fax: +92 (221) 771 303
Year instruction started: **1951**
Language of instruction: **English**
Duration of basic medical degree course, including practical training: **5 years**
Entrance examination: **No**
Foreign students eligible: **Yes**

AGA KHAN MEDICAL COLLEGE
AGA KHAN UNIVERSITY
STADIUM ROAD
PO BOX 3500
KARACHI
Year instruction started: **1983**

KARACHI MEDICAL AND DENTAL COLLEGE AND ABBASI SHAHEED
    HOSPITAL[1]
KARACHI METROPOLITAN CORPORATION
F. B. AREA BLOCK 16
KARACHI 75950
Tel.: +92 (21) 632 0020/632 0021/632 0022
Year instruction started: **1991**

BAQAI MEDICAL COLLEGE[1]
UNIVERSITY OF KARACHI
51 DEH TOR
TOLL PLAZA
PO BOX 2407
KARACHI 18
Tel.: +92 (21) 635 0433/635 0434
Fax: +92 (21) 661 7968
E-mail: bih@cyber.net.pk
Year instruction started: **1988**
Language of instruction: **English**
Duration of basic medical degree course, including practical training: **5 years**
Entrance examination: **Yes**
Foreign students eligible: **Yes**

DOW MEDICAL COLLEGE
UNIVERSITY OF KARACHI
BABA-E-URDU ROAD
KARACHI 74400
Year instruction started: **1945**

SIND MEDICAL COLLEGE
UNIVERSITY OF KARACHI
RAFIQUE H.I. SHAHEED ROAD
KARACHI 77510
Tel.: +92 (21) 519 006/519 007/519 008
Year instruction started: **1973**
Language of instruction: **English**
Duration of basic medical degree course, including practical training: **5 years**
Entrance examination: **No**
Foreign students eligible: **Yes**

---

[1] Provisional recognition.

ALLAMA IQBAL MEDICAL COLLEGE
UNIVERSITY OF PUNJAB
6 BIRDWOOD ROAD
LAHORE
Year instruction started: **1975**

FATIMA JINNAH MEDICAL COLLEGE FOR WOMEN
UNIVERSITY OF PUNJAB
LAHORE
Year instruction started: **1948**

KING EDWARD MEDICAL COLLEGE
UNIVERSITY OF PUNJAB
NILA GUMBAND
LAHORE
Year instruction started: **1860**

CHANDKA MEDICAL COLLEGE
UNIVERSITY OF SIND JAMSHORO
LARKANA

NISHTAR MEDICAL COLLEGE
BAHUDDIN ZAKARIA UNIVERSITY
MULTAN
Year instruction started: **1951**

NAWABSHAH MEDICAL COLLEGE FOR GIRLS
UNIVERSITY OF SIND
NAWABSHAH

KHYBER MEDICAL COLLEGE
UNIVERSITY OF PESHAWAR
UNIVERSITY CAMPUS
PESHAWAR
Tel.: +92 (521) 841 425
Fax: +92 (521) 841 598
Year instruction started: **1954**
Language of instruction: **English**
Duration of basic medical degree course, including practical training: **5 years**
Entrance examination: **Yes**
Foreign students eligible: **Yes**

BOLAN MEDICAL COLLEGE
UNIVERSITY OF BALUCHISTAN
QUETTA
Year instruction started: **1972**

ARMY MEDICAL COLLEGE
QUAID-E-AZAM UNIVERSITY
ABID MAJID ROAD
RAWALPINDI 46000
Tel.: +92 (51) 584 780
Fax: +92 (51) 581 085
Year instruction started: **1977**
Language of instruction: **English**
Duration of basic medical degree course, including practical training: **5 years**
Entrance examination: **Yes**
Foreign students eligible: **Yes**

RAWALPINDI MEDICAL COLLEGE
UNIVERSITY OF PUNJAB
TIPU ROAD
RAWALPINDI 46000
Tel.: +92 (51) 552 819
Fax: +92 (51) 502 148
Year instruction started: **1973**
Language of instruction: **English**
Duration of basic medical degree course, including practical training: **5 years**
Entrance examination: **No**
Foreign students eligible: **Yes**

PALAU

Total population in 1995: —
Number of physicians per 100 000 population (1993): —
Number of medical schools: **None**
Medical registration/licence to practise: **Registration is obligatory with the Ministry of Health, PO Box 6027, Koror 96940. The licence to practise medicine is granted to graduates of a recognized medical school who hold a current licence.**
Work in government service after graduation: **Not obligatory**
Agreements with other countries: **None**

PANAMA

Total population in 1995: **2 677 000**
Number of physicians per 100 000 population (1993): **119**
Number of medical schools: **2**
Duration of basic medical degree course, including practical training: **6 years**
Title of degree awarded: *Doctor en Medicina* **(Doctor of Medicine)**
Medical registration/licence to practise: **Registration is obligatory with the Ministry of Education. The licence to practise medicine is granted by the** *Consejo Técnico de Salud, Ministry of Health, Avenida Cuba y Calle 34, Panama.* **Applicants should make their request through a lawyer. They should submit the originals and one copy of their degree certificate, as well as evidence to certify that they have successfully completed a 2-year internship. Those with foreign medical qualifications must have their degree certified by the Panamanian consular authorities in the country concerned. Foreigners are not entitled to practise.**
Work in government service after graduation: **Not obligatory**
Agreements with other countries: —

FACULTAD DE MEDICINA
UNIVERSIDAD DE PANAMA
VIA TRANSISTMICA
APDO 3368
PANAMA
Tel.: +507 223 8512
Fax: +507 223 8512
Year instruction started: **1951**
Language of instruction: **Spanish**
Duration of basic medical degree course, including practical training: **6 years**
Entrance examination: **Yes**
Foreign students eligible: **Yes**

FACULTAD DE CIENCIAS MEDICAS Y DE LA SALUD
UNIVERSIDAD LATINA DE PANAMA
CALLE 55 EL CANGREJO
APDO 87-0887
BELLA VISTA
PANAMA
Tel.: +507 263 2038/263 3409
Fax: +507 263 3376

E-mail: fac-med@ns.ulat.ac.pa
Year instruction started: **1994**
Language of instruction: **Spanish, English**
Duration of basic medical degree course, including practical training: **6 years**
Entrance examination: **Yes**
Foreign students eligible: **Yes**

PAPUA NEW GUINEA

Total population in 1995: **4 400 000**
Number of physicians per 100 000 population (1993): **18**
Number of medical schools: **1**
Duration of basic medical degree course, including practical training: **6 years**
Title of degree awarded: **Bachelor of Medicine and Bachelor of Surgery**
Medical registration/licence to practise: —
Work in government service after graduation: —
Agreements with other countries: —

FACULTY OF MEDICINE
UNIVERSITY OF PAPUA NEW GUINEA
PO BOX 5623
BOROKO
Year instruction started: **1959**

PARAGUAY

Total population in 1995: **4 957 000**
Number of physicians per 100 000 population (1993): **67**
Number of medical schools: **1**
Duration of basic medical degree course, including practical training: **6 years**
Title of degree awarded: ***Médico Cirujano*** **(Physician and Surgeon)**
Medical registration/licence to practise: —
Work in government service after graduation: —
Agreements with other countries: —

FACULTAD DE CIENCIAS MEDICAS
UNIVERSIDAD NACIONAL DE ASUNCION
AVENIDA DE MONTERO 658
CASILLA 1102
ASUNCION
Year instruction started: **1898**
Duration of basic medical degree course, including practical training: **6 years**

PERU

Total population in 1995: **23 944 000**
Number of physicians per 100 000 population (1993): **73**
Number of medical schools: **17**
Duration of basic medical degree course, including practical training: **6–8 years (a further year of supervised clinical practice in the four basic subjects is required before the degree is awarded)**
Title of degree awarded: ***Médico Cirujano*** (**Physician and Surgeon**)
Medical registration/licence to practise: **Registration is obligatory with the *Colegio Médico del Perú, Malecon Almendaríz, Miraflores, Lima.* The licence to practise medicine is granted to graduates of a recognized medical school who have successfully completed a 1-year internship and 1 year of service in a rural area.**
Work in government service after graduation: **Obligatory (1 year in a rural area)**
Agreements with other countries: —

FACULTAD DE MEDICINA HUMANA
UNIVERSIDAD CATOLICA DE SANTA MARIA
URBANIZACION SAN JOSE
APDO 1350
AREQUIPA
Tel.: +51 (54) 251 213/251 210
Fax: +51 (54) 251 144
Year instruction started: **1988**
Language of instruction: **Spanish**
Duration of basic medical degree course, including practical training: **7 years**
Entrance examination: **Yes**
Foreign students eligible: **Yes**

FACULTAD DE MEDICINA
UNIVERSIDAD NACIONAL DE SAN AGUSTIN
DANIEL A. CARRION 101 CERCADO
APDO 1365
AREQUIPA
Tel.: +51 (54) 233 803
Fax: +51 (54) 233 803
E-mail: cd.fm@medic.unsa.edu.pe
Year instruction started: **1958**
Language of instruction: **Spanish**
Duration of basic medical degree course, including practical training: **7 years**
Entrance examination: **Yes**
Foreign students eligible: **Yes**

FACULTAD DE CIENCIAS DE LA SALUD
UNIVERSIDAD NACIONAL DE CAJAMARCA
CAJAMARCA
Year instruction started: **1991**

FACULTAD DE MEDICINA HUMANA
UNIVERSIDAD NACIONAL DE SAN ANTONIO ABAD DEL CUSCO
AVENIDA DE LA CULTURA S/N
CIUDAD UNIVERSITARIA
APDO 367
CUSCO
Tel.: +51 (84) 224 905
Fax: +51 (84) 226 048
E-mail: famehum@unsaac.edu.pe
Year instruction started: **1980**
Language of instruction: **Spanish**
Duration of basic medical degree course, including practical training: **7 years**
Entrance examination: **Yes**
Foreign students eligible: **Yes**

FACULTAD DE MEDICINA HUMANA
UNIVERSIDAD NACIONAL "JOSE FAUSTINO SANCHEZ CARRION"
AVENIDA MERCEDES INDACOCHEA
HUACHO
Tel.: +51 (1) 312 395
Year instruction started: **1990**
Language of instruction: **Spanish**
Duration of basic medical degree course, including practical training: **7 years**
Entrance examination: **Yes**
Foreign students eligible: **Yes**

FACULTAD DE ENFERMERIA Y MEDICINA HUMANA
UNIVERSIDAD NACIONAL DEL CENTRO DE PERU
HUANCAYO
Year instruction started: **1991**

PROGRAMA ACADEMICO DE MEDICINA HUMANA
UNIVERSIDAD "SAN LUIS GONZAGA"
JR DOS DE MAYO 187
APDO 187
ICA
Year instruction started: **1963**

FACULTAD DE MEDICINA HUMANA "RAFAEL DONAYRE ROJAS"
UNIVERSIDAD NACIONAL DE LA AMAZONIA PERUANA
AVENIDA COLONIAL S/N
MORONILLO
PUNCHANA
APDO 613
IQUITOS
Tel.: +51 (94) 251 780
Year instruction started: **1982**
Language of instruction: **Spanish**
Duration of basic medical degree course, including practical training: **7 years**
Entrance examination: **Yes**
Foreign students eligible: **Yes**

FACULTAD DE MEDICINA HUMANA
UNIVERSIDAD NACIONAL PEDRO RUIZ GALLO
LAMBAYEQUE
Year instruction started: **1982**

PROGRAMA ACADEMICO DE MEDICINA HUMANA
UNIVERSIDAD NACIONAL FEDERICO VILLARREAL
COLMENA 412
LIMA
Year instruction started: **1966**

ESCUELA DE MEDICINA HUMANA
UNIVERSIDAD NACIONAL MAYOR DE SAN MARCOS
AVENIDA GRAU 755
APDO 529
LIMA 100
Tel.: +51 (1) 328 3237
Fax: +51 (1) 328 3231
E-mail: decano@sanfer.edu.pe
Year instruction started: **1856**
Language of instruction: **Spanish**
Duration of basic medical degree course, including practical training: **7 years**
Entrance examination: **Yes**
Foreign students eligible: **Yes**

PROGRAMA ACADEMICO DE MEDICINA
UNIVERSIDAD PERUANA CAYETANO HEREDIA
AVENIDA HONORIO DELGADO 932
SAN MARTIN DE PORRES
APDO 5045
LIMA
Year instruction started: **1962**

FACULTAD DE MEDICINA HUMANA
UNIVERSIDAD NACIONAL DE PIURA
APDO 295
PIURA
Tel.: +51 (74) 328 491
Fax: +51 (74) 331 683
E-mail: medicina@unpiur.edu.pe
Year instruction started: **1982**
Language of instruction: **Spanish**
Duration of basic medical degree course, including practical training: **6 years**
Entrance examination: **Yes**
Foreign students eligible: **Yes**

FACULTAD DE CIENCIAS DE LA SALUD
UNIVERSIDAD NACIONAL DEL ALTIPLANO
PUNO
Year instruction started: **1983**

FACULTAD DE MEDICINA HUMANA
UNIVERSIDAD DE SAN MARTIN DE PORRES
AVENIDA LAS CALANDRIAS S/N
SANTA ANITA 44
Tel.: +51 (4) 362 1293
Fax: +51 (4) 362 1293
Year instruction started: **1983**
Language of instruction: **Spanish**
Duration of basic medical degree course, including practical training: **7 years**
Entrance examination: **Yes**
Foreign students eligible: **Yes**

FACULTAD DE MEDICINA HUMANA
UNIVERSIDAD PRIVADA DE TACNA
AVENIDA 28 AGOSTO 275 (POCOLLAY)
APDO 746
TACNA

Tel.: +51 (54) 743 378
Fax: +51 (54) 726 881/727 212
E-mail: famh@heroica.upt.edu.pe
Year instruction started: **1994**
Language of instruction: **Spanish**
Duration of basic medical degree course, including practical training: **7 years**
Entrance examination: **Yes**
Foreign students eligible: **Yes**

PROGRAMA ACADEMICO DE MEDICINA HUMANA
UNIVERSIDAD NACIONAL DE TRUJILLO
INDEPENDENCIA 431
OF. 203
TRUJILLO
Year instruction started: **1958**

PHILIPPINES

Total population in 1995: **69 282 000**
Number of physicians per 100 000 population (1993): **11**
Number of medical schools: **28**
Duration of basic medical degree course, including practical training: **4–7 years**
Title of degree awarded: ***Manggagamot* (Doctor of Medicine)**
Medical registration/licence to practise: **Registration is obligatory with the Professional Regulation Commission, P. Parades Street, Manila. The licence to practise medicine is granted to graduates of a recognized medical school in the Philippines who have completed 1 year as an intern before taking the licensing examination. The licence must be renewed every 5 years. Foreigners and nationals with foreign medical qualifications are allowed to practise only if they are from a country that has a reciprocal agreement with the Philippines.**
Work in government service after graduation: **Not obligatory**
Agreements with other countries: —

COLLEGE OF MEDICINE
ANGELES UNIVERSITY FOUNDATION
MACARTHUR HIGHWAY
ANGELES CITY 2009
PAMPANGA
Tel.: +63 (455) 602 8882/602 8883/602 8884
Fax: +63 (455) 888 2725

Year instruction started: **1983**
Language of instruction: **English**
Duration of basic medical degree course, including practical training: **4 years**
Entrance examination: **Yes**
Foreign students eligible: **Yes**

COLLEGE OF MEDICINE
SAINT LOUIS UNIVERSITY
BONIFACIO STREET
BAGUIO CITY 2600
BENGUET
Tel.: +63 (74) 442 2793/442 3043/443 2001
Fax: +63 (74) 442 2842
Year instruction started: **1976**
Language of instruction: **English**
Duration of basic medical degree course, including practical training: **4 years**
Entrance examination: **No**
Foreign students eligible: **Yes**

COLLEGE OF MEDICINE
UNIVERSITY OF PERPETUAL HELP SYSTEM
SANTO NINO
BINAN 4024
LAGUNA
Tel.: +63 (049) 511 8636
Year instruction started: **1977**
Language of instruction: **English**
Duration of basic medical degree course, including practical training: **4 years**
Entrance examination: **Yes**
Foreign students eligible: **Yes**

DR JOSE P. RIZAL COLLEGE OF MEDICINE
XAVIER UNIVERSITY
CORRALES AVENUE
CAGAYAN DE ORO CITY 9000
MISAMIS ORIENTAL
Tel.: +63 (8822) 722 678
E-mail: jprcm@xu.edu.ph
Year instruction started: **1983**
Language of instruction: **English**
Duration of basic medical degree course, including practical training: **4 years**
Entrance examination: **Yes**
Foreign students eligible: **Yes**

COLLEGE OF MEDICINE
MANILA CENTRAL UNIVERSITY
FILEMON D. TANCHOCO MEDICAL FOUNDATION
EDSA STREET
CALOOCAN CITY 1400
RIZAL
Tel.: +63 (2) 362 1046/362 1047/362 1048
Fax: +63 (2) 361 4664
Year instruction started: **1947**
Language of instruction: **English**
Duration of basic medical degree course, including practical training: **4 years**
Entrance examination: **Yes**
Foreign students eligible: **Yes**

CEBU DOCTORS COLLEGE OF MEDICINE
KAMUNING STREET
OSMENA BOULEVARD
CEBU CITY 6000
CEBU
Tel.: +63 (32) 536 92
Fax: +63 (32) 253 0976
E-mail: records@cdc-cdh.edu
Year instruction started: **1977**
Language of instruction: **English**
Duration of basic medical degree course, including practical training: **4 years**
Entrance examination: **Yes**
Foreign students eligible: **Yes**

CEBU INSTITUTE OF MEDICINE
79 F. RAMOS STREET
CEBU CITY 6000
CEBU
Tel.: +63 (32) 253 7413
Fax: +63 (32) 253 9127
Year instruction started: **1957**
Language of instruction: **English**
Duration of basic medical degree course, including practical training: **4 years**
Entrance examination: **No**
Foreign students eligible: **Yes**

MATIAS H. AZNAR MEMORIAL COLLEGE OF MEDICINE
URGELLO PRIVATE ROAD
CEBU CITY 6000
CEBU

Tel.: +63 (32) 611 44/255 6469
Fax: +63 (32) 527 99
Year instruction started: **1946**
Language of instruction: **English**
Duration of basic medical degree course, including practical training: **4 years**
Entrance examination: **Yes**
Foreign students eligible: **Yes**

COLLEGE OF MEDICINE
DR FRANCISCO Q. DUQUE MEDICAL FOUNDATION
LYCEUM NORTHWESTERN
TAPUAC DISTRICT
DAGUPAN CITY 2400
PANGASINAN
Tel.: +63 (75) 522 0296
Fax: +63 (75) 522 0296
Year instruction started: **1975**
Language of instruction: **English**
Duration of basic medical degree course, including practical training: **4 years**
Entrance examination: **Yes**
Foreign students eligible: **Yes**

COLLEGE OF MEDICINE
DE LA SALLE UNIVERSITY
CONGRESSIONAL AVENUE
DASMARINAS 4114
CAVITE
Tel.: +63 (46) 6226/6704/6705
Fax: +63 (46) 6465
Year instruction started: **1979**
Language of instruction: **English**
Duration of basic medical degree course, including practical training: **4 years**
Entrance examination: **Yes**
Foreign students eligible: **Yes**

DAVAO MEDICAL SCHOOL FOUNDATION
MEDICAL SCHOOL DRIVE
BAJADA
PO BOX 80712
DAVAO CITY 8000
DAVAO
Tel.: +63 (82) 623 44
Fax: +63 (82) 768 86

Year instruction started: **1977**
Language of instruction: **English**
Duration of basic medical degree course, including practical training: **4 years**
Entrance examination: **Yes**
Foreign students eligible: **Yes**

COLLEGE OF MEDICINE
MINDANAO STATE UNIVERSITY
MSU-IIT CAMPUS
TIBANGA
ILIGAN CITY 9200
MINDANAO
Tel.: +63 (88) 138 35
Fax: +63 (88) 153 84
Year instruction started: **1984**
Language of instruction: **English**
Duration of basic medical degree course, including practical training: **4 years**
Entrance examination: **Yes**
Foreign students eligible: **No**

ILOILO DOCTORS COLLEGE OF MEDICINE
WEST AVENUE
MOLO
ILOILO CITY 5901
ILOILO
Tel.: +63 (33) 777 55
Year instruction started: **1981**
Language of instruction: **English**
Duration of basic medical degree course, including practical training: **4 years**
Entrance examination: **Yes**
Foreign students eligible: **Yes**

COLLEGE OF MEDICINE
WEST VISAYAS STATE UNIVERSITY
LUNA STREET
ILOILO CITY 5000
ILOILO
Tel.: +63 (33) 320 0881/320 0870
Fax: +63 (33) 202 631
Year instruction started: **1975**
Language of instruction: **English**
Duration of basic medical degree course, including practical training: **4 years**
Entrance examination: **Yes**
Foreign students eligible: **Yes**

BICOL CHRISTIAN COLLEGE OF MEDICINE
RIZAL STREET
LEGASPI CITY 4500
ALBAY
Tel.: +63 (5221) 447 83
Year instruction started: **1980**
Language of instruction: **English**
Duration of basic medical degree course, including practical training: **4 years**
Entrance examination: **Yes**
Foreign students eligible: **Yes**

GULLAS COLLEGE OF MEDICINE
UNIVERSITY OF VISAYAS
BANILAD
MANDAUE CITY 6433
CEBU
Tel.: +63 (32) 839 25
Year instruction started: **1977**
Language of instruction: **English**
Duration of basic medical degree course, including practical training: **4 years**
Entrance examination: **Yes**
Foreign students eligible: **Yes**

DR NICANOR REYES MEDICAL FOUNDATION INSTITUTE OF MEDICINE
FAR EASTERN UNIVERSITY
NICANOR REYES SR STREET
PO BOX 616
MANILA 2801
Year instruction started: **1952**

FACULTY OF MEDICINE AND SURGERY
UNIVERSITY OF SANTO TOMAS
ESPANA STREET
MANILA 2801
Tel.: +63 (2) 741 5314/731 3126
Fax: +63 (2) 731 3126
Year instruction started: **1871**
Language of instruction: **English**
Duration of basic medical degree course, including practical training: **4 years**
Entrance examination: **Yes**
Foreign students eligible: **Yes**

COLLEGE OF MEDICINE
UNIVERSITY OF THE CITY OF MANILA
GENERAL MURALLA STREET
INTRAMUROS
MANILA 1002
Tel.: +63 (2) 527 7941/527 7942/527 7943
Fax: +63 (2) 527 7949
Year instruction started: **1983**
Language of instruction: **English**
Duration of basic medical degree course, including practical training: **4 years**
Entrance examination: **Yes**
Foreign students eligible: **No**

COLLEGE OF MEDICINE
UNIVERSITY OF THE PHILIPPINES SYSTEM
547 PEDRO GIL STREET
ERMITA
PO BOX 593
MANILA 1000
Tel.: +63 (2) 526 4256
Fax: +63 (2) 526 0371
Year instruction started: **1908**
Language of instruction: **English**
Duration of basic medical degree course, including practical training: **7 years**
Entrance examination: **Yes**
Foreign students eligible: **Yes**

INSTITUTE OF HEALTH SCIENCES
UNIVERSITY OF THE PHILIPPINES SYSTEM
PALO 7101
LEYTE
Year instruction started: **1976**

COLLEGE OF MEDICINE
RAMON MAGSAYSAY MEMORIAL MEDICAL CENTER
UNIVERSITY OF THE EAST
QUEZON CITY 3008
Year instruction started: **1956**

ST LUKE'S COLLEGE OF MEDICINE
WILLIAM H. QUASHA MEMORIAL
CATHEDRAL HEIGHTS
279 E. RODRIGUEZ SR BOULEVARD
PO BOX 780
QUEZON CITY 1099

Tel.: +63 (2) 723 0101
Year instruction started: **1994**
Language of instruction: **Pilipino, English**
Duration of basic medical degree course, including practical training: **5 years**
Entrance examination: **Yes**
Foreign students eligible: **Yes**

COLLEGE OF MEDICINE
VIRGEN MILAGROSA UNIVERSITY FOUNDATION
TALOY STREET
SAN CARLOS CITY 2420
PANGASINAN
Tel.: +63 (75) 532 2380
Fax: +63 (75) 695 477
Year instruction started: **1975**
Language of instruction: **English**
Duration of basic medical degree course, including practical training: **4 years**
Entrance examination: **Yes**
Foreign students eligible: **Yes**

COLLEGE OF MEDICINE
REMEDIOS T. ROMUALDEZ MEDICAL FOUNDATION
TACLOBAN CITY 7101
LEYTE
Tel.: +63 (53) 321 2345/325 7074
Fax: +63 (53) 325 8353
Year instruction started: **1980**
Language of instruction: **English**
Duration of basic medical degree course, including practical training: **4 years**
Entrance examination: **Yes**
Foreign students eligible: **Yes**

COLLEGE OF MEDICINE
CAGAYAN STATE UNIVERSITY
TUGUEGARAO
CAGAYAN

FATIMA COLLEGE OF MEDICINE
FATIMA MEDICAL SCIENCE FOUNDATION
120 MACARTHUR HIGHWAY
VALENZUELA 2627
MANILA
Tel.: +63 (2) 293 2703

Year instruction started: **1979**
Language of instruction: **English**
Duration of basic medical degree course, including practical training: **4 years**
Entrance examination: **Yes**
Foreign students eligible: **Yes**

COLLEGE OF MEDICINE
ATENEO DE ZAMBOANGA
ZAMBOANGA CITY

POLAND

Total population in 1995: **38 601 000**
Number of physicians per 100 000 population (1993): **—**
Number of medical schools: **14**
Duration of basic medical degree course, including practical training: **4 or 6 years**
Title of degree awarded: *Lekarz* **(Doctor of Medicine)**
Medical registration/licence to practise: **Registration is obligatory with the**
    Naczelna Izba Lekarska, Ulica Grojecka 65A, 02-094 Warsaw. **The licence to**
    practise medicine is granted to graduates of a recognized medical school
    who have completed a 1-year internship. Foreigners must hold a residence
    permit. They should apply to the Minister of Health and Social Welfare
    and provide original or certified documents to the Supreme Medical
    Council. They may only practise for a limited period and must have an
    adequate command of the Polish language.
Work in government service after graduation: **Not obligatory**
Agreements with other countries: **Bilateral and multilateral agreements exist**
    with a number of countries.

BIALYSTOK AKADEMIA MEDYCZNA
ULICA KILINSKIEGO 1
PL-15-230 BIALYSTOK
Year instruction started: **1950**

AKADEMIA MEDYCZNA IM. LUDWIKA RYDYGIERA
ULICA JAGIELLONSKA 13
PL-85-067 BYDGOSZCZ
Tel.: +48 (52) 211 818
Telex: 562138 amb pl
Year instruction started: **1987**
Language of instruction: **Polish**
Duration of basic medical degree course, including practical training: **6 years**
Entrance examination: **Yes**
Foreign students eligible: **Yes**

AKADEMIA MEDYCZNA W GDANSKU
ULICA SKLODOWSKIEJ CURIE-3A
PL-80-210 GDANSK
Tel.: +48 (58) 478 222
Fax: +48 (58) 316 115
Telex: 512997 amg pl
Year instruction started: **1945**
Language of instruction: **Polish**
Duration of basic medical degree course, including practical training: **6 years**
Entrance examination: **Yes**
Foreign students eligible: **Yes**

SLASKA AKADEMIA MEDYCZNA
ULICA PONIATOWSKIEGO 15
PL-40-952 KATOWICE
Tel.: +48 (32) 514 964
Fax: +48 (32) 511 410
Telex: 0315338 slam pl
Year instruction started: **1948**
Language of instruction: **Polish**
Duration of basic medical degree course, including practical training: **6 years**
Entrance examination: **Yes**
Foreign students eligible: **Yes**

COLLEGIUM MEDICUM
UNIWERSYTET JAGIELLONSKI
ULICA SW. ANNY 12
PL-31-008 KRAKOW
Year instruction started: **1364**

LODZ AKADEMIA MEDYCZNA
ULICA KOSCIUSZKI 4
PL-90-419 LODZ
Year instruction started: **1945**

FACULTY OF MEDICINE
MILITARY MEDICAL ACADEMY
PL-90-001 LODZ
Year instruction started: **1956**

AKADEMIA MEDYCZNA W LUBLINIE
AL. RACLAWICKIE 1
PL-20-950 LUBLIN
Tel.: +48 (81) 209 21
Fax: +48 (81) 289 03
Year instruction started: **1944**
Language of instruction: **Polish**
Duration of basic medical degree course, including practical training: **6 years**
Entrance examination: **Yes**

AKADEMIA MEDYCZNA IM. KAROLA MARCINKOWSKIEGO W. POZNANIU
FACULTY I
ULICA FREDRY 10
PL-61-701 POZNAN
Tel.: +48 (61) 852 1161
Fax: +48 (61) 852 0455
Year instruction started: **1919**
Language of instruction: **Polish, English**
Duration of basic medical degree course, including practical training: **6 years**
Entrance examination: **Yes**
Foreign students eligible: **Yes**

AKADEMIA MEDYCZNA IM. KAROLA MARCINKOWSKIEGO W. POZNANIU
FACULTY II
ULICA DABROWSKIEGO 79
PL-60-529 POZNAN
Tel.: +48 (61) 847 7458
Fax: +48 (61) 847 7489
Year instruction started: **1993**[1]
Language of instruction: **Polish, English**
Duration of basic medical degree course, including practical training: **4 or 6 years**
Entrance examination: **Yes**
Foreign students eligible: **Yes**[2]

POMORSKA AKADEMIA MEDYCZNA
ULICA RYBACKA 1
PL-70-204 SZCZECIN
Tel.: +48 (91) 347 524
Fax: +48 (91) 335 660

---

[1] Refers to the 4-year course. The 6-year course started in 1995.
[2] Only foreign students are accepted.

Telex: 425677 pam pl
Year instruction started: **1948**
Language of instruction: **Polish, English**
Duration of basic medical degree course, including practical training: **6 years**
Entrance examination: **Yes**
Foreign students eligible: **Yes**

AKADEMIA MEDYCZNA W WARSZAWIE
ULICA FILTROWA 30
PL-02-032 WARSZAWA
Year instruction started: **1818**

AKADEMIA MEDYCZNA W WROCLAWIU
ULICA PASTEURA I
PL-50-364 WROCLAW
Tel.: +48 (71) 221 891
Fax: +48 (71) 215 729
Year instruction started: **1992**
Language of instruction: **Polish**
Entrance examination: **Yes**
Foreign students eligible: **Yes**

AKADEMIA MEDYCZNA W WROCLAWIU IM. PIASTOW SLASKICH
MIKULICZA-RADECKIEGO 5
PL-50-368 WROCLAW
Tel.: +48 (71) 229 525
Fax: +48 (71) 216 454
Year instruction started: **1946**
Language of instruction: **Polish**
Duration of basic medical degree course, including practical training: **6 years**
Entrance examination: **Yes**
Foreign students eligible: **Yes**

PORTUGAL

Total population in 1995: **9 808 000**
Number of physicians per 100 000 population (1993): **291**
Number of medical schools: **5**
Duration of basic medical degree course, including practical training: **6 years (a further 18 months of supervised practice is required before the degree is awarded)**
Title of degree awarded: *Licenciatura em Medicina* (Licence in Medicine)
Medical registration/licence to practise: **Registration is obligatory with the *Ordem***

dos Médicos, Avenida Almirante Gago Coutinho 151, P-1700 Lisboa. The licence to practise medicine is granted to graduates of a recognized medical school who have completed an 18-month internship.

Work in government service after graduation: **Not obligatory**

Agreements with other countries: **An agreement exists with other countries of the European Union (Directive 93/16/EEC governing the employment of doctors).**

FACULDADE DE MEDICINA
UNIVERSIDADE DE COIMBRA
P-3000 COIMBRA
Year instruction started: **1290**

FACULDADE DE MEDICINA DE LISBOA
UNIVERSIDADE DE LISBOA
AVENIDA PROFESSOR EGAS MONIZ
P-1699 LISBOA CODEX
Tel.: +351 (1) 797 2988
Fax: +351 (1) 795 5380
Year instruction started: **1911**
Language of instruction: **Portuguese**
Duration of basic medical degree course, including practical training: **6 years**
Entrance examination: **Yes**
Foreign students eligible: **Yes**

FACULDADE DE CIENCIAS MEDICAS
UNIVERSIDADE NOVA DE LISBOA
CAMPO DOS MARTIRES DA PATRIA 130
P-1198 LISBOA CODEX
Tel.: +351 (1) 885 3000
Fax: +351 (1) 885 1920
E-mail: bibfacmed-unl@telepac.pt
Year instruction started: **1973**
Language of instruction: **Portuguese**
Duration of basic medical degree course, including practical training: **6 years**
Entrance examination: **Yes**
Foreign students eligible: **Yes**

FACULDADE DE MEDICINA
UNIVERSIDADE DE PORTO
ALAMEDA PROFESSOR HERNANI MONTEIRO
P-4200 PORTO
Tel.: +351 (2) 550 3997
Fax: +351 (2) 551 0119

Year instruction started: **1836**
Language of instruction: **Portuguese**
Duration of basic medical degree course, including practical training: **6 years**
Entrance examination: **No**
Foreign students eligible: **Yes**

INSTITUTO DE CIENCIAS BIOMEDICAS ABEL SALAZAR
UNIVERSIDADE DE PORTO
LARGO DA ESCOLA MEDICA
P-4100 PORTO CODEX
Year instruction started: **1976**

PUERTO RICO

Total population in 1995: —
Number of physicians per 100 000 population (1993): —
Number of medical schools: **4**
Duration of basic medical degree course, including practical training: **4–5 years**
Title of degree awarded: —
Medical registration/licence to practise: —
Work in government service after graduation:—
Agreements with other countries: —

UNIVERSIDAD CENTRAL DEL CARIBE
SCHOOL OF MEDICINE
PO BOX 60327
BAYAMON 00621-6032
Year instruction started: **1976**

ESCUELA DE MEDICINA SAN JUAN BAUTISTA
AVENIDA LUIS MUNOZ MARIN
APDO 71365
CAGUAS 00936-8465
Tel.: +1 (787) 743 3038
Fax: +1 (787) 746 3093
Year instruction started: **1979**
Language of instruction: **Spanish, English**
Duration of basic medical degree course, including practical training: **4 years**
Entrance examination: **Yes**
Foreign students eligible: **Yes**

PONCE SCHOOL OF MEDICINE
DR ANA D. PEREZ MARCHAND STREET
PO BOX 7004
PONCE 00732
Tel.: +1 (787) 844 3710
Fax: +1 (787) 840 9756
E-mail: psm004@caribe.net
Year instruction started: **1977**
Language of instruction: **Spanish, English**
Duration of basic medical degree course, including practical training: **4 years**
Entrance examination: **Yes**
Foreign students eligible: **Yes**

ESCUELA DE MEDICINA
UNIVERSIDAD DE PUERTO RICO
APDO 365067
RIO PIEDRAS 00936-5067
Tel.: +1 (787) 758 4029
Fax: +1 (787) 758 4029
Year instruction started: **1950**
Language of instruction: **Spanish, English**
Duration of basic medical degree course, including practical training: **5 years**
Entrance examination: **Yes**
Foreign students eligible: **Yes**

REPUBLIC OF KOREA

Total population in 1995: **45 314 000**
Number of physicians per 100 000 population (1993): **127**
Number of medical schools: **48**
Duration of basic medical degree course, including practical training: **6 years**
Title of degree awarded: ***Euihaksa* (Bachelor in Medicine)**
Medical registration/licence to practise: **Registration is obligatory with the
    Ministry of Health and Welfare, Government Complex 2, Kwachon, Kyung
    Ki Do Province. All graduates must take the government licensure exami-
    nation to obtain the licence to practise medicine.**
Work in government service after graduation: **Not obligatory**
Agreements with other countries: **None**

COLLEGE OF MEDICINE
SOONCHUNHYANG UNIVERSITY
SAN 53-1 EUPNAE-RI
SHINCHANG-MYUN
ASAN-GUN
CHOONGCHUN
Year instruction started: **1978**

COLLEGE OF MEDICINE
CHEJU NATIONAL UNIVERSITY
1 ARAI-DONG
CHEJU-SHI
CHEJU-DO
Year instruction started: **1996**

COLLEGE OF MEDICINE
DANKOOK UNIVERSITY
29 SAN ANSEO-DONG
CHEONAN 330-714
CHOONGNAM-DO
Tel.: +82 (417) 550 3900
Fax: +82 (417) 550 3905
Year instruction started: **1990**
Language of instruction: **Korean**
Duration of basic medical degree course, including practical training: **6 years**
Entrance examination: **Yes**
Foreign students eligible: **Yes**

COLLEGE OF MEDICINE
CHUNGBUK NATIONAL UNIVERSITY
48 SAN GAESHIN-DONG
HUNGDOK-GU
CHEONGJU-SI 361-763
CHUNGBUK
Tel.: +82 (431) 61 2830
Fax: +82 (431) 272 1603
E-mail: office@med.chungbuk.ac.kr
Year instruction started: **1985**
Language of instruction: **Korean**
Duration of basic medical degree course, including practical training: **6 years**
Entrance examination: **Yes**
Foreign students eligible: **Yes**

COLLEGE OF MEDICINE
CHONBUK NATIONAL UNIVERSITY
2-20 SAN KEUMAM-DONG
CHONJU 560-182
CHONBUK
Tel.: +82 (652) 703 055/703 051
Fax: +82 (652) 703 053
Year instruction started: **1971**
Language of instruction: **Korean**
Duration of basic medical degree course, including practical training: **6 years**
Entrance examination: **Yes**
Foreign students eligible: **Yes**

COLLEGE OF MEDICINE
HALLYM UNIVERSITY
1 OKCHON-DONG
CHUNCHON 200-702
KANGWON-DO
Tel.: +82 (361) 581 600
Fax: +82 (361) 563 426
Year instruction started: **1982**
Language of instruction: **Korean**
Duration of basic medical degree course, including practical training: **6 years**
Entrance examination: **Yes**
Foreign students eligible: **Yes**

COLLEGE OF MEDICINE
KANG-WON UNIVERSITY
192-1 HYOJA-DONG
CHUNCHON
KANGWON-DO
Year instruction started: **1995**

COLLEGE OF MEDICINE
KON-KUK UNIVERSITY
CHUNGJOO CAMPUS
322 DANWOL-DONG
CHUNGJOO-SHI 380-701
CHUNGCHUNGBUK-DO
Year instruction started: **1986**

COLLEGE OF MEDICINE
INHA UNIVERSITY
253 YOUNG HYEON-DONG
INCHON
Year instruction started: **1985**

COLLEGE OF ORIENTAL MEDICINE
WONKWANG UNIVERSITY
344-2 SHINYONG-DONG
IRI 570-749
CHONBUK
Year instruction started: **1972**

SCHOOL OF MEDICINE
WONKWANG UNIVERSITY
344-2 SHINYONG-DONG
IRI 570-749
CHONBUK
Fax: +82 (653) 506 752
Year instruction started: **1982**
Language of instruction: **Korean**
Duration of basic medical degree course, including practical training: **6 years**
Entrance examination: **Yes**
Foreign students eligible: **Yes**

COLLEGE OF ORIENTAL MEDICINE
SAE-MYUNG UNIVERSITY
421-1 SHINWOL-DONG
JECHON-SHI
CHUNGCHUNGBUK-DO
Year instruction started: **1991**

COLLEGE OF MEDICINE
CHONNAM NATIONAL UNIVERSITY
5 HAK-DONG
DONG-KU
KWANGJU 501-190
CHONLANAM-DO
Tel.: +82 (62) 220 4000
Fax: +82 (62) 227 9976
Year instruction started: **1944**
Language of instruction: **Korean**
Duration of basic medical degree course, including practical training: **6 years**
Entrance examination: **No**
Foreign students eligible: **Yes**

COLLEGE OF MEDICINE
CHOSUN UNIVERSITY
375 SEOSEOK-DONG
KWANGJU 500
CHONLANAM-DO
Year instruction started: **1967**

DEPARTMENT OF ORIENTAL MEDICINE
KYUNGJU COLLEGE
DONGGUK UNIVERSITY
691 SEOKSANG-DONG
KYOUNGJI-SHI
KYUNGSANGPUK-DO
Year instruction started: **1979**

DONGGUK UNIVERSITY MEDICAL COLLEGE
1090-1 SUKJANG-DONG
KYUNGJU-SI
KYUNGBUK
Tel.: +82 (562) 770 2397
Year instruction started: **1986**
Language of instruction: **Korean**
Duration of basic medical degree course, including practical training: **6 years**
Entrance examination: **Yes**
Foreign students eligible: **Yes**

COLLEGE OF MEDICINE
GYEONGSANG NATIONAL UNIVERSITY
92 CHILAM-DONG
CHINJU-SHI
KYUNGNAM 660-280
Year instruction started: **1983**

COLLEGE OF ORIENTAL MEDICINE
KYUNGSAN UNIVERSITY
75 GEOMCHEON-DONG
MOUTAIN
KYUNGSAN 712-240
KYUNGBUK
Tel.: +82 (53) 813 5555
Fax: +82 (53) 813 5554

Year instruction started: **1981**
Language of instruction: **Korean**
Duration of basic medical degree course, including practical training: **6 years**
Entrance examination: **Yes**
Foreign students eligible: **Yes**

COLLEGE OF ORIENTAL MEDICINE
DONG-SHIN UNIVERSITY
252 DAEHO-DONG
NAJU-SHI
CHONLANAM-DO
Year instruction started: **1991**

COLLEGE OF MEDICINE
SEONAM UNIVERSITY
KWANGCHI-DONG
NAMWON CITY
CHONBUK
Year instruction started: **1995**

COLLEGE OF MEDICINE
KONYANG UNIVERSITY
30 SAN NAEDONGRI
NONSAN 320-800
CHUNGNAM
Year instruction started: **1995**

COLLEGE OF MEDICINE
DONG-A UNIVERSITY
1 TONGDAESIN-DONG 3-GA
SEO-KU
PUSAN 602-103
Tel.: +82 (51) 240 2903
Fax: +82 (51) 243 0116
Year instruction started: **1987**
Language of instruction: **Korean**
Duration of basic medical degree course, including practical training: **6 years**
Entrance examination: **Yes**
Foreign students eligible: **Yes**

COLLEGE OF ORIENTAL MEDICINE
DONG-EUI UNIVERSITY
SAN 45-1 YANGJEONG
JIN-GU
PUSAN
Year instruction started: **1986**

IN-JE COLLEGE SCHOOL OF MEDICINE
633-165 KAEGUM-DONG
PUSANJIN-KU
PUSAN
Year instruction started: **1979**

KOSIN MEDICAL COLLEGE
34 AMNAM-DONG
SEO-KU
PUSAN
Year instruction started: **1981**

COLLEGE OF MEDICINE
PUSAN NATIONAL UNIVERSITY
10 AMI-DONG 1 GA
SEO-KU
PUSAN 602-739
Tel.: +82 (51) 256 0273/240 7701/240 7702
Fax: +82 (51) 254 1930
Year instruction started: **1955**
Language of instruction: **Korean**
Duration of basic medical degree course, including practical training: **6 years**
Entrance examination: **Yes**
Foreign students eligible: **Yes**

COLLEGE OF ORIENTAL MEDICINE
KYOUNG-WON UNIVERSITY
65 SAN BACKJEONG-DONG
SUJEONG-GU
SEONGNAM-SHI
KYOUNGGI-DO
Year instruction started: **1990**

CATHOLIC MEDICAL COLLEGE
505 BANPO-DONG
KANGNAM-KU
SEOUL 135
Year instruction started: **1954**

COLLEGE OF MEDICINE
CHUNGANG UNIVERSITY
221 HEUKSUK-DONG
DONGJAK-KU
SEOUL 151-756
Year instruction started: **1971**

COLLEGE OF MEDICINE
EWHA WOMEN'S UNIVERSITY
11-1 DAEHYUN-DONG
SOEDAEMOON-KU
SEOUL
Year instruction started: **1945**

COLLEGE OF MEDICINE
HANYANG UNIVERSITY
17 HYANGDANG-DONG
SEONGDONG-KU
SEOUL
Year instruction started: **1968**

COLLEGE OF MEDICINE
KOREA UNIVERSITY
42ND STREET
MYUNGYUN-DONG
CHONGNO-KU
SEOUL
Year instruction started: **1938**

COLLEGE OF MEDICINE
KYUNGHEE UNIVERSITY
HOIKI-DONG
DONGDAEMOON-KU
SEOUL
Year instruction started: **1967**

COLLEGE OF ORIENTAL MEDICINE
KYUNGHEE UNIVERSITY
HOIKI-DONG
DONGDAEMOON-KU
SEOUL 130-701
Tel.: +82 (2) 961 0321
Fax: +82 (2) 966 0535

Year instruction started: **1965**
Language of instruction: **Korean**
Duration of basic medical degree course, including practical training: **6 years**
Entrance examination: **Yes**
Foreign students eligible: **Yes**

COLLEGE OF MEDICINE
SEOUL NATIONAL UNIVERSITY
28 YONGON-DONG
CHONGNO-KU
SEOUL 110-799
Tel.: +82 (2) 740 8001
Fax: +82 (2) 742 5947
Year instruction started: **1899**
Language of instruction: **Korean**
Duration of basic medical degree course, including practical training: **6 years**
Entrance examination: **Yes**
Foreign students eligible: **Yes**

COLLEGE OF MEDICINE
UNIVERSITY OF ULSAN
388-1 POONGNAP-DONG
SONGPA-KU
SEOUL 138-040
Tel.: +82 (2) 224 4209/224 4210/224 4211
Fax: +82 (2) 224 4220
Year instruction started: **1990**
Language of instruction: **Korean**
Duration of basic medical degree course, including practical training: **6 years**
Entrance examination: **Yes**
Foreign students eligible: **Yes**

COLLEGE OF MEDICINE
YONSEI UNIVERSITY
134 SHINCHON-DONG
SEODAEMOON-KU
PO BOX 8044
SEOUL
Tel.: +82 (2) 361 5051
Fax: +82 (2) 312 5370
Year instruction started: **1896**
Language of instruction: **Korean**
Duration of basic medical degree course, including practical training: **6 years**
Entrance examination: **Yes**
Foreign students eligible: **Yes**

AJOU UNIVERSITY SCHOOL OF MEDICINE
5 WONCHON DONG
PALDAL-KU
SUWON 442-749
KYUNGGI
Tel.: +82 (331) 219 5018
Fax: +82 (331) 219 5019
Year instruction started: **1988**
Language of instruction: **Korean**
Duration of basic medical degree course, including practical training: **6 years**
Entrance examination: **Yes**
Foreign students eligible: **Yes**

SCHOOL OF MEDICINE
CATHOLIC UNIVERSITY OF TAEGU-HYOSUNG
3056-6 DAEMYUNG-4 DONG
NAM-GU
TAEGU 705-034
Tel.: +82 (53) 650 4455
Fax: +82 (53) 621 4106
E-mail: medi@cuth.cataegu.ac.kr
Year instruction started: **1991**
Language of instruction: **Korean**
Duration of basic medical degree course, including practical training: **6 years**
Entrance examination: **Yes**
Foreign students eligible: **Yes**

COLLEGE OF MEDICINE
KEIMYUNG UNIVERSITY
194 DONGSAN-DONG
TAEGU
Year instruction started: **1979**

SCHOOL OF MEDICINE
KYUNGPOOK NATIONAL UNIVERSITY
CHUNGU DONGIN-DONG 2-KA
TAEGU 700-422
Tel.: +82 (53) 423 0981
Fax: +82 (53) 421 6585
Year instruction started: **1923**
Language of instruction: **Korean**
Duration of basic medical degree course, including practical training: **6 years**
Entrance examination: **Yes**
Foreign students eligible: **Yes**

COLLEGE OF MEDICINE
YEUNGNAM UNIVERSITY
317-1 DAEMYUNG-DONG
TAEGU
Year instruction started: **1979**

COLLEGE OF MEDICINE
CHUNGNAM NATIONAL UNIVERSITY
6 MUNHWA-1 DONG
JUNG-KU
TAEJEON 301-131
Tel.: +82 (42) 580 8100
Fax: +82 (42) 584 2846
Year instruction started: **1968**
Language of instruction: **Korean**
Duration of basic medical degree course, including practical training: **6 years**
Entrance examination: **Yes**
Foreign students eligible: **No**

ORIENTAL MEDICAL COLLEGE
TAEJON UNIVERSITY
96-3 YONGWOONDONG
DONG-KU
TAEJEON 300-716
Tel.: +82 (42) 280 2615/280 2602/280 2600
Fax: +82 (42) 274 2600
Year instruction started: **1981**
Language of instruction: **Korean**
Duration of basic medical degree course, including practical training: **6 years**
Entrance examination: **Yes**
Foreign students eligible: **Yes**

COLLEGE OF ORIENTAL MEDICINE
WOO-SEOK UNIVERSITY
490 HOOJEONG-RI
SAMRYE-HEE
WANJU-KUN
CHONLANAM-DO
Year instruction started: **1987**

WONJU MEDICAL COLLEGE
YONSEI UNIVERSITY
162 ILSAN-DONG
WONJU
KANGWON-DO
Year instruction started: **1978**

COLLEGE OF ORIENTAL MEDICINE
SANG-JI UNIVERSITY
SAN 41 WOOSAN-DONG
WONJU-SHI
KWANGWON-DO
Year instruction started: **1987**

COLLEGE OF MEDICINE
KWANDONG UNIVERSITY
7 IMCHUN-LI
YANGYANG-EUP
YANGWANG-GUN
KANGWON-DO
Year instruction started: **1995**

REPUBLIC OF MOLDOVA

Total population in 1995: **4 444 000**
Number of physicians per 100 000 population (1993): **356**
Number of medical schools: **1**
Duration of basic medical degree course, including practical training: **6 years**
Title of degree awarded: **Doctor of Medicine**
Medical registration/licence to practise: —
Work in government service after graduation: **Not obligatory**
Agreements with other countries: —

STATE MEDICAL AND PHARMACEUTICAL UNIVERSITY "NICOLAE
    TESTEMITANU" OF THE REPUBLIC OF MOLDOVA[1]
165 STEFAN CEL MARE BOULEVARD
CHISINAU 2004
Tel.: +373 (2) 243 408
Fax: +373 (2) 242 344

---

[1] Formerly known as the Kishinev State Medical University (1945–91) and the State Medical University "N. Testemitanu" (1991–96).

Year instruction started: **1945**
Language of instruction: **Romanian, Russian**
Duration of basic medical degree course, including practical training: **6 years**
Entrance examination: **Yes**
Foreign students eligible: **Yes**

ROMANIA

Total population in 1995: **22 655 000**
Number of physicians per 100 000 population (1993): **176**
Number of medical schools: **11**
Duration of basic medical degree course, including practical training: **6 years**
Title of degree awarded: ***Doctor–medic* (Doctor of Medicine)**
Medical registration/licence to practise: **The licence to practise medicine is granted by the Ministry of Health, 1–3 Ministerului Street, Sector 1, Bucharest, to graduates of a recognized medical school, provided they are resident in Romania. Foreigners may practise only if they are from a country with a reciprocal agreement with Romania.**
Work in government service after graduation: **Not obligatory**
Agreements with other countries: **—**

FACULTATEA DE MEDICINA
UNIVERSITATEA DE VEST "VASILE GOLDIS"
BULVARDUL REVOLUTIEI 81
R-2900 ARAD
Tel.: +40 (57) 280 335
Fax: +40 (57) 280 810
Year instruction started: **1992**
Language of instruction: **Romanian**
Duration of basic medical degree course, including practical training: **6 years**
Entrance examination: **Yes**
Foreign students eligible: **Yes**

FACULTATEA DE MEDICINA GENERALA
UNIVERSITATEA TRANSILVANIA
STR. CIBINULUI 1 BIS
R-2200 BRASOV
Tel.: +40 (68) 142 343/410 286
Fax: +40 (68) 150 274/144 634
Year instruction started: **1992**
Language of instruction: **Romanian**
Duration of basic medical degree course, including practical training: **6 years**
Entrance examination: **Yes**
Foreign students eligible: **Yes**

UNIVERSITATEA DE MEDICINA SI FARMACIE "CAROL DAVILA"
STR. DIONISIE LUPU 37
R-70000 BUCURESTI
Year instruction started: **1869**
Language of instruction: **Romanian**
Duration of basic medical degree course, including practical training: **6 years**
Entrance examination: **Yes**
Foreign students eligible: **Yes**

FACULTATEA DE MEDICINA
UNIVERSITATEA DE MEDICINA SI FARMACIE "IULIU HATIEGANU"
STR. EMIL ISAC 13
R-3400 CLUJ-NAPOCA
Tel.: +40 (64) 195 524
Fax: +40 (64) 197 257
Year instruction started: **1872**
Language of instruction: **Romanian**
Duration of basic medical degree course, including practical training: **6 years**
Entrance examination: **Yes**
Foreign students eligible: **Yes**

FACULTATEA DE MEDICINA SI FARMACIE
UNIVERSITATEA "OVIDUS"
STR. IOAN VODA 54
R-8700 CONSTANTA
Tel.: +40 (41) 612 257
Fax: +40 (41) 612 257
Year instruction started: **1990**
Language of instruction: **Romanian, French, English**
Duration of basic medical degree course, including practical training: **6 years**
Entrance examination: **Yes**
Foreign students eligible: **Yes**

FACULTATEA DE MEDICINA
UNIVERSITATEA DIN CRAIOVA
STR. PETRU RARES 4
R-1100 CRAIOVA
Tel.: +40 (51) 122 458
Fax: +40 (51) 122 770
Year instruction started: **1970**
Language of instruction: **Romanian**
Duration of basic medical degree course, including practical training: **6 years**
Entrance examination: **Yes**
Foreign students eligible: **Yes**

UNIVERSITATEA DE MEDICINA SI FARMACIE "GRIGORE T. POPA"
STR. UNIVERSITATII 16
R-6600 IASI
Year instruction started: **1879**
Language of instruction: **Romanian**
Duration of basic medical degree course, including practical training: **6 years**
Entrance examination: **Yes**
Foreign students eligible: **Yes**

FACULTATEA DE MEDICINA
UNIVERSITATEA DIN ORADEA
STR. 1 DECEMBRIE 10
R-3700 ORADEA
Tel.: +40 (59) 412 834
Fax: +40 (59) 418 266
Year instruction started: **1991**
Language of instruction: **Romanian, English**
Duration of basic medical degree course, including practical training: **6 years**
Entrance examination: **Yes**
Foreign students eligible: **Yes**

FACULTATEA DE MEDICINA "VICTOR PAPILIAN"
UNIVERSITATEA "LUCIAN BLAGA"
DIN SIBIU
BD. VICTORIEI 10
R-2400 SIBIU
Tel.: +40 (69) 217 989
Fax: +40 (69) 210 512
Year instruction started: **1990**
Language of instruction: **Romanian**
Duration of basic medical degree course, including practical training: **6 years**
Entrance examination: **Yes**
Foreign students eligible: **Yes**

UNIVERSITATEA DE MEDICINA SI FARMACIE
PIATA EFTIMIE MURGU 2
R-1900 TIMISOARA
Year instruction started: **1948**
Language of instruction: **Romanian**
Duration of basic medical degree course, including practical training: **6 years**
Entrance examination: **Yes**
Foreign students eligible: **Yes**

FACULTATEA DE MEDICINA
UNIVERSITATEA DE MEDICINA SI FARMACIE
STR. GH. MARINESCU 38
R-4300 TIRGU MURES
Tel.: +40 (65) 113 127
Fax: +40 (65) 164 407
Year instruction started: **1945**
Language of instruction: **Romanian, Hungarian**
Duration of basic medical degree course, including practical training: **6 years**
Entrance examination: **Yes**
Foreign students eligible: **Yes**

RUSSIAN FEDERATION

Total population in 1995: **148 126 000**
Number of physicians per 100 000 population (1993): **380**
Number of medical schools: **53**
Duration of basic medical degree course, including practical training: **6 or 7 years**
Title of degree awarded: **Doctor of Medicine**
Medical registration/licence to practise: **The licence to practise medicine is granted by the Licensing Commissions of government bodies within the Russian Federation to holders of a diploma of medical education. Applicants should provide a certificate showing their area of specialization (Doctor of Medicine, Paediatrician, Master of Pharmacy, Physician–Hygienist, Epidemiologist, Doctor of Stomatology). Foreign medical degrees must be recognized as equivalent.**
Work in government service after graduation: **Obligatory (1–5 years)**
Agreements with other countries: **Agreements exist with over 60 countries.**

ARKHANGELSK STATE MEDICAL ACADEMY
51 TROITZKY AVENUE
ARKHANGELSK 163061
Tel.: +7 (8182) 432 160
Fax: +7 (8182) 263 226/493 972
Year instruction started: **1932**
Language of instruction: **Russian**
Duration of basic medical degree course, including practical training: **6 years**
Entrance examination: **Yes**
Foreign students eligible: **Yes**

ASTRAKHAN STATE MEDICAL ACADEMY
ULICA BAKINSKAJA 121
ASTRAKHAN 414000
Year instruction started: **1918**

ALTAI STATE MEDICAL UNIVERSITY
PROSPEKT LENINA 40
BARNAUL 656099
Tel.: +7 (385) 225 3027
Fax: +7 (385) 222 1421
Year instruction started: **1954**
Language of instruction: **Russian**
Duration of basic medical degree course, including practical training: **6 years**
Entrance examination: **Yes**
Foreign students eligible: **Yes**

AMUR STATE MEDICAL ACADEMY
ULICA GORKOGO 95
BLAGOVESTCHENSK 675006
Year instruction started: **1952**

CUVASSIA STATE UNIVERSITY MEDICAL FACULTY
MOSKOVSKIJ PR. 15
CEBOKSARY 428015
Tel.: +7 (8352) 440 379
Year instruction started: **1967**

CELJABINSK STATE MEDICAL ACADEMY
ULICA VOROVSKOGO 64
CELJABINSK 454092
Year instruction started: **1944**

CITA STATE MEDICAL ACADEMY
ULICA GORKOGO 39A
CITA 672090
Year instruction started: **1953**

URAL STATE MEDICAL ACADEMY
ULICA REPINA 3
EKATERINBURG 620219
Tel.: +7 (3432) 511 490
Fax: +7 (3432) 516 400
Year instruction started: **1939**
Language of instruction: **Russian**
Duration of basic medical degree course, including practical training: **6 years**
Entrance examination: **Yes**
Foreign students eligible: **Yes**

MEDICAL FACULTY
CECENJA STATE UNIVERSITY
ULICA A. SERIPOVA 32
GROZNIJ 364907
Tel.: +7 (3432) 319 463
Year instruction started: **1930**

HABAROVSK STATE MEDICAL INSTITUTE
ULICA K. MARKSA 35
HABAROVSK 680013
Year instruction started: **1930**

IRKUTSK STATE MEDICAL UNIVERSITY
ULICA KRASNOGO VOSSTANIJA 1
IRKUTSK 664003
Year instruction started: **1930**

IVANOVO STATE MEDICAL ACADEMY
ULICA F. ENGELSA 8
IVANOVO 153462
Year instruction started: **1930**

IZEVSK STATE MEDICAL ACADEMY
ULICA REVOLJUCIONNAJA 199
IZEVSK 426034
Year instruction started: **1933**

MEDICAL FACULTY
JAKUTSK STATE UNIVERSITY
KULAKOVSKOGO 34
JAKUTSK 677891
Tel.: +7 (4112) 263 344
Year instruction started: **1957**

JAROSLAVL STATE MEDICAL ACADEMY
ULICA REVOLJUCIONNAJA 5
JAROSLAVL 150000
Year instruction started: **1944**

KAZAN STATE MEDICAL UNIVERSITY
ULICA BUTLEROVA 49
KAZAN 420012
Tel.: +7 (8432) 360 652
Fax: +7 (8432) 360 393

E-mail: office@intdept.kcn.ru
Year instruction started: **1814**
Language of instruction: **Russian**
Duration of basic medical degree course, including practical training: **6 years**
Entrance examination: **Yes**
Foreign students eligible: **Yes**

KEMEROVO STATE MEDICAL ACADEMY
ULICA VOROSILOVA 22A
KEMEROVO 650029
Tel.: +7 (3842) 557 889
Fax: +7 (3842) 557 889
Year instruction started: **1956**
Language of instruction: **Russian**
Duration of basic medical degree course, including practical training: **7 years**
Entrance examination: **Yes**
Foreign students eligible: **Yes**

KIROV STATE MEDICAL INSTITUTE
ULICA K. MARSKA 88
KIROV 610000
Year instruction started: **1994**

KUBAN STATE MEDICAL ACADEMY
ULICA SEDINA 4
KRASNODAR 350640
Year instruction started: **1920**

KRASNOJARSK MEDICAL ACADEMY
ULICA PARTIZANA ZELEZNJAKA 1
KRASNOJARSK 660022
Tel.: +7 (3912) 274 924
Fax: +7 (3912) 237 835
Year instruction started: **1942**
Language of instruction: **Russian**
Duration of basic medical degree course, including practical training: **6 years**
Entrance examination: **Yes**
Foreign students eligible: **Yes**

KURSK STATE MEDICAL UNIVERSITY
ULICA K. MARKSA 3
KURSK 305033
Year instruction started: **1935**

DAGESTAN STATE MEDICAL ACADEMY
PLOSCAD LENINA 6
MAHACKALA 367012
Year instruction started: **1932**

I.M. SECHENOV MOSCOW MEDICAL ACADEMY
ULICA BOLSHAYA PIROGOVSKAYA 2/6
MOSCOW 119881
Tel.: +7 (95) 248 0553
Fax: +7 (95) 248 0214
Year instruction started: **1765**
Language of instruction: **Russian**
Duration of basic medical degree course, including practical training: **6 years**
Entrance examination: **Yes**
Foreign students eligible: **Yes**

MEDICAL FACULTY
JEWISH STATE ACADEMY (MOSCOW)
ULICA B. BRONNAJA 6
MOSCOW 103104
Tel.: +7 (95) 122 3336
Year instruction started: **1960**

MOSCOW MEDICAL STOMATOLOGY INSTITUTE
ULICA DELEGATSKAJA 20/1
MOSCOW 103473
Tel.: +7 (95) 978 0569
Fax: +7 (95) 973 3559
E-mail: mmsi@glas.apc.org
Year instruction started: **1935**
Language of instruction: **Russian**
Duration of basic medical degree course, including practical training: **6 years**
Entrance examination: **Yes**
Foreign students eligible: **Yes**

MEDICAL FACULTY
RUSSIAN "PEOPLE'S FRIENDSHIP" UNIVERSITY
ULICA MIKLUHO-MAKLAJA 6
MOSCOW 117198
Tel.: +7 (95) 434 7027
Year instruction started: **1960**

RUSSIAN STATE MEDICAL UNIVERSITY (RSMU)
ULICA OSTROVITJANOVA 1
MOSCOW 117869
Tel.: +7 (95) 434 1422
Fax: +7 (95) 434 1411
Year instruction started: **1906**
Language of instruction: **Russian, English**
Duration of basic medical degree course, including practical training: **6 years**
Entrance examination: **Yes**
Foreign students eligible: **Yes**

MEDICAL FACULTY
KABARDINO–BALKARIA STATE UNIVERSITY
ULICA CERNYSEVSKOGO 173
NALCHIK 360004
Tel.: +7 (866) 222 2560/222 2562
Year instruction started: **1966**
Language of instruction: **Russian**
Duration of basic medical degree course, including practical training: **6 years**
Entrance examination: **Yes**
Foreign students eligible: **Yes**

NIZHNI NOVGOROD STATE MEDICAL ACADEMY
PLOSCAD MININA I POZARSKOGO 10/1
NIZHNI NOVGOROD 603005
Year instruction started: **1920**

NOVOSIBIRSK MEDICAL INSTITUTE
KRASNIJ PROSPEKT 52
NOVOSIBIRSK 630021
Tel.: +7 (3832) 209 405
Fax: +7 (3832) 209 405
Year instruction started: **1935**
Language of instruction: **Russian**
Duration of basic medical degree course, including practical training: **6 years**
Entrance examination: **Yes**
Foreign students eligible: **Yes**

OMSK STATE MEDICAL ACADEMY
ULICA LENINA 12
OMSK 644099
Year instruction started: **1921**

ORENBURG STATE MEDICAL ACADEMY
ULICA SOVETSKAJA 6
ORENBURG 460014
Tel.: +7 (3532) 776 103
Fax: +7 (3532) 779 408
Year instruction started: **1944**
Language of instruction: **Russian, English**
Duration of basic medical degree course, including practical training: **6 years**
Entrance examination: **Yes**
Foreign students eligible: **Yes**

PERM STATE MEDICAL ACADEMY
ULICA KUJBISKEVA 39
PO BOX 7019
PERM 614600
Tel.: +7 (3422) 337 527
Fax: +7 (3422) 332 441
Year instruction started: **1917**
Language of instruction: **Russian**
Duration of basic medical degree course, including practical training: **7 years**
Entrance examination: **Yes**
Foreign students eligible: **Yes**

MEDICAL FACULTY
PETROZAVODSK STATE UNIVERSITY
PROSPEKT LENINA 33
PETROZAVODSK 185640
Tel.: +7 (8142) 775 140
Year instruction started: **1960**

RJAZAN STATE MEDICAL UNIVERSITY
ULICA VYSOKOVOLTNAJA 9
RJAZAN 391000
Year instruction started: **1950**

ROSTOV STATE MEDICAL UNIVERSITY
NAHICEVANSKIJ PEREULOK 29
ROSTOV 344700
Year instruction started: **1930**

MILITARY MEDICAL ACADEMY
ULICA LEBEDEVA 6
PO BOX K-175
SAINT PETERSBURG 194175
Tel.: +7 (812) 542 2139
Fax: +7 (812) 541 8486
Year instruction started: **1798**
Language of instruction: **Russian**
Duration of basic medical degree course, including practical training: **7 years**
Entrance examination: **Yes**
Foreign students eligible: **Yes**

SAINT PETERSBURG STATE I.P. PAVLOV MEDICAL UNIVERSITY
ULICA TOLSTOGO 6/8
SAINT PETERSBURG 197089
Tel.: +7 (812) 238 7153
Fax: +7 (812) 234 0125
E-mail: provost@spmu.rssi.ru
Year instruction started: **1897**
Language of instruction: **Russian**
Duration of basic medical degree course, including practical training: **6 years**
Entrance examination: **Yes**
Foreign students eligible: **Yes**

SAINT PETERSBURG STATE MEDICAL ACADEMY
PISKAREVSKIJ PROSPEKT 47
SAINT PETERSBURG 195067
Tel.: +7 (812) 543 9609
Fax: +7 (812) 543 1571
Telex: 122292 sanhig ru
Year instruction started: **1911**
Language of instruction: **Russian**
Duration of basic medical degree course, including practical training: **6 years**
Entrance examination: **Yes**
Foreign students eligible: **Yes**

SAINT PETERSBURG STATE PEDIATRIC MEDICAL ACADEMY
ULICA LITOVSKAJA 2
SAINT PETERSBURG 194100
Tel.: +7 (812) 542 6733
Fax: +7 (812) 542 6733

Year instruction started: **1925**
Language of instruction: **Russian**
Duration of basic medical degree course, including practical training: **6 years**
Entrance examination: **Yes**
Foreign students eligible: **Yes**

SAMARA STATE MEDICAL UNIVERSITY
ULICA CAPAEVSKAJA 89
SAMARA 443099
Tel.: +7 (8462) 321 634
Fax: +7 (8462) 322 907
Year instruction started: **1918**
Language of instruction: **Russian**
Duration of basic medical degree course, including practical training: **6 years**
Entrance examination: **Yes**
Foreign students eligible: **Yes**

MEDICAL FACULTY
MORDOVIA STATE UNIVERSITY
ULICA ULJANOVA 26
SARANSK 430032
Tel.: +7 (834) 330 983
Year instruction started: **1967**
Language of instruction: **Russian**
Duration of basic medical degree course, including practical training: **6 years**
Entrance examination: **Yes**
Foreign students eligible: **Yes**

SARATOV STATE MEDICAL UNIVERSITY
ULICA B. KAZACJA 112
SARATOV 410710
Year instruction started: **1909**

SMOLENSK STATE MEDICAL ACADEMY
ULICA KRUPSKOJ 28
SMOLENSK 214019
Year instruction started: **1920**

STAVROPOL STATE MEDICAL ACADEMY
ULICA MIRA 310
STAVROPOL 355017
Tel.: +7 (8652) 352 331
Fax: +7 (8652) 352 487

Year instruction started: **1937**
Language of instruction: **Russian**
Duration of basic medical degree course, including practical training: **6 years**
Entrance examination: **No**
Foreign students eligible: **Yes**

TJUMEN STATE MEDICAL ACADEMY
ULICA ODESSKAJA 52
TJUMEN 625023
Tel.: +7 (3452) 226 200
Fax: +7 (3452) 226 200
Year instruction started: **1963**
Language of instruction: **Russian**
Duration of basic medical degree course, including practical training: **6 years**
Entrance examination: **Yes**
Foreign students eligible: **No**

SIBERIAN STATE MEDICAL UNIVERSITY
MOSKOVSKIJ TRAKT 2
TOMSK 634050
Year instruction started: **1888**

TVER STATE MEDICAL ACADEMY
ULICA SOVETSKAJA 4
TVER 170642
Year instruction started: **1954**

BASKIRIAN STATE MEDICAL UNIVERSITY
ULICA LENINA 3
UFA 450000
Year instruction started: **1932**

NORTH OSSETIAN STATE MEDICAL ACADEMY
ULICA PUSHKINSKAJA 40
VLADIKAVKAZ 362019
Tel.: +7 (423) 233 4221
Fax: +7 (423) 233 0321
Year instruction started: **1939**
Language of instruction: **Russian**
Duration of basic medical degree course, including practical training: **6 years**
Entrance examination: **Yes**
Foreign students eligible: **Yes**

VLADIVOSTOK STATE MEDICAL UNIVERSITY
OSTRYAKOVA PROSPEKT 2
VLADIVOSTOK 690600
Tel.: +7 (4232) 251 624
Fax: +7 (4232) 251 719
Year instruction started: **1958**
Language of instruction: **Russian**
Duration of basic medical degree course, including practical training: **6 years**
Entrance examination: **Yes**
Foreign students eligible: **Yes**

VOLGOGRAD MEDICAL ACADEMY
PLOSCAD PAVSIH BORTSOV 1
VOLGOGRAD 400066
Tel.: +7 (8442) 339 830
Fax: +7 (8442) 367 144
Year instruction started: **1935**
Language of instruction: **Russian**
Duration of basic medical degree course, including practical training: **6 years**
Entrance examination: **Yes**
Foreign students eligible: **Yes**

VORONEZ STATE MEDICAL ACADEMY
ULICA STUDENCESKAJA 10
VORONEZ 394622
Year instruction started: **1918**

RWANDA

Total population in 1995: **5 397 000**
Number of physicians per 100 000 population (1993): —
Number of medical schools: **1**
Duration of basic medical degree course, including practical training: **7 years**
Title of degree awarded: *Docteur en Médecine* (**Doctor of Medicine**)
Medical registration/licence to practise: —
Work in government service after graduation: —
Agreements with other countries: —

FACULTE DE MEDECINE
UNIVERSITE NATIONALE DE RWANDA
BP 30
BUTARE

Tel.: +250 303 28
Fax: +250 303 28
Year instruction started: **1963**
Language of instruction: **French, English**
Duration of basic medical degree course, including practical training: **7 years**
Entrance examination: **Yes**
Foreign students eligible: **Yes**

SAINT KITTS AND NEVIS

Total population in 1995: —
Number of physicians per 100 000 population (1993): **89**
Number of medical schools: **2**
Duration of basic medical degree course, including practical training: —
Title of degree awarded: —
Medical registration/licence to practise: —
Obligation to work in government service: —
Agreements with other countries: —

MEDICAL UNIVERSITY OF THE AMERICAS
POTSWORKS ESTATES
WHITEHALL
NEVIS
Tel.: +1 (978) 630 5122[1]
Fax: +1 (978) 632 2168[1]
Year instruction started: **1998**

INTERNATIONAL UNIVERSITY OF THE HEALTH SCIENCES
SAINT KITTS
Year instruction started: **1998**

SAINT LUCIA

Total population in 1995: —
Number of physicians per 100 000 population (1993): **35**
Number of medical schools: **None**
Medical registration/licence to practise: **Registration is obligatory with the**

---

[1] Administrative office in the USA.

Medical Council, c/o Ministry of Health, Castries. The licence to practise medicine is granted to graduates of a recognized medical school. Applicants must provide a certificate of good standing from their current Medical Council. Foreigners must hold a work permit.

Agreements with other countries: **An agreement exists with the University of the West Indies.**

SAINT VINCENT AND THE GRENADINES

Total population in 1995: —

Number of physicians per 100 000 population (1993): **46**

Number of medical schools: **1**

Duration of basic medical degree course, including practical training: **4.5 years (a further 2 years of supervised clinical practice are required before the degree is awarded)**

Title of degree awarded: **Doctor of Medicine (MD)**

Medical registration/licence to practise: **Registration is obligatory with the Medical Board, Ministry of Health, Kingstown. The licence to practise medicine is granted to graduates of a recognized medical school who can provide proof of having completed a 2-year internship and have an adequate command of English. Those who have qualified abroad must provide proof of registration in their country of training.**

Work in government service after graduation: **Obligatory (2 years prior to full registration)**

Agreements with other countries: **An agreement exists with Grenada.**

KINGSTOWN MEDICAL COLLEGE[1]

PO BOX 585

RATHO MILL

SAINT VINCENT

Tel.: +1809 458 4832

Fax: +1809 456 9670

E-mail: sgu_info@mssl.com

Year instruction started: **1979**

Language of instruction: **English**

Duration of basic medical degree course, including practical training: **4.5 years**

Entrance examination: **Yes**

Foreign students eligible: **Yes**

---

[1] Kingstown Medical College offers instruction only in the fifth and sixth terms. Students study at St George's University School of Medicine, Grenada, from the first to fourth and seventh to eleventh terms and receive a degree granted by that institution.

SAMOA

Total population in 1995: **166 000**
Number of physicians per 100 000 population (1993): **38**
Number of medical schools: **None**
Medical registration/licence to practise: **Registration is obligatory with the Samoa Medical Association, c/o National Hospital, Private Bag, Apia. The licence to practise medicine is granted to graduates of a recognized medical school following 3 years' work in government service.**
Work in government service after graduation: **Obligatory (3 years)**
Agreements with other countries: **Agreements exist with Commonwealth countries and the USA.**

SAUDI ARABIA

Total population in 1995: **18 836 000**
Number of physicians per 100 000 population (1993): **166**
Number of medical schools: **6**
Duration of basic medical degree course, including practical training: **6 years (a further year of supervised clinical practice is required before the degree is awarded)**
Title of degree awarded: **Bachelor of Medicine and Bachelor of Surgery (MB, BS)**
Medical registration/licence to practise: **The licence to practise medicine is granted by the Ministry of Health, Riyadh, to graduates of a recognized medical school who have completed 1 year as an intern. Foreigners must receive authorization to practise.**
Work in government service after graduation: **Not obligatory**
Agreements with other countries: **—**

ABHA COLLEGE OF MEDICINE
KING SAUD UNIVERSITY
PO BOX 641
ABHA
Tel.: +966 (7) 226 0711
Fax: +966 (7) 224 7570
Year instruction started: **1981**
Language of instruction: **English**
Duration of basic medical degree course, including practical training: **6 years**
Entrance examination: **Yes**
Foreign students eligible: **No**

COLLEGE OF MEDICINE AND MEDICAL SCIENCES
KING FAISAL UNIVERSITY
PO BOX 2208
AL KHOBAR 31952

COLLEGE OF MEDICINE AND MEDICAL SCIENCES
KING FAISAL UNIVERSITY
PO BOX 2114
DAMMAM 31451
Tel.: +966 (3) 857 5307/857 5528
Fax: +966 (3) 857 5329
Telex: 870020 faisal sj
Year instruction started: **1975**
Language of instruction: **English**
Duration of basic medical degree course, including practical training: **6 years**
Entrance examination: **Yes**
Foreign students eligible: **Yes**

COLLEGE OF MEDICINE AND ALLIED SCIENCES
KING ABDUL AZIZ UNIVERSITY
PO BOX 9029
JEDDAH 21413
Tel.: +966 (2) 695 2082/695 2036
Fax: +966 (2) 640 0855
Telex: 601141 kauni sj
Year instruction started: **1975**
Language of instruction: **English**
Duration of basic medical degree course, including practical training: **6 years**
Entrance examination: **Yes**
Foreign students eligible: **No**

FACULTY OF MEDICINE,
UMM AL QURA UNIVERSITY
PO BOX 7607
MECCA
Tel.: +966 (2) 528 1189
Fax: +966 (2) 528 1189
Year instruction started: **1996**
Language of instruction: **English**
Duration of basic medical degree course, including practical training: **6 years**
Entrance examination: **Yes**
Foreign students eligible: **No**

COLLEGE OF MEDICINE
KING SAUD UNIVERSITY
PO BOX 2925
RIYADH 11461
Tel.: +966 (1) 467 0878
Fax: +966 (1) 467 2650
Year instruction started: **1967**
Language of instruction: **English**
Duration of basic medical degree course, including practical training: **6 years**
Entrance examination: **Yes**
Foreign students eligible: **Yes**

SENEGAL

Total population in 1995: **8 532 000**
Number of physicians per 100 000 population (1993): **7**
Number of medical schools: **1**
Duration of basic medical degree course, including practical training: **8 years**
Title of degree awarded: ***Doctorat d'État en Médecine* (Doctor of Medicine)**
Medical registration/licence to practise: **Registration is obligatory with the**
   Conseil national de l'Ordre des Médecins du Sénégal, Institut d'Hygiène
   ***sociale, Dakar.* The licence to practise medicine is granted to graduates**
   from a recognized medical school in France. Graduates from medical
   schools in other countries must have their degree validated.
Work in government service after graduation: **Not obligatory**
Agreements with other countries: **An agreement exists with countries of the**
   ***Conseil Africain et Malagache de l'Enseignement Supérieur* (CAMES).**

FACULTE DE MEDECINE ET DE PHARMACIE
UNIVERSITE DE DAKAR
81 BOULEVARD DE LA REPUBLIQUE
BP 5005
DAKAR
Tel.: +221 245 588/249 591/258 593
Year instruction started: **1950**
Language of instruction: **French**
Duration of basic medical degree course, including practical training: **8 years**
Foreign students eligible: **Yes**

SIERRA LEONE

Total population in 1995: **4 297 000**
Number of physicians per 100 000 population (1993): —
Number of medical schools: **1**
Duration of basic medical degree course, including practical training: **5.5 years**
Title of degree awarded: **Bachelor of Medicine and Bachelor of Surgery (MB, ChB)**
Medical registration/licence to practise: —
Work in government service after graduation: —
Agreements with other countries: —

COLLEGE OF MEDICINE AND ALLIED HEALTH SCIENCES
UNIVERSITY OF SIERRA LEONE
PRIVATE MAIL BAG
FREETOWN
Tel.: +232 (22) 240 583/240 884
Fax: +232 (22) 222 161
E-mail: comahs@srl.healthnet.org
Year instruction started: **1988**
Language of instruction: **English**
Duration of basic medical degree course, including practical training: **5.5 years**
Entrance examination: **No**
Foreign students eligible: **Yes**

SINGAPORE

Total population in 1995: **3 384 000**
Number of physicians per 100 000 population (1993): **147**
Number of medical schools: **1**
Duration of basic medical degree course, including practical training: **5 years**
Title of degree awarded: **Bachelor of Medicine and Bachelor of Surgery (MB, BS)**
Medical registration/licence to practise: **Registration is obligatory with the Singapore Medical Council, Ministry of Health, 16 College Road, Singapore 169854. The licence to practise medicine is granted to graduates of a recognized medical school who have satisfactorily completed a 1-year internship. Graduates of.foreign medical schools are granted temporary registration only.**
Work in government service after graduation: **Obligatory (1 year prior to full registration)**
Agreements with other countries: **None**

FACULTY OF MEDICINE
NATIONAL UNIVERSITY OF SINGAPORE
10 KENT RIDGE CRESCENT
SINGAPORE 119260
Tel.: +65 772 3297
Fax: +65 778 5743
Year instruction started: **1905**
Language of instruction: **English**
Duration of basic medical degree course, including practical training: **5 years**
Entrance examination: **Yes**
Foreign students eligible: **Yes**

SLOVAKIA

Total population in 1995: **5 347 000**
Number of physicians per 100 000 population (1993): **325**
Number of medical schools: **3**
Duration of basic medical degree course, including practical training: **6 years**
Title of degree awarded: ***Medicinae Universae Doctor*** **(MUDr) (Doctor of Medicine)**
Medical registration/licence to practise: **Registration is obligatory with the Slovak Medical Board,** *26 Lazaretská, 811 09 Bratislava.* **The licence to practise medicine is granted to graduates of a recognized medical school who hold a specialization diploma. They must also provide a recent certificate of good conduct. Foreigners must hold a residence and a work permit.**
Work in government service after graduation: **Not obligatory**
Agreements with other countries: **Agreements exist with Bulgaria, the Czech Republic, Hungary, Mongolia, Poland, Viet Nam and countries of the former USSR and former Yugoslavia.**

LEKARSKA FAKULTA
UNIVERSITA KOMENSKEHO
SPITALSKA 24
BRATISLAVA 811 08
Tel.: +421 (7) 361 736
Fax: +421 (7) 325 574
Year instruction started: **1919**
Language of instruction: **Slovak, English**
Duration of basic medical degree course, including practical training: **6 years**
Entrance examination: **Yes**
Foreign students eligible: **Yes**

LEKARSKA FAKULTA
UNIVERZITY P.J. SAFARIKA
TRADA SNP C. 1
KOSICE 040 66
Tel.: +421 (95) 428 151
Fax: +421 (95) 425 460
E-mail: office@central.medic.upjs.sk
Year instruction started: **1948**
Language of instruction: **Slovak, English**
Duration of basic medical degree course, including practical training: **6 years**

JESENIOVA LEKARSKA FAKULTA
UNIVERZITY KOMENSKEHO
ZABORSKEHO 2
MARTIN 036 45
Tel.: +421 (842) 333 05
Fax: +421 (842) 363 32
E-mail: sd@jfmed.uniba.sk
Year instruction started: **1969**
Language of instruction: **Slovak, English**
Duration of basic medical degree course, including practical training: **6 years**
Entrance examination: **Yes**
Foreign students eligible: **Yes**

SLOVENIA

Total population in 1995: **1 924 000**
Number of physicians per 100 000 population (1993): **219**
Number of medical schools: **1**
Duration of basic medical degree course, including practical training: **6 years (a further 2 years of supervised work in designated departments of a teaching hospital is required before the degree is awarded)**
Title of degree awarded: *Doktor Medicine* (*dr med.*, **Doctor of Medicine**)
Medical registration/licence to practise: **Registration is obligatory with the Medical Chamber of Slovenia, *10 Dalmatinova, 1000 Ljubljana*. Graduates must complete 2 years as an intern and pass a licensure examination before they are granted a licence to practise medicine. They must also provide a certificate of competence. Those with foreign medical qualifications must have their degree validated. Foreigners must become citizens of Slovenia and have an adequate command of Slovenian.**
Work in government service after graduation: **Not obligatory**
Agreements with other countries: —

MEDICINSKA FAKULTETA
UNIVERZA V LJUBLJANI
VRAZOV TRG 2
LJUBLJANA 1000
Tel.: +386 (61) 312 669
Fax: +386 (61) 321 755
E-mail: dekanat@mf.uni-lj.si
Year instruction started: **1919**
Language of instruction: **Slovenian**
Duration of basic medical degree course, including practical training: **6 years**
Entrance examination: **No**
Foreign students eligible: **Yes**

SOLOMON ISLANDS

Total population in 1995: **391 000**
Number of physicians per 100 000 population (1993): —
Number of medical schools: **None**
Medical registration/licence to practise: **Registration is obligatory with the Medical and Dental Board, Ministry of Health and Medical Services, PO Box 349, Honiara. The licence to practise medicine is granted to graduates of a recognized medical school. Applicants should not have a criminal record. Foreigners require a work permit.**
Work in government service after graduation: **Not obligatory**
Agreements with other countries: —

SOUTH AFRICA

Total population in 1995: **42 393 000**
Number of physicians per 100 000 population (1993): **59**
Number of medical schools: **8**
Duration of basic medical degree course, including practical training: **6 years**
Title of degree awarded: **Bachelor of Medicine and Surgery (MB, ChB)**
Medical registration/licence to practise: **Registration is obligatory with the South African Medical and Dental Council, PO Box 205, Pretoria. The licence to practise medicine is granted to graduates who have completed a 1-year internship and received a certificate of competence. Foreigners are granted temporary registration only.**
Work in government service after graduation: **Obligatory**
Agreements with other countries: **Agreements exist with Belgium, Ireland and the United Kingdom.**

FACULTY OF MEDICINE
UNIVERSITY OF THE ORANGE FREE STATE
ZASTRONSTREET
PO BOX 339
BLOEMFONTEIN 9300
FREE STATE
Tel.: +27 (51) 405 3013/401 2847
Fax: +27 (51) 448 0967
E-mail: gndklt@med.uovs.ac.za
Year instruction started: **1969**
Language of instruction: **Afrikaans, English**
Duration of basic medical degree course, including practical training: **6 years**
Entrance examination: **No**
Foreign students eligible: **No**

FACULTY OF MEDICINE
UNIVERSITY OF CAPE TOWN
ANZIO ROAD
OBSERVATORY
CAPE TOWN 7925
CAPE PROVINCE
Tel.: +27 (21) 406 6107
Fax: +27 (21) 478 955
E-mail: medbk@medicine.uct.ac.za
Year instruction started: **1900**
Language of instruction: **English**
Duration of basic medical degree course, including practical training: **6 years**
Entrance examination: **No**
Foreign students eligible: **Yes**

FACULTY OF MEDICINE
UNIVERSITY OF NATAL
719 UMBILO ROAD
PRIVATE BAG 7
CONGELLA
DURBAN 4013
KWAZULU/NATAL
Tel.: +27 (31) 260 4232
Fax: +27 (31) 260 4410

Telex: 621231 undad sa
E-mail: meddean@med.und.ac.za
Year instruction started: **1951**
Language of instruction: **English**
Duration of basic medical degree course, including practical training: **6 years**
Entrance examination: **No**
Foreign students eligible: **Yes**

FACULTY OF HEALTH SCIENCES
UNIVERSITY OF THE WITWATERSRAND
7 YORK ROAD
PARK TOWN
JOHANNESBURG 2193
GAUTENG
Tel.: +27 (11) 647 1111
Fax: +27 (11) 643 4318
E-mail: 081prim@chiron.wits.ac.za
Year instruction started: **1921**
Language of instruction: **English**
Duration of basic medical degree course, including practical training: **6 years**
Entrance examination: **No**
Foreign students eligible: **Yes**

FACULTY OF MEDICINE
MEDICAL UNIVERSITY OF SOUTH AFRICA (MEDUNSA)
PO BOX 210
PRETORIA 0204
Tel.: +27 (12) 529 4321
Fax: +27 (12) 529 5811
Year instruction started: **1977**
Language of instruction: **English**
Duration of basic medical degree course, including practical training: **6 years**
Entrance examination: **No**
Foreign students eligible: **Yes**

FACULTEIT GENEESKUNDE
UNIVERSITEIT VAN PRETORIA
DR SAVAGE WEG
RIVIERA
PO BOX 667
PRETORIA 0001
GAUTENG
Tel.: +27 (12) 319 2541
Fax: +27 (12) 329 1351

E-mail: dekoon@medic.up.ac.za
Year instruction started: **1943**
Language of instruction: **Afrikaans, English**
Duration of basic medical degree course, including practical training: **6 years**
Entrance examination: **No**
Foreign students eligible: **Yes**

FACULTEIT GENEESKUNDE
UNIVERSITEIT VAN STELLENBOSCH
FRANCIE VAN ZIJLRYLAAN
PAROWVALLEI
PO BOX 19063
TYGERBERG 7505
WESTERN CAPE
Tel.: +27 (21) 938 9111
Fax: +27 (21) 931 7810
Year instruction started: **1956**
Language of instruction: **Afrikaans, English**
Duration of basic medical degree course, including practical training: **6 years**
Entrance examination: **No**
Foreign students eligible: **No**

FACULTY OF MEDICINE AND HEALTH SCIENCES
UNIVERSITY OF TRANSKEI
2 EAST LONDON ROAD
PRIVATE BAG 11
UMTATA 5100
EASTERN CAPE
Tel.: +27 (471) 302 233
Fax: +27 (471) 302 235
E-mail: medicine@gebafix.utr.ac.za
Year instruction started: **1986**
Language of instruction: **English**
Duration of basic medical degree course, including practical training: **6 years**
Entrance examination: **No**
Foreign students eligible: **Yes**

SPAIN

Total population in 1995: **39 674 000**
Number of physicians per 100 000 population (1993): **400**
Number of medical schools: **26**
Duration of basic medical degree course, including practical training: **6 years**

Title of degree awarded: *Licenciado en Medicina y Cirugía* (Licentiate in Medicine and Surgery)
Medical registration/licence to practise: —
Work in government service after graduation: —
Agreements with other countries: **An agreement exists with other countries of the European Union (Directive 93/16/EEC governing the employment of doctors).**

FACULTAD DE MEDICINA
UNIVERSIDAD DE ALCALA DE HENARES
CAMPUS UNIVERSITARIO
CARRETERA DE BARCELONA KM 3
E-28800 ALCALA DE HENARES
Tel.: +34 (1) 885 4000
Year instruction started: **1975**

FACULTAD DE MEDICINA
UNIVERSIDAD DE ALICANTE
CARRETERA SAN VICENTE S/N
APDO 374
E-03080 ALICANTE
Tel.: +34 (6) 565 8529
Fax: +34 (6) 565 8513
Year instruction started: **1980**
Language of instruction: **Spanish**
Duration of basic medical degree course, including practical training: **6 years**
Entrance examination: **Yes**
Foreign students eligible: **Yes**

FACULTAD DE MEDICINA
UNIVERSIDAD DE EXTREMADURA
AVENIDA DE ELVAS S/N
E-06071 BADAJOZ
Year instruction started: **1973**

FACULTAD DE MEDICINA
UNIVERSIDAD AUTONOMA DE BARCELONA
CAMPUS UNIVERSITARIO
BELLATERRA
E-08193 BARCELONA
Tel.: +34 (3) 581 1921
Year instruction started: **1968**

FACULTAT DE MEDICINA
UNIVERSITAT DE BARCELONA
CALLE CASANOVA 143
E-08036 BARCELONA
Tel.: +34 (3) 451 1389/323 3622
Fax: +34 (3) 451 1802
Year instruction started: **1845**
Language of instruction: **Catalan, Spanish**
Duration of basic medical degree course, including practical training: **6 years**
Entrance examination: **Yes**
Foreign students eligible: **Yes**

FACULTAD DE MEDICINA
UNIVERSIDAD DEL PAIS VASCO
APDO 1397
E-48080 BILBAO
Year instruction started: **1968**

FACULTAD DE MEDICINA
UNIVERSIDAD DE CADIZ
PLAZA DE FRAGELA S/N
E-11003 CADIZ
Tel.: +34 (56) 213 921
Year instruction started: **1748**

FACULTAD DE MEDICINA
UNIVERSIDAD DE CORDOBA
AVENIDA MENENDEZ PIDAL S/N
E-14004 CORDOBA
Tel.: +34 (57) 218 227
Fax: +34 (57) 218 287
E-mail: infomed@lucano.uco.es
Year instruction started: **1973**
Language of instruction: **Spanish**
Duration of basic medical degree course, including practical training: **6 years**
Entrance examination: **No**
Foreign students eligible: **Yes**

FACULTAD DE MEDICINA
UNIVERSIDAD DE GRANADA
AVENIDA DE MADRID 11
E-18071 GRANADA
Tel.: +34 (58) 243 505
Fax: +34 (58) 291 843

Year instruction started: **1531**
Language of instruction: **Spanish**
Duration of basic medical degree course, including practical training: **6 years**
Entrance examination: **Yes**
Foreign students eligible: **Yes**

FACULTAD DE MEDICINA
UNIVERSIDAD DE LA LAGUNA
CAMPUS DE OFRA
E-38071 LA LAGUNA
Tel.: +34 (22) 603 405
Fax: +34 (22) 603 407
Year instruction started: **1968**
Language of instruction: **Spanish**
Duration of basic medical degree course, including practical training: **6 years**
Entrance examination: **No**
Foreign students eligible: **Yes**

CENTRO SUPERIOR DE CIENCIAS Y DE LA SALUD
UNIVERSIDAD DE LAS PALMAS DE GRAN CANARIA
AVENIDA MARITIMA DEL SUR S/N
E-35016 LAS PALMAS DE GRAN CANARIA
Tel.: +34 (28) 451 400
Year instruction started: **1989**

FACULTAT DE MEDICINA
UNIVERSITAT DE LLEIDA
AVENIDA ALCALDE ROVIRA ROURE 44
E-25198 LLEIDA
Tel.: +34 (73) 702 400
Fax: +34 (73) 702 425
Year instruction started: **1977**
Language of instruction: **Catalan, Spanish**
Duration of basic medical degree course, including practical training: **6 years**
Entrance examination: **No**
Foreign students eligible: **Yes**

FACULTAD DE MEDICINA
UNIVERSIDAD AUTONOMA DE MADRID
ARZOBISPO MORCILLO 4
E-28029 MADRID
Tel.: +34 (1) 397 5486
Fax: +34 (1) 397 5353

Year instruction started: **1968**
Language of instruction: **Spanish**
Duration of basic medical degree course, including practical training: **6 years**
Entrance examination: **Yes**
Foreign students eligible: **Yes**

FACULTAD DE MEDICINA
UNIVERSIDAD COMPLUTENSE DE MADRID
CIUDAD UNIVERSITARIA
E-28040 MADRID
Tel.: +34 (1) 394 1325
Year instruction started: **1949**

FACULTAD DE MEDICINA
UNIVERSIDAD DE MALAGA
CAMPUS DE TEATINOS
COLONIA DE SANTA INES
E-29071 MALAGA
Tel.: +34 (5) 213 1542/213 1543
Year instruction started: **1972**

FACULTAD DE MEDICINA
UNIVERSIDAD DE MURCIA
CAMPUS DE ESPINARDO
E-30100 MURCIA
Tel.: +34 (68) 307 100
Year instruction started: **1968**

FACULTAD DE MEDICINA
UNIVERSIDAD DE OVIEDO
JULIAN CLAVERIA S/N
E-33006 OVIEDO
Tel.: +34 (8) 510 3531
Fax: +34 (8) 523 2255
Year instruction started: **1969**
Language of instruction: **Spanish**
Duration of basic medical degree course, including practical training: **6 years**
Entrance examination: **Yes**
Foreign students eligible: **Yes**

FACULTAD DE MEDICINA
UNIVERSIDAD DE NAVARRA
IRUNLARREA S/N
APDO 31080
E-31008 PAMPLONA

Tel.: +34 (48) 425 600
Fax: +34 (48) 425 649
Telex: 37917 unav e
Year instruction started: **1954**
Language of instruction: **Spanish**
Duration of basic medical degree course, including practical training: **6 years**
Entrance examination: **Yes**
Foreign students eligible: **No**

FACULTAD DE MEDICINA Y CIENCIAS DE LA SALUD
UNIVERSIDAD ROVIRA I VIRGILI
CALLE SAN LORENZO 21
E-43201 REUS
Tel.: +34 (77) 759 300
Fax: +34 (77) 759 322
E-mail: secmed@fmcs.urv.es
Year instruction started: **1977**
Language of instruction: **Catalan, Spanish**
Duration of basic medical degree course, including practical training: **6 years**
Entrance examination: **Yes**
Foreign students eligible: **Yes**

FACULTAD DE MEDICINA
UNIVERSIDAD DE SALAMANCA
CAMPUS MIGUEL DE UNAMUNO
AVENIDA CAMPO CHARRO S/N
E-37007 SALAMANCA
Tel.: +34 (23) 294 541
Fax: +34 (23) 294 510
Year instruction started: **1944**
Language of instruction: **Spanish**
Duration of basic medical degree course, including practical training: **6 years**
Entrance examination: **Yes**
Foreign students eligible: **Yes**

FACULTAD DE MEDICINA
UNIVERSIDAD DE CANTABRIA
CARDENAL HERRERA ONA S/N
E-39009 SANTANDER
Tel.: +34 (42) 201 911
Year instruction started: **1974**

FACULTAD DE MEDICINA Y ODONTOLOGIA
UNIVERSIDAD DE SANTIAGO
CALLE SAN FRANCISCO 1
E-15705 SANTIAGO DE COMPOSTELA
Tel.: +34 (81) 563 100
Year instruction started: **17th century**

FACULTAD DE MEDICINA
UNIVERSIDAD DE SEVILLA
AVENIDA SANCHEZ PIZJUAN 4
E-41009 SEVILLA
Tel.: +34 (5) 455 9822
Fax: +34 (5) 455 9827
Year instruction started: **1748**
Language of instruction: **Spanish**
Duration of basic medical degree course, including practical training: **6 years**
Entrance examination: **Yes**
Foreign students eligible: **Yes**

FACULTAD DE MEDICINA Y ODONTOLOGIA
UNIVERSIDAD DE VALENCIA
AVENIDA BLASCO IBANEZ 17
E-46010 VALENCIA
Tel.: +34 (6) 386 4150
Fax: +34 (6) 386 4173
E-mail: facultat.medicina@uv.es
Year instruction started: **1498**
Language of instruction: **Spanish**
Duration of basic medical degree course, including practical training: **6 years**
Entrance examination: **Yes**
Foreign students eligible: **Yes**

FACULTAD DE MEDICINA
UNIVERSIDAD DE ESTUDI VALLADOLID
AVENIDA RAMON Y CAJAL 7
E-47005 VALLADOLID
Tel.: +34 (83) 423 000
Year instruction started: **1944**

FACULTAD DE MEDICINA
UNIVERSIDAD DE ZARAGOZA
DOMINGO MIRAL S/N
E-50009 ZARAGOZA
Tel.: +34 (76) 761 000
Fax: +34 (76) 761 664

Year instruction started: **1893**
Language of instruction: **Spanish**
Duration of basic medical degree course, including practical training: **6 years**
Entrance examination: **Yes**
Foreign students eligible: **Yes**

SRI LANKA

Total population in 1995: **18 100 000**
Number of physicians per 100 000 population (1993): **23**
Number of medical schools: **6**
Duration of basic medical degree course, including practical training: **5 years**
Title of degree awarded: **Bachelor of Medicine and Bachelor of Surgery (MB, BS)**
Medical registration/licence to practise: **Registration is obligatory with the Sri Lankan Medical Council, 6 *Wijerama Mawatha, Colombo* 7. The licence to practise medicine is granted to graduates who have completed a 1-year internship in general medicine. Nationals who have qualified abroad must take a special examination. Foreigners who have qualified abroad may practise temporarily by special invitation only.**
Work in government service after graduation: **Not obligatory**
Agreements with other countries: —

FACULTY OF MEDICINE
UNIVERSITY OF COLOMBO
KINSEY ROAD
COLOMBO
Year instruction started: **1870**

FACULTY OF MEDICINE
UNIVERSITY OF RUHUNA
KARAPITIYA
PO BOX 70
GALLE
Tel.: +94 (9) 348 01/348 03/347 30
Fax: +94 (9) 223 14
Year instruction started: **1980**
Language of instruction: **English**
Duration of basic medical degree course, including practical training: **5 years**
Entrance examination: **Yes**
Foreign students eligible: **Yes**

FACULTY OF MEDICINE
UNIVERSITY OF JAFFNA
ADIYAPATHAM ROAD
KOKUVIL
JAFFNA
Tel.: +94 (21) 238 38
Year instruction started: **1978**
Language of instruction: **English**
Duration of basic medical degree course, including practical training: **5 years**
Entrance examination: **Yes**
Foreign students eligible: **Yes**

FACULTY OF MEDICAL SCIENCES
UNIVERSITY OF SRI JAYEWARDENEPURA
GANGODAWILA
NUGEGODA
Tel.: +94 (8) 114 80
Fax: +94 (8) 526 04
E-mail: postmaster@sjp.ac.lk
Year instruction started: **1993**
Language of instruction: **English**
Duration of basic medical degree course, including practical training: **5 years**
Entrance examination: **Yes**
Foreign students eligible: **Yes**

FACULTY OF MEDICINE
UNIVERSITY OF PERADENIYA
PERADENIYA
Year instruction started: **1962**

FACULTY OF MEDICINE
UNIVERSITY OF KELANIYA
PO BOX 6
TALAGOLLA ROAD
RAGAMA
Tel.: +94 (1) 538 219/538 039
Fax: +94 (1) 538 251
Year instruction started: **1991**
Language of instruction: **English**
Duration of basic medical degree course, including practical training: **5 years**
Entrance examination: **No**
Foreign students eligible: **Yes**

SUDAN

Total population in 1995: **27 291 000**
Number of physicians per 100 000 population (1993): **10**
Number of medical schools: **14**
Duration of basic medical degree course, including practical training: **5 or 6 years**
Title of degree awarded: **Bachelor of Medicine and Bachelor of Surgery (MB, BS)**
Medical registration/licence to practise: **Registration is obligatory with the Sudanese Medical Council, Khartoum. The licence to practise medicine is granted by the Provincial Ministry of Health to graduates of a recognized medical school. Graduates of foreign medical schools must have their degree validated by the Medical Council. Foreigners are granted temporary registration if they hold a work permit issued by the Ministry of the Interior.**
Work in government service after graduation: **Obligatory (3 years)**
Agreements with other countries: **None**

FACULTY OF MEDICINE AND HEALTH SCIENCES
UNIVERSITY OF EL ZAEEM
EL AZHARI

FACULTY OF MEDICINE AND HEALTH SCIENCES
EL FASHER UNIVERSITY
PO BOX 321
EL FASHER 49
Year instruction started: **1991**
Language of instruction: **Arabic**
Duration of basic medical degree course, including practical training: **6 years**
Entrance examination: **Yes**
Foreign students eligible: **Yes**

FACULTY OF MEDICINE AND HEALTH SCIENCES
UNIVERSITY OF KORDOFAN
PO BOX 160/517
EL OBIED 51111
Tel.: +249 (81) 3307
Year instruction started: **1991**
Language of instruction: **Arabic, English**
Duration of basic medical degree course, including practical training: **6 years**

FACULTY OF MEDICINE AND HEALTH SCIENCES
KASSALA UNIVERSITY
KASSALA WEST BANK OF CASH RIVER
PO BOX 266
KASSALA
Tel.: +249 (20) 772 095
Year instruction started: **1990**
Language of instruction: **Arabic**
Duration of basic medical degree course, including practical training: **6 years**

ACADEMY OF MEDICAL SCIENCES AND TECHNOLOGY
PO BOX 12810
KHARTOUM
Tel.: +249 (11) 724 762/723 385
Fax: +249 (11) 724 799
Year instruction started: **1996**
Language of instruction: **English**
Duration of basic medical degree course, including practical training: **5 years**
Foreign students eligible: **Yes**

COLLEGE OF MEDICINE
UNIVERSITY OF JUBA
PO BOX 321/1
KHARTOUM
Tel.: +249 (11) 451 353/451 352
Fax: +249 (11) 451 351
Year instruction started: **1978**
Language of instruction: **English**
Duration of basic medical degree course, including practical training: **6 years**
Entrance examination: **No**
Foreign students eligible: **Yes**

FACULTY OF MEDICINE
UNIVERSITY OF KHARTOUM
PO BOX 102
KHARTOUM
Tel.: +249 (11) 772 224
Year instruction started: **1924**
Language of instruction: **Arabic, English**
Duration of basic medical degree course, including practical training: **6 years**
Entrance examination: **No**
Foreign students eligible: **Yes**

FACULTY OF MEDICINE AND HEALTH SCIENCES
UPPER NILE UNIVERSITY
PO BOX 1660
KHARTOUM
Year instruction started: **1994**

FACULTY OF MEDICINE
UNIVERSITY OF EL IMAM EL MAHDI
PO BOX 209
KOSTI
Tel.: +249 (71) 220 022
Language of instruction: **Arabic**
Duration of basic medical degree course, including practical training: **6 years**
Entrance examination: **No**
Foreign students eligible: **Yes**

SCHOOL OF MEDICINE
AHFAD UNIVERSITY FOR WOMEN
PO BOX 167
OMDURMAN
Year instruction started: **1990**

FACULTY OF MEDICINE AND HEALTH SCIENCES
OMDURMAN ISLAMIC UNIVERSITY
PO BOX 382
OMDURMAN
Tel.: +249 (11) 554 989
Fax: +249 (11) 778 113
Telex: 22527 oiu sd
Year instruction started: **1989**
Language of instruction: **Arabic, English**
Duration of basic medical degree course, including practical training: **5 years**
Entrance examination: **No**
Foreign students eligible: **Yes**

FACULTY OF MEDICINE AND HEALTH SCIENCES
SHENDI UNIVERSITY
PO BOX 10
SHENDI
Year instruction started: **1990**

FACULTY OF MEDICINE
UNIVERSITY OF GEZIRA
WAD MEDANI
Year instruction started: **1978**

FACULTY OF MEDICINE AND HEALTH SCIENCES
BAHR EL GHAZAL UNIVERSITY
PO BOX 30
WAU
Year instruction started: **1994**

SURINAME

Total population in 1995: **432 000**
Number of physicians per 100 000 population (1993): **40**
Number of medical schools: **1**
Duration of basic medical degree course, including practical training: **7 years**
Title of degree awarded: *Arts* **(Physician)**
Medical registration/licence to practise: **Registration is obligatory with the Medical Inspectorate in the Ministry of Health, Gravenstraat 64 Boven, Paramaribo. The licence to practise medicine is granted to graduates of Suriname University or a recognized medical school who have completed a 1-year internship in Suriname.**
Work in government service after graduation: **Obligatory (1 year)**
Agreements with other countries: **An agreement exists with other Caribbean countries.**

FACULTEIT DER MEDISCHE WETENSHAPPEN
ANTON DE KOM UNIVERSITEIT VAN SURINAME
KERNKAMPWEG 5
PARAMARIBO
Tel.: +597 441 071
Fax: +597 441 071
Year instruction started: **1892**
Language of instruction: **Dutch, English**
Duration of basic medical degree course, including practical training: **7 years**
Entrance examination: **No**
Foreign students eligible: **No**

SWEDEN

Total population in 1995: **8 819 000**
Number of physicians per 100 000 population (1993): **299**
Number of medical schools: **6**
Duration of basic medical degree course, including practical training: **5.5 years**
Title of degree awarded: *Läkarexamen* **(Physician's examination)**
Medical registration/licence to practise: **Registration is obligatory with the National Board of Health and Welfare (Socialstyrelsen), S-106 30 Stock-**

holm. The licence to practise medicine is granted to graduates of a recognized medical school who have completed 21 months as an intern. Those with foreign medical qualifications must take an examination and a language proficiency test. They must also have a knowledge of Swedish medical legislation.

Work in government service after graduation: **Obligatory (21 months prior to full registration)**

Agreements with other countries: **Agreements exist with other countries of the European Union (Directive 93/16/EEC governing the employment of doctors), and with Iceland, Liechtenstein and Norway.**

MEDICINSKA FAKULTETEN
GOETEBORGS UNIVERSITET
MEDICINAREGATAN 16
S-413 90 GOETEBORG
Tel.: +46 (31) 773 1000
Fax: +46 (31) 773 3866
E-mail: info@medkan.gu.se
Year instruction started: **1945**
Language of instruction: **Swedish, English**
Duration of basic medical degree course, including practical training: **5.5 years**
Entrance examination: **No**
Foreign students eligible: **Yes**

MEDICINSKA FAKULTETEN
LINKOEPING UNIVERSITET
REGIONSJUKHUSET
S-581 85 LINKOEPING
Year instruction started: **1970**

MEDICINSKA FAKULTETEN
LUND UNIVERSITET
PARADISGATAN 5
BOX 117
S-221 00 LUND
Tel.: +46 (46) 222 7219
Fax: +46 (46) 222 4170
E-mail: medschool@kanslim.lu.se
Year instruction started: **1667**
Language of instruction: **Swedish, English**
Duration of basic medical degree course, including practical training: **5.5 years**
Entrance examination: **No**
Foreign students eligible: **Yes**

MEDICINSKA FAKULTETEN
KAROLINSKA INSTITUTET
SOLNAVAGEN 1
S-171 77 STOCKHOLM
Tel.: +46 (8) 728 6400
Fax: +46 (8) 310 343
Year instruction started: **1810**
Language of instruction: **Swedish**
Duration of basic medical degree course, including practical training: **5.5 years**
Entrance examination: **Yes**
Foreign students eligible: **Yes**

MEDICINSKA FAKULTETEN
UMEA UNIVERSITET
S-901 87 UMEA
Tel.: +46 (90) 165 000
Fax: +46 (90) 167 660
Year instruction started: **1956**
Language of instruction: **Swedish**
Duration of basic medical degree course, including practical training: **5.5 years**
Entrance examination: **No**
Foreign students eligible: **Yes**

MEDICINSKA FAKULTETEN
UPPSALA UNIVERSITET
ST OLOFSGATAN 10B
BOX 256
S-751 05 UPPSALA
Tel.: +46 (18) 182 500
Fax: +46 (18) 181 858
Telex: 76024 univups s
E-mail: ulf.heyman@uadm.uu.se
Year instruction started: **1477**
Language of instruction: **Swedish**
Duration of basic medical degree course, including practical training: **5.5 years**
Entrance examination: **No**
Foreign students eligible: **Yes**

SWITZERLAND

Total population in 1995: **7 224 000**
Number of physicians per 100 000 population (1993): **301**
Number of medical schools: **5**
Duration of basic medical degree course, including practical training: **6 years**
Title of degree awarded: *Eidgenössisches Arztdiplom* or *Diplôme fédéral de médecin* (**Federal Diploma of Physician**)
Medical registration/licence to practise: **Registration is obligatory with the health authorities in the individual cantons. The licence to practise medicine is granted to holders of the Federal Diploma of Physician. Applicants must provide proof of their legal status and of good conduct. Nationals with foreign medical qualifications require special authorization to practise. Foreigners require a residence permit and may only enter private practice if they have qualified in Switzerland.**
Work in government service after graduation: **Not obligatory**
Agreements with other countries: **None**

MEDIZINISCHE FAKULTAET
UNIVERSITAET BASEL
HEBELSTRASSE 25
CH-4031 BASEL
Year instruction started: **1460**

MEDIZINISCHE FAKULTAET
UNIVERSITAET BERN
MURTENSTRASSE 11
POSTFACH 7
CH-3010 BERN
Tel.: +41 (31) 632 3553
Fax: +41 (31) 632 4994
Year instruction started: **1805**
Language of instruction: **German, French**
Duration of basic medical degree course, including practical training: **6 years**
Entrance examination: **No**
Foreign students eligible: **Yes**

FACULTE DE MEDECINE
UNIVERSITE DE GENEVE
RUE MICHEL-SERVET 1
CH-1211 GENEVE 4
Tel.: +41 (22) 702 5111
Fax: +41 (22) 347 3334

Year instruction started: **1876**
Language of instruction: **French**
Duration of basic medical degree course, including practical training: **6 years**
Entrance examination: **No**
Foreign students eligible: **Yes**

FACULTE DE MEDECINE
UNIVERSITE DE LAUSANNE
LE CHAMP DE L'AIR
RUE DU BUGNON 21
CH-1005 LAUSANNE
Year instruction started: **1890**

MEDIZINISCHE FAKULTAET
UNIVERSITAET ZUERICH
RAEMISTRASSE 100
CH-8091 ZUERICH
Tel.: +41 (1) 257 2029
Fax: +41 (1) 255 4565
Year instruction started: **1833**
Language of instruction: **German**
Duration of basic medical degree course, including practical training: **6 years**
Entrance examination: **No**

SYRIAN ARAB REPUBLIC

Total population in 1995: **14 574 000**
Number of physicians per 100 000 population (1993): **109**
Number of medical schools: **3**
Duration of basic medical degree course, including practical training: **6 years**
Title of degree awarded: **Doctor of Medicine**
Medical registration/licence to practise: —
Work in government service after graduation: —
Agreements with other countries: —

FACULTY OF MEDICINE
UNIVERSITY OF ALEPPO
ALEPPO
Year instruction started: **1967**

FACULTY OF HUMAN MEDICINE
UNIVERSITY OF DAMASCUS
MAZEH STREET AUTOSTRADE
DAMASCUS
Tel.: +963 (11) 212 3664
Year instruction started: **1919**
Language of instruction: **Arabic, French, English**
Duration of basic medical degree course, including practical training: **6 years**
Entrance examination: **No**
Foreign students eligible: **Yes**

FACULTY OF MEDICINE
UNIVERSITY OF TICHREEN
LATTAKIA
Year instruction started: **1974**

TAJIKISTAN

Total population in 1995: **5 935 000**
Number of physicians per 100 000 population (1993): **210**
Number of medical schools: **1**
Duration of basic medical degree course, including practical training: —
Title of degree awarded: —
Medical registration/licence to practise: —
Work in government service after graduation: —
Agreements with other countries: —

TADZHIK MEDICAL INSTITUTE IM. ABU-ALI'IBN SINA
PROSPEKT LENINA 48
DUSHANBE 734017
Year instruction started: **1939**

THAILAND

Total population in 1995: **58 703 000**
Number of physicians per 100 000 population (1993): **24**
Number of medical schools: **12**
Duration of basic medical degree course, including practical training: **5 or 6 years**
Title of degree awarded: **Doctor of Medicine (MD)**
Medical registration/licence to practise: **Registration is obligatory with the**

Medical Council, Office of Permanent Secretary Building, Ministry of Public Health, Nonthaburi 11000, which grants the licence to practise medicine to graduates from public medical faculties. Graduates from private medical faculties and those with foreign medical qualifications must take a licensing examination.

Work in government service after graduation: **Obligatory (3 years in a rural area)**
Agreements with other countries: **None**

FACULTY OF MEDICINE
CHULALONGKORN UNIVERSITY
1873 RAMA IV ROAD
BANGKOK 10330
Tel.: +66 (2) 256 4244
Fax: +66 (2) 252 4963
Year instruction started: **1947**
Language of instruction: **Thai**
Duration of basic medical degree course, including practical training: **6 years**
Entrance examination: **Yes**
Foreign students eligible: **No**

BANGKOK METROPOLITAN MEDICAL COLLEGE
MAHIDOL UNIVERSITY
681 SAMSEN ROAD
DUSIT
BANGKOK 10300
Tel.: +66 (2) 241 5129
Fax: +66 (2) 241 5129
Year instruction started: **1993**
Language of instruction: **Thai**
Duration of basic medical degree course, including practical training: **6 years**
Entrance examination: **Yes**
Foreign students eligible: **No**

FACULTY OF MEDICINE
MAHIDOL UNIVERSITY
RAMATHIBODI HOSPITAL
270 RAMA VI ROAD
BANGKOK 10400
Tel.: +66 (2) 245 5704/245 8822
Fax: +66 (2) 246 2123
Year instruction started: **1969**
Language of instruction: **Thai, English**
Duration of basic medical degree course, including practical training: **6 years**
Entrance examination: **Yes**
Foreign students eligible: **No**

FACULTY OF MEDICINE
MAHIDOL UNIVERSITY
SIRIRAJ HOSPITAL
2 PRAN-NOK ROAD
BANGKOK 10700
Tel.: +66 (2) 411 1429/419 7676
Fax: +66 (2) 412 1371
Telex: 84770 unimahi th
Year instruction started: **1890**
Language of instruction: **Thai**
Duration of basic medical degree course, including practical training: **6 years**
Entrance examination: **Yes**
Foreign students eligible: **No**

PRAMONGKUTKLAO COLLEGE OF MEDICINE
315 RAJAVITHI ROAD
RAJATHEVEE DISTRICT
BANGKOK 10400
Tel.: +66 (2) 248 3391/245 8279
Fax: +66 (2) 247 9559/245 8277
Year instruction started: **1975**
Language of instruction: **Thai**
Duration of basic medical degree course, including practical training: **6 years**
Entrance examination: **Yes**
Foreign students eligible: **No**

FACULTY OF MEDICINE
RANGSIT UNIVERSITY
PHYA THAI 2 HOSPITAL
943 PAHALYOTHIN ROAD
BANGKOK 10440
Tel.: +66 (2) 270 1847
Fax: +66 (2) 271 2306
Year instruction started: **1989**
Language of instruction: **Thai, English**
Duration of basic medical degree course, including practical training: **6 years**
Entrance examination: **Yes**
Foreign students eligible: **Yes**

FACULTY OF MEDICINE
SRINAKHARINWIROT UNIVERSITY
PRASARNMIT CAMPUS
SUKHUMVIT 23
BANGKOK 10110

Tel.: +66 (2) 260 2124
Fax: +66 (2) 260 0125
Year instruction started: **1985**
Language of instruction: **Thai**
Duration of basic medical degree course, including practical training: **6 years**
Entrance examination: **Yes**
Foreign students eligible: **No**

FACULTY OF MEDICINE
CHIANG MAI UNIVERSITY
110 INTAVAROROS AMPHUR MUANG
CHIANG MAI 50200
Tel.: +66 (53) 221 122
Fax: +66 (53) 217 144
Year instruction started: **1958**
Language of instruction: **Thai, English**
Duration of basic medical degree course, including practical training: **6 years**
Entrance examination: **Yes**
Foreign students eligible: **No**

FACULTY OF MEDICINE
KHON KAEN UNIVERSITY
123 MITRAPARP HIGHWAY
MAUNG
KHON KAEN 40002
Tel.: +66 (43) 237 909
Fax: +66 (43) 348 375
Telex: 72173 unikhan th
E-mail: pisaln-m@medlib2.kku.ac.th
Year instruction started: **1974**
Language of instruction: **Thai**
Duration of basic medical degree course, including practical training: **6 years**
Entrance examination: **Yes**
Foreign students eligible: **Yes**

FACULTY OF MEDICINE
THAMMASAT UNIVERSITY
RANGSIT CAMPUS
KLONG-LUANG
PATHUMTHANI 12121
Tel.: +66 (2) 516 1020/516 1021/516 1022
Fax: +66 (2) 516 9403

Year instruction started: **1991**
Language of instruction: **Thai**
Duration of basic medical degree course, including practical training: **5 years**
Entrance examination: **Yes**
Foreign students eligible: **No**

FACULTY OF MEDICINE
NARESUAN UNIVERSITY
AMPHUR MUANG
PHITSANULOK 65000
Tel.: +66 (55) 261 071
Fax: +66 (55) 261 057
Year instruction started: **1995**
Duration of basic medical degree course, including practical training: **6 years**

FACULTY OF MEDICINE
PRINCE OF SONGKLA UNIVERSITY
71/7 KANCHANAVANICH ROAD
HAADYAI
SONGKHLA 90110
Tel.: +66 (74) 212 070
Fax: +66 (74) 212 900/212 903
E-mail: mededu@ratree.psu.ac.th, med_ed@medicine.psu.ac.th
Year instruction started: **1973**
Language of instruction: **Thai**
Duration of basic medical degree course, including practical training: **6 years**
Entrance examination: **Yes**
Foreign students eligible: **No**

THE FORMER YUGOSLAV REPUBLIC OF MACEDONIA

Total population in 1995: **2 174 000**
Number of physicians per 100 000 population (1993): **219**
Number of medical schools: **1**
Duration of basic medical degree course, including practical training: **6 years (a
    further period of supervised practice is required before the degree is
    awarded)**
Title of degree awarded: **Doctor of Medicine**
Medical registration/licence to practise: **Registration is obligatory with the
    Doctors' Chamber of Macedonia, Naroden Front 21, Skopje. The licence to
    practise medicine is granted to graduates of a recognized medical school
    who have passed a specialist examination. Nationals and foreigners
    who have graduated abroad must have their degree validated and take**

additional examinations. Foreigners must also hold a residence and a work permit.
Work in government service after graduation: **Obligatory (1 year)**
Agreements with other countries: —

MEDICINSKI FAKULTET
UNIVERZITET "SV KIRIL I METODIJ" SKOPJE
50 DIVIZIJA BR. 6
SKOPJE 91000
Tel.: +389 (91) 235 155
Fax: +389 (91) 220 935
Year instruction started: **1947**
Language of instruction: **Macedonian**
Duration of basic medical degree course, including practical training: **6 years**
Entrance examination: **Yes**
Foreign students eligible: **Yes**

TOGO

Total population in 1995: **4 201 000**
Number of physicians per 100 000 population (1993): **6**
Number of medical schools: **1**
Duration of basic medical degree course, including practical training: **7 years**
Title of degree awarded: ***Docteur en Médecine (Diplôme d'État)* (Doctor of Medicine (State Diploma))**
Medical registration/licence to practise: —
Work in government service after graduation: —
Agreements with other countries: —

FACULTE MIXTE DE MEDECINE ET DE PHARMACIE
UNIVERSITE DE BENIN
BP 1515
LOME
Tel.: +228 252 787
Fax: +228 258 784
Telex: 5258 ub tg
Year instruction started: **1973**
Language of instruction: **French**
Duration of basic medical degree course, including practical training: **7 years**
Entrance examination: **No**
Foreign students eligible: **Yes**

TONGA

Total population in 1995: —
Number of physicians per 100 000 population (1993): —
Number of medical schools: **None**
Medical registration/licence to practise: **Graduates must register with the Registrar, Health Practitioners' Registration Council, Ministry of Health, PO Box 59, Nuku'alofer. Applicants must have qualified at a recognized medical school. They should be proficient in Tongan or English and provide evidence of good character and professional competence.**
Work in government service after graduation: **Not obligatory**
Agreements with other countries: **None**

TRINIDAD AND TOBAGO

Total population in 1995: **1 297 000**
Number of physicians per 100 000 population (1993): **90**
Number of medical schools: **1**
Duration of basic medical degree course, including practical training: **5 years**
Title of degree awarded: **Bachelor of Medicine and Bachelor of Surgery (MB, BS)**
Medical registration/licence to practise: **Registration is obligatory with the Medical Board of Trinidad and Tobago, Eric Williams Medical Sciences Complex, Uriah Butler Highway, Champs Fleurs, Trinidad. The licence to practise medicine is granted to graduates of a recognized medical school who have completed an 18-month internship.**
Work in government service after graduation: **Obligatory for holders of a government scholarship**
Agreements with other countries: **An agreement exists with the General Medical Council of the United Kingdom.**

FACULTY OF MEDICAL SCIENCES – ST AUGUSTINE
UNIVERSITY OF THE WEST INDIES
ERIC WILLIAMS MEDICAL SCIENCES COMPLEX
CHAMPS FLEURS
Tel.: +1868 645 2640/645 2649
Fax: +1868 663 9836
Telex: 24520 uwi wg
E-mail: fms@medsci.uwi.tt
Year instruction started: **1967**
Language of instruction: **English**
Duration of basic medical degree course, including practical training: **5 years**
Entrance examination: **No**
Foreign students eligible: **Yes**

TUNISIA

Total population in 1995: **9 156 000**
Number of physicians per 100 000 population (1993): **67**
Number of medical schools: **4**
Duration of basic medical degree course, including practical training: **7 years**
Title of degree awarded: ***Doctorat en Médecine*** (Doctor of Medicine)
Medical registration/licence to practise: **Registration is obligatory with the**
Conseil national de l'Ordre des Médecins, 16 rue Touraine, Tunis. **Graduates**
of foreign medical schools must have their degree validated. Foreigners
require authorization from the Ministry of Public Health to practise.
Work in government service after graduation: **Not obligatory**
Agreements with other countries: **Agreements exist with Algeria, the Libyan**
Arab Jamahiriya, Mauritania and Morocco.

FACULTE DE MEDECINE DE MONASTIR
AVICENNE
MONASTIR 5019
Tel.: +216 (3) 462 200
Fax: +216 (3) 460 737
Year instruction started: **1980**
Language of instruction: **French**
Duration of basic medical degree course, including practical training: **7 years**
Entrance examination: **Yes**
Foreign students eligible: **Yes**

FACULTE DE MEDECINE DE SFAX
RUE MAGIDA BOULILA
BP 96
SFAX 3029
Tel.: +216 (4) 241 888
Fax: +216 (4) 246 217
Year instruction started: **1974**
Language of instruction: **French**
Duration of basic medical degree course, including practical training: **7 years**
Entrance examination: **No**
Foreign students eligible: **Yes**

FACULTE DE MEDECINE "IBN EL JAZZAR" DE SOUSSE
AVENUE MOHAMED KAROUI
BP 126
SOUSSE 4002
Tel.: +216 (3) 222 600
Fax: +216 (3) 224 899

Telex: 30988 famso tn
Year instruction started: **1974**
Language of instruction: **French**
Duration of basic medical degree course, including practical training: **7 years**
Entrance examination: **No**
Foreign students eligible: **Yes**

FACULTE DE MEDECINE ET DE PHARMACIE DE TUNIS
9 AVENUE ZOUHAIER ESSAFI
TUNIS 1006
Tel.: +216 (1) 263 709/263 710
Fax: +216 (1) 569 427
Year instruction started: **1964**
Language of instruction: **French**
Duration of basic medical degree course, including practical training: **7 years**
Entrance examination: **No**
Foreign students eligible: **Yes**

TURKEY

Total population in 1995: **61 797 000**
Number of physicians per 100 000 population (1993): **103**
Number of medical schools: **33**
Duration of basic medical degree course, including practical training: **6 or 7 years**
Title of degree awarded: ***Tip Doktoru*** (Doctor of Medicine)
Medical registration/licence to practise: **Registration is obligatory for private practice with the Turkish Medical Association, Mithatpasa Caddesi No. 62/15–18, 06420 Yonisehir, Ankara. Graduates with foreign qualifications must validate their degree with the Ministry of Health. A licence is not required for practice in the governmental or private sector, except for physicians who wish to have their own clinics.**
Work in government service after graduation: **Not obligatory**
Agreements with other countries: —

TIP FAKULTESI
YEDITEPE UNIVERSITESI
IBRAHIMAGA MAH. KOFTUNCU SOKAK
ACIBADEM-KADIKOY 81001
ISTANBUL
Tel.: +90 (216) 327 6860
Fax: +90 (216) 327 6473
Year instruction started: **1996**

TIP FAKULTESI
ANKARA UNIVERSITESI
DEKANLIK BINASI
SIHHIYE
ANKARA 06100
Tel.: +90 (312) 312 4834
Fax: +90 (312) 310 6370
E-mail: skemahli@neuron.ato.org.tr
Year instruction started: **1945**
Language of instruction: **Turkish**
Duration of basic medical degree course, including practical training: **6 years**
Entrance examination: **Yes**
Foreign students eligible: **Yes**

TIP FAKULTESI
GAZI UNIVERSITESI
BESEVLER
ANKARA 06500
Tel.: +90 (312) 223 7467
Fax: +90 (312) 212 4647
Year instruction started: **1979**
Language of instruction: **Turkish**
Duration of basic medical degree course, including practical training: **6 years**
Entrance examination: **Yes**
Foreign students eligible: **Yes**

TIP FAKULTESI
HACETTEPE UNIVERSITESI
ANKARA 06100
Tel.: +90 (312) 324 3286
Fax: +90 (312) 310 0580
Telex: 42237 htk tr
Year instruction started: **1963**
Language of instruction: **Turkish, English**
Duration of basic medical degree course, including practical training: **6 years**
Entrance examination: **Yes**
Foreign students eligible: **Yes**

TIP FAKULTESI
AKDENIZ UNIVERSITESI
DUMLUPINAR CADDESI
ARAPSUYU 07070
ANTALYA

Tel.: +90 (242) 227 4480
Fax: +90 (242) 227 4482
Year instruction started: **1978**
Language of instruction: **Turkish**
Duration of basic medical degree course, including practical training: **6 years**
Entrance examination: **Yes**
Foreign students eligible: **Yes**

TIP FAKULTESI
CUKUROVA UNIVERSITESI
BALCALI 01330
ADANA
Tel.: +90 (322) 338 6404
Fax: +90 (322) 338 6572
Year instruction started: **1972**
Language of instruction: **Turkish**
Duration of basic medical degree course, including practical training: **6 years**
Entrance examination: **Yes**
Foreign students eligible: **Yes**

CERRAHPASA TIP FAKULTESI
ISTANBUL UNIVERSITESI
KOCAMUSTAFA PASA CADDESI
AKSARAY 34303
ISTANBUL
Tel.: +90 (212) 588 4800
Fax: +90 (212) 632 0050
Year instruction started: **1967**
Language of instruction: **Turkish**
Duration of basic medical degree course, including practical training: **6 years**
Entrance examination: **Yes**
Foreign students eligible: **Yes**

TIP FAKULTESI
EGE UNIVERSITESI
BORNOVA 35100
IZMIR
Year instruction started: **1956**
Language of instruction: **Turkish, English**
Duration of basic medical degree course, including practical training: **6 years**
Entrance examination: **Yes**
Foreign students eligible: **Yes**

TIP FAKULTESI
ULUDAG UNIVERSITESI
GORUKLE KAMPUSU
BURSA 21900
Tel.: +90 (224) 442 8048
Fax: +90 (224) 442 8018
Year instruction started: **1975**
Language of instruction: **Turkish**
Duration of basic medical degree course, including practical training: **6 years**
Entrance examination: **Yes**
Foreign students eligible: **Yes**

ISTANBUL TIP FAKULTESI
ISTANBUL UNIVERSITESI
MILLET CADDESI
CAPA 34390
ISTANBUL
Tel.: +90 (212) 631 1349/631 0276
Fax: +90 (212) 631 1350/632 6066
Year instruction started: **1827**
Language of instruction: **Turkish**
Duration of basic medical degree course, including practical training: **6 years**
Entrance examination: **Yes**
Foreign students eligible: **Yes**

TIP FAKULTESI
KOCAELI UNIVERSITESI
IBNI-SINA BULVARI
DERINCE 41900
KOCAELI
Tel.: +90 (262) 239 4466
Fax: +90 (262) 239 4465
Year instruction started: **1992**
Language of instruction: **Turkish**
Duration of basic medical degree course, including practical training: **6 years**
Entrance examination: **Yes**
Foreign students eligible: **Yes**

TIP FAKULTESI
DICLE UNIVERSITESI
DIYARBAKIR 21280
Tel.: +90 (412) 248 8141
Fax: +90 (412) 248 8440
Year instruction started: **1968**

Language of instruction: **Turkish**
Duration of basic medical degree course, including practical training: **6 years**
Entrance examination: **Yes**
Foreign students eligible: **No**

DUZCE TIP FAKULTESI DEKANLIGI
ABANT IZZET BAYSAL UNIVERSITESI
ESKI TEKEL BINASI
DUZCE 14500
BOLU
Tel.: +90 (374) 524 1732/524 2028
Fax: +90 (374) 524 1736
Year instruction started: **1996**

TIP FAKULTESI
TRAKYA UNIVERSITESI
EDIRNE 22030
Tel.: +90 (289) 235 7641/235 7642/235 7643
Fax: +90 (289) 235 7540
Year instruction started: **1982**
Language of instruction: **Turkish**
Duration of basic medical degree course, including practical training: **6 years**
Entrance examination: **Yes**
Foreign students eligible: **Yes**

TIP FAKULTESI
FIRAT UNIVERSITESI
ELAZIG 23100
Tel.: +90 (424) 212 8500
Fax: +90 (424) 237 9138
Year instruction started: **1982**
Language of instruction: **Turkish**
Duration of basic medical degree course, including practical training: **6 years**
Entrance examination: **Yes**
Foreign students eligible: **Yes**

TIP FAKULTESI
ATATURK UNIVERSITESI
ERZURUM 25240
Tel.: +90 (442) 218 7985
Fax: +90 (442) 234 9013
Year instruction started: **1966**

Language of instruction: **Turkish**
Duration of basic medical degree course, including practical training: **6 years**
Entrance examination: **Yes**
Foreign students eligible: **Yes**

GATA ASKERI TIP FAKULTESI
GULHANE ASKERI TIP AKADEMISI
ETLIK
ANKARA
Tel.: +90 (312) 321 0657
Fax: +90 (312) 321 3106
Year instruction started: **1981**
Language of instruction: **Turkish**
Duration of basic medical degree course, including practical training: **6 years**
Entrance examination: **Yes**
Foreign students eligible: **Yes**

TIP FAKULTESI
GAZIANTEP UNIVERSITESI
GAZIANTEP 27310
Tel.: +90 (342) 360 0753
Fax: +90 (342) 360 1617
Year instruction started: **1988**
Language of instruction: **Turkish**
Duration of basic medical degree course, including practical training: **6 years**
Entrance examination: **Yes**
Foreign students eligible: **No**

TIP FAKULTESI
SULEYMAN DEMIREL UNIVERSITESI
ISPARTA 32040
Tel.: +90 (246) 232 6657
Fax: +90 (246) 232 9422
Year instruction started: **1993**
Language of instruction: **Turkish**
Duration of basic medical degree course, including practical training: **6 years**
Entrance examination: **Yes**

FACULTY OF MEDICINE
MARMARA UNIVERSITY
TIBBIYE CADDESI
HAYDARPASA
ISTANBUL 81010
Tel.: +90 (216) 336 0212
Fax: +90 (216) 414 4731

Year instruction started: **1983**
Language of instruction: **English**
Duration of basic medical degree course, including practical training: **6 years**
Entrance examination: **Yes**
Foreign students eligible: **No**

TIP FAKULTESI
DOKUZ EYLUL UNIVERSITESI
MITHATPASA
INCIRALTI
IZMIR 35340
Tel.: +90 (232) 277 7777
Fax: +90 (232) 259 0541
Year instruction started: **1978**
Language of instruction: **Turkish, English**
Duration of basic medical degree course, including practical training: **6 years**
Entrance examination: **Yes**
Foreign students eligible: **Yes**

TIP FAKULTESI
ERCIYES UNIVERSITESI
TALAS YOLU
KAYSERI 38039
Tel.: +90 (352) 437 4910
Fax: +90 (352) 437 4911
Year instruction started: **1975**
Language of instruction: **Turkish**
Duration of basic medical degree course, including practical training: **7 years**
Entrance examination: **Yes**
Foreign students eligible: **Yes**

TIP FAKULTESI
PAMUKKALE UNIVERSITESI
KINIKLI 20020
DENIZLI
Tel.: +90 (258) 266 3045
Fax: +90 (258) 266 1817
Year instruction started: **1987**
Language of instruction: **Turkish**
Duration of basic medical degree course, including practical training: **6 years**
Entrance examination: **Yes**
Foreign students eligible: **Yes**

TIP FAKULTESI
SELCUK UNIVERSITESI
KONYA 42080
Tel.: +90 (332) 323 2642
Fax: +90 (332) 323 2643
Year instruction started: **1983**
Language of instruction: **Turkish**
Duration of basic medical degree course, including practical training: **6 years**
Entrance examination: **Yes**
Foreign students eligible: **Yes**

TIP FAKULTESI
INONU UNIVERSITESI
ELAZIG YOLU KAMPUS
PO BOX 326
MALATYA 44100
Tel.: +90 (422) 341 0036/341 0045
Fax: +90 (422) 341 0036
E-mail: inonu01@vm.ege.edu.tr
Year instruction started: **1988**
Language of instruction: **Turkish, English**
Duration of basic medical degree course, including practical training: **7 years**
Entrance examination: **Yes**
Foreign students eligible: **No**

TIP FAKULTESI
MALTEPE UNIVERSITESI
FEYZULLAH CADDESI 39
MALTEPE 81530
ISTANBUL
Tel.: +90 (216) 399 0060
Fax: +90 (216) 370 2230
Year instruction started: **1997**

TIP FAKULTESI
CELAL BAYAR UNIVERSITESI
GAZIOSMANPASA CADDESI 47
MANISA 45020
Tel.: +90 (236) 237 6440/237 6441/237 6442
Fax: +90 (236) 237 2442

Year instruction started: **1995**
Language of instruction: **Turkish**
Duration of basic medical degree course, including practical training: **6 years**
Entrance examination: **Yes**
Foreign students eligible: **Yes**

TIP FAKULTESI
OSMANGAZI UNIVERSITESI
MESELIK 26480
ESKISEHIR
Tel.: +90 (222) 239 3770
Fax: +90 (222) 239 3772
Year instruction started: **1980**
Language of instruction: **Turkish**
Duration of basic medical degree course, including practical training: **6 years**
Entrance examination: **Yes**
Foreign students eligible: **Yes**

TIP FAKULTESI
ONDOKUZ MAYIS UNIVERSITESI
BAFRA CADDESI
SAMSUN 55139
Tel.: +90 (362) 457 6070
Fax: +90 (362) 457 6041
Year instruction started: **1973**
Language of instruction: **Turkish**
Duration of basic medical degree course, including practical training: **6 years**
Entrance examination: **Yes**
Foreign students eligible: **Yes**

TIP FAKULTESI
HARRAN UNIVERSITESI
SANLIURFA 63300
Tel.: +90 (414) 314 8414
Fax: +90 (414) 313 9615
Year instruction started: **1992**
Language of instruction: **Turkish**
Duration of basic medical degree course, including practical training: **6 years**
Entrance examination: **Yes**
Foreign students eligible: **No**

TIP FAKULTESI
CUMHURIYET UNIVERSITESI
KAMPUS
SIVAS 58140
Tel.: +90 (346) 226 1517
Fax: +90 (346) 226 1556
Year instruction started: **1974**
Language of instruction: **Turkish**
Duration of basic medical degree course, including practical training: **6 years**
Entrance examination: **Yes**
Foreign students eligible: **Yes**

TIP FAKULTESI
KARADENIZ TEKNIK UNIVERSITESI
TRABZON 61080
Tel.: +90 (462) 325 1609
Fax: +90 (462) 325 2270
Year instruction started: **1981**
Language of instruction: **Turkish**
Duration of basic medical degree course, including practical training: **6 years**
Entrance examination: **Yes**
Foreign students eligible: **Yes**

TIP FAKULTESI
YUZUNCU YIL UNIVERSITESI
VAN 680
Tel.: +90 (432) 216 7325
Fax: +90 (432) 216 7519
Year instruction started: **1992**
Language of instruction: **Turkish**
Duration of basic medical degree course, including practical training: **6 years**
Entrance examination: **Yes**
Foreign students eligible: **No**

TURKMENISTAN

Total population in 1995: **4 155 000**
Number of physicians per 100 000 population (1993): **353**
Number of medical schools: **1**
Duration of basic medical degree course, including practical training: —
Title of degree awarded: —
Medical registration/licence to practise: —
Work in government service after graduation: —
Agreements with other countries: —

TURKMEN DRUZBI NARODOV MEDICAL INSTITUTE
ULICA SAUMJANA 58
ASHKHABAT 744000
Year instruction started: **1932**

TUVALU

Total population in 1995: —
Number of physicians per 100 000 population (1993): **89**
Number of medical schools: **None**
Medical registration/licence to practise: **Registration is obligatory with the
Ministry of Health, PO Box 41, Funafuti.**
Work in government service after graduation: **Not obligatory**
Agreements with other countries: **None**

UGANDA

Total population in 1995: **20 256 000**
Number of physicians per 100 000 population (1993): **4**
Number of medical schools: **3**
Duration of basic medical degree course, including practical training: **4 or 5 years**
Title of degree awarded: **Bachelor of Medicine and Bachelor of Surgery (MB,
ChB)**
Medical registration/licence to practise: **Registration is obligatory with the
Registrar, Uganda Medical Council, PO Box 16115 Wandegeya, Kampala.
The licence to practise medicine is granted to graduates of a recognized
medical school who have successfully completed a 1-year internship.
Foreigners require a work permit.**
Work in government service after graduation: **Obligatory (at least 2 years)**
Agreements with other countries: **None**

KIGEZI INTERNATIONAL SCHOOL OF MEDICINE
KABALE HOSPITAL
PO BOX 7
KABALE
Tel.: +256 (248) 220 06/+44 (1223) 355 076
Fax: +44 (1223) 327 292
E-mail: kigezi.med@dial.pipex.com
Year instruction started: **1996**
Language of instruction: **English**
Duration of basic medical degree course, including practical training: **4 or 5 years**
Entrance examination: **Yes**
Foreign students eligible: **Yes**

FACULTY OF MEDICINE
MAKERERE UNIVERSITY MEDICAL SCHOOL
PO BOX 7072
KAMPALA
Tel.: +256 (41) 530 020
Fax: +256 (41) 531 091
Year instruction started: **1923**
Language of instruction: **English**
Duration of basic medical degree course, including practical training: **5 years**
Entrance examination: **No**
Foreign students eligible: **Yes**

FACULTY OF MEDICINE
MBARARA UNIVERSITY OF SCIENCE AND TECHNOLOGY
PO BOX 1410
MBARARA
Tel.: +256 (485) 207 82/200 07
Year instruction started: **1990**
Language of instruction: **English**
Duration of basic medical degree course, including practical training: **5 years**
Entrance examination: **No**
Foreign students eligible: **Yes**

UKRAINE

Total population in 1995: **51 608 000**
Number of physicians per 100 000 population (1993): **429**
Number of medical schools: **15**
Duration of basic medical degree course, including practical training: **6–8 years**
Title of degree awarded: ***Vrač-spetsialist*** (**Doctor of Medicine**)
Medical registration/licence to practise: **Registration is obligatory with the Health Administration of the province in which the physician wishes to work. The licence to practise medicine is granted by the Ministry of Health, Ulica Groushevskovo 7, 252021 Kiev, to graduates of a recognized medical school with training in a specialization. They should provide a copy of their diploma as well as any certificates of further training obtained during the previous 5 years. Evidence of competence to work and of a formal offer of employment must also be provided. Requirements are being drawn up for graduates of foreign medical schools.**
Work in government service after graduation: **Obligatory during specialist training**
Agreements with other countries: **Bilateral agreements exist with a number of countries, including Belarus, the Czech Republic, Poland, the Republic of Moldova, the Russian Federation, Slovakia and Uzbekistan.**

BUKOVYNIAN STATE MEDICAL ACADEMY
TEATRALNA SQUARE 2
CHERNOVTSY 274000
Tel.: +380 (372) 553 754
Fax: +380 (372) 221 910
E-mail: luchak@ctd.ite.chernovtsy.ua
Year instruction started: **1944**
Language of instruction: **Ukrainian, Russian, English**
Duration of basic medical degree course, including practical training: **6 years**
Entrance examination: **Yes**
Foreign students eligible: **Yes**

DNIEPROPETROVSK STATE MEDICAL ACADEMY
ULICA DZERZHINSKY 9
DNIEPROPETROVSK 320044
Tel.: +380 (562) 451 565
Fax: +380 (562) 464 191
E-mail: root@dma.dnepropetrovsk.ua
Year instruction started: **1916**
Language of instruction: **Ukrainian, Russian**
Duration of basic medical degree course, including practical training: **8 years**
Entrance examination: **Yes**
Foreign students eligible: **Yes**

DONECK MEDICAL UNIVERSITY
PROSPEKT ILICA 26
DONECK 340098
Year instruction started: **1930**

IVANO-FRANKOVSK STATE MEDICAL ACADEMY
2 HALYTSKA STREET
PO BOX 368
IVANO-FRANKOVSK 284000
Tel.: +380 (34) 242 95
Fax: +380 (34) 242 95
Year instruction started: **1945**
Language of instruction: **Ukrainian**
Duration of basic medical degree course, including practical training: **6 years**
Entrance examination: **Yes**
Foreign students eligible: **Yes**

KHARKOV MEDICAL UNIVERSITY
PROSPEKT LENINA 4
KHARKOV 310022
Year instruction started: **1805**

NATIONAL MEDICAL UNIVERSITY
BULVAR SEVCENKO 13
KIEV 252004
Year instruction started: **1841**

LUGANSK MEDICAL UNIVERSITY
KV. IM 50-LET. OB. LUGANSKA 1
LUGANSK 348045
Year instruction started: **1956**

DANYLO HALYTSKY LVIV STATE MEDICAL UNIVERSITY
PEKARSKAYA STREET 69
LVIV 290000
Tel.: +380 (322) 767 818/722 660
Fax: +380 (322) 767 818/767 973
E-mail: lutsyk@meduniv.lviv.ua
Year instruction started: **1896**
Entrance examination: **No**
Foreign students eligible: **Yes**

ODESSA MEDICAL UNIVERSITY
PROUL. N. NARIMANOVA 2
ODESSA 270100
Year instruction started: **1901**

UKRAINIAN MEDICAL AND DENTAL ACADEMY
ULICA SEVCENKO 23
POLTAVA 314034
Year instruction started: **1921**

CRIMEAN MEDICAL INSTITUTE
BULVAR LENINA 5/7
SIMFEROPOL 333670
Year instruction started: **1931**

TERNOPOL MEDICAL INSTITUTE
MAYDAN VOLI 1
TERNOPOL 282001
Tel.: +380 (3522) 244 92
Fax: +380 (3522) 214 64
Year instruction started: **1957**
Language of instruction: **Ukrainian**
Duration of basic medical degree course, including practical training: **6 years**
Entrance examination: **Yes**
Foreign students eligible: **Yes**

MEDICAL FACULTY
UZGOROD STATE UNIVERSITY
ULICA GORKOGO 40
UZGOROD 294000
Year instruction started: **1945**

VINNICA MEDICAL UNIVERSITY
ULICA PIROGOVA 56
VINNICA 280028
Year instruction started: **1934**

ZAPOROZHYE STATE MEDICAL UNIVERSITY
ULICA MAJAKOVSKI 26
ZAPOROZHYE 330035
Tel.: +380 (612) 335 007/335 008
Fax: +380 (612) 330 125
Year instruction started: **1903**
Language of instruction: **Russian**
Duration of basic medical degree course, including practical training: **6 years**
Entrance examination: **Yes**
Foreign students eligible: **Yes**

UNITED ARAB EMIRATES

Total population in 1995: **2 260 000**
Number of physicians per 100 000 population (1993): **168**
Number of medical schools: **2**
Duration of basic medical degree course, including practical training: **6 or 7 years**
Title of degree awarded: —
Medical registration/licence to practise: —
Work in government service after graduation: —
Agreements with other countries: —

FACULTY OF MEDICINE AND HEALTH SCIENCES
UNITED ARAB EMIRATES UNIVERSITY
PO BOX 17666
AL AIN
ABU DHABI
Tel.: +971 (2) 631 341
Fax: +971 (2) 631 945

Year instruction started: **1986**
Language of instruction: **English**
Duration of basic medical degree course, including practical training: **7 years**
Entrance examination: **Yes**
Foreign students eligible: **No**

DUBAI MEDICAL COLLEGE FOR GIRLS
PO BOX 20170
DUBAI
Tel.: +971 (4) 646 465/646 130
Fax: +971 (4) 646 030
Telex: 45923 slotah em
Year instruction started: **1986**
Language of instruction: **English**
Duration of basic medical degree course, including practical training: **6 years**
Entrance examination: **No**
Foreign students eligible: **Yes**

UNITED KINGDOM OF GREAT BRITAIN AND NORTHERN IRELAND

Total population in 1995: **58 144 000**
Number of physicians per 100 000 population (1993): **164**
Number of medical schools: **27**
Duration of basic medical degree course, including practical training: **5–7 years**
Title of degree awarded: **Bachelor of Medicine and Bachelor of Surgery (MB, ChB)**
Medical registration/licence to practise: **Registration is obligatory with the General Medical Council, 178 Great Portland Street, London W1N 6JE, after postgraduate general clinical training.**
Work in government service after graduation: **Not obligatory**
Agreements with other countries: **An agreement exists with other countries of the European Union (Directive 93/16/EEC governing the employment of doctors).**

■ ENGLAND
THE MEDICAL SCHOOL
UNIVERSITY OF BIRMINGHAM
EDGBASTON
BIRMINGHAM B15 2TT
Tel.: +44 (121) 414 6886
Fax: +44 (121) 414 4036

E-mail: medschool-enquiries@bham.ac.uk
Year instruction started: **1825**
Language of instruction: **English**
Duration of basic medical degree course, including practical training: **5 years**
Entrance examination: **No**
Foreign students eligible: **Yes**

THE MEDICAL SCHOOL
UNIVERSITY OF BRISTOL
SENATE HOUSE
TYNDALL AVENUE
BRISTOL BS8 1TH
Tel.: +44 (117) 928 9000
Fax: +44 (117) 925 1424
Year instruction started: **1833**
Language of instruction: **English**
Duration of basic medical degree course, including practical training: **5 years**
Entrance examination: **No**
Foreign students eligible: **Yes**

SCHOOL OF CLINICAL MEDICINE
UNIVERSITY OF CAMBRIDGE
ADDENBROOKES HOSPITAL
HILLS ROAD
CAMBRIDGE CB2 2QQ
Year instruction started: **1453**

SCHOOL OF MEDICINE
UNIVERSITY OF LEEDS
WORSLEY MEDICAL AND DENTAL BUILDING
THORESBY PLACE
LEEDS LS2 9NL
Tel.: +44 (113) 233 4364
Fax: +44 (113) 233 4373
Year instruction started: **1831**
Language of instruction: **English**
Duration of basic medical degree course, including practical training: **5 years**
Entrance examination: **No**
Foreign students eligible: **Yes**

SCHOOL OF MEDICINE
UNIVERSITY OF LEICESTER
MAURICE SHOCK MEDICAL SCIENCES BUILDING
UNIVERSITY ROAD
PO BOX 138
LEICESTER LE1 9HN
Tel.: +44 (116) 252 2966
Fax: +44 (116) 252 3013
Year instruction started: **1975**
Language of instruction: **English**
Duration of basic medical degree course, including practical training: **5 years**
Entrance examination: **No**
Foreign students eligible: **Yes**

FACULTY OF MEDICINE
UNIVERSITY OF LIVERPOOL
DUNCAN BUILDING
DAULBY STREET
LIVERPOOL L69 3GA
Tel.: +44 (151) 706 4268
Fax: +44 (151) 706 5667
Year instruction started: **1834**
Language of instruction: **English**
Duration of basic medical degree course, including practical training: **5 years**
Entrance examination: **No**
Foreign students eligible: **Yes**

CHARING CROSS AND WESTMINSTER MEDICAL SCHOOL
IMPERIAL COLLEGE SCHOOL OF MEDICINE
UNIVERSITY OF LONDON
THE REYNOLDS BUILDING
ST DUNSTAN'S ROAD
LONDON W6 8RP
Tel.: +44 (181) 846 1234
Fax: +44 (181) 846 7222
Year instruction started: **1984**[1]
Language of instruction: **English**
Duration of basic medical degree course, including practical training: **5 years**
Entrance examination: **No**
Foreign students eligible: **Yes**

---

[1] Merger of Charing Cross Hospital Medical School and Westminster Medical School, both of which began instruction in 1834.

KING'S COLLEGE SCHOOL OF MEDICINE AND DENTISTRY
UNIVERSITY OF LONDON
BESSEMER ROAD
LONDON SE5 9PJ
Tel.: +44 (171) 312 5622
Fax: +44 (171) 312 5621
Year instruction started: **1831**
Language of instruction: **English**
Entrance examination: **No**
Foreign students eligible: **Yes**

ROYAL FREE HOSPITAL SCHOOL OF MEDICINE
UNIVERSITY OF LONDON
ROWLAND HILL STREET
LONDON NW3 2PF
Tel.: +44 (171) 794 0500
Fax: +44 (171) 794 3505
Year instruction started: **1874**
Language of instruction: **English**
Duration of basic medical degree course, including practical training: **5 years**
Entrance examination: **No**
Foreign students eligible: **Yes**

ST BARTHOLOMEW'S AND THE ROYAL LONDON SCHOOL OF MEDICINE
    AND DENTISTRY
QUEEN MARY AND WESTFIELD COLLEGE
UNIVERSITY OF LONDON
47 TURNER STREET
LONDON E1 2AD
Tel.: +44 (171) 377 7603/377 7604
Fax: +44 (171) 377 7612
E-mail: d.marshall@qmw.ac.uk
Year instruction started: **1995**[1]
Language of instruction: **English**
Duration of basic medical degree course, including practical training: **5 years**
Entrance examination: **No**
Foreign students eligible: **Yes**

---

[1] Merger of St Bartholomew's Hospital Medical College and the London Hospital Medical College, which began instruction in 1123 and 1785, respectively, and Queen Mary and Westfield College, which began instruction in 1989.

ST GEORGE'S HOSPITAL MEDICAL SCHOOL
UNIVERSITY OF LONDON
CRANMER TERRACE
LONDON SW17 0RE
Tel.: +44 (181) 672 9944
Fax: +44 (181) 672 6940
Year instruction started: **1751**
Language of instruction: **English**
Duration of basic medical degree course, including practical training: **5 years**
Entrance examination: **No**
Foreign students eligible: **Yes**

ST MARY'S HOSPITAL MEDICAL SCHOOL
IMPERIAL COLLEGE SCHOOL OF MEDICINE
UNIVERSITY OF LONDON
NORFOLK PLACE
LONDON W2 1PG
Year instruction started: **1854**

UNITED MEDICAL AND DENTAL SCHOOLS OF GUY'S AND ST THOMAS'S
    HOSPITALS
KING'S COLLEGE
UNIVERSITY OF LONDON
LAMBETH PALACE ROAD
LONDON SE1 7EH
Year instruction started: **1982**[1]

SCHOOL OF MEDICINE
UNIVERSITY COLLEGE
UNIVERSITY OF LONDON
GOWER STREET
LONDON WC1E 6BT
Tel.: +44 (171) 209 6300
Fax: +44 (171) 383 2462
Year instruction started: **1828**
Language of instruction: **English**
Duration of basic medical degree course, including practical training: **5 years**
Entrance examination: **No**
Foreign students eligible: **Yes**

---

[1] Merger of Guy's Hospital Medical School, which began instruction in 1769, and St Thomas's Hospital Medical School, which began instruction in 1553.

FACULTY OF MEDICINE
UNIVERSITY OF MANCHESTER
MANCHESTER M13 9PL
Tel.: +44 (161) 275 5027
Fax: +44 (161) 275 5584
Year instruction started: **1814**
Language of instruction: **English**
Duration of basic medical degree course, including practical training: **5 years**
Entrance examination: **No**
Foreign students eligible: **Yes**

FACULTY OF MEDICINE
UNIVERSITY OF NEWCASTLE-UPON-TYNE
FRAMLINGTON PLACE
NEWCASTLE-UPON-TYNE NE2 4HH
Tel.: +44 (191) 222 6000
Fax: +44 (191) 222 6621
E-mail: dean-of-medicine@ncl.ac.uk
Year instruction started: **1834**
Language of instruction: **English**
Duration of basic medical degree course, including practical training: **5 years**
Entrance examination: **No**
Foreign students eligible: **Yes**

MEDICAL SCHOOL
THE UNIVERSITY OF NOTTINGHAM
QUEEN'S MEDICAL CENTRE
NOTTINGHAM NG7 2UH
Tel.: +44 (115) 970 9379
Fax: +44 (115) 970 9922
Year instruction started: **1970**
Language of instruction: **English**
Duration of basic medical degree course, including practical training: **5 years**

OXFORD UNIVERSITY MEDICAL SCHOOL
JOHN RADCLIFFE HOSPITAL
HEADINGTON
OXFORD OX3 9DU
Tel.: +44 (1865) 221 689
Fax: +44 (1865) 750 750
E-mail: medschool@ox.ac.uk

Year instruction started: **13th century**
Language of instruction: **English**
Duration of basic medical degree course, including practical training: **5.8 years**
Entrance examination: **No**
Foreign students eligible: **Yes**

FACULTY OF MEDICINE AND DENTISTRY
UNIVERSITY OF SHEFFIELD MEDICAL SCHOOL
BEECH HILL ROAD
SHEFFIELD S10 2RX
Year instruction started: **1828**
Language of instruction: **English**
Duration of basic medical degree course, including practical training: **5 years**
Entrance examination: **No**
Foreign students eligible: **Yes**

FACULTY OF MEDICINE
UNIVERSITY OF SOUTHAMPTON
MEDICAL AND BIOLOGICAL SCIENCES BUILDING
BASSETT CRESCENT EAST
SOUTHAMPTON SO9 1AA
Year instruction started: **1971**

■ **NORTHERN IRELAND**
COLLEGE OF MEDICINE AND HEALTH SCIENCES
THE QUEEN'S UNIVERSITY OF BELFAST
71 UNIVERSITY ROAD
BELFAST BT7 1NF
Tel.: +44 (1232) 245 133
Fax: +44 (1232) 330 571
E-mail: coll.med@qub.ac.uk
Year instruction started: **1849**
Language of instruction: **English**
Duration of basic medical degree course, including practical training: **5 years**
Entrance examination: **No**
Foreign students eligible: **Yes**

■ **SCOTLAND**
FACULTY OF MEDICINE AND MEDICAL SCIENCES
UNIVERSITY OF ABERDEEN
POLWARTH BUILDING
FORESTERHILL
ABERDEEN AB9 2ZD

Tel.: +44 (1224) 681 818
Fax: +44 (1224) 840 708
E-mail: g.catto@admin.abdn.ac.uk
Year instruction started: **1497**
Language of instruction: **English**
Duration of basic medical degree course, including practical training: **5 years**
Entrance examination: **No**
Foreign students eligible: **Yes**

FACULTY OF MEDICINE AND DENTISTRY
UNIVERSITY OF DUNDEE
NINEWELLS HOSPITAL AND MEDICAL SCHOOL
DUNDEE DD1 9SY
Tel.: +44 (1382) 660 111
Fax: +44 (1382) 644 267
E-mail: medshoff@dundee.ac.uk
Year instruction started: **1882**
Language of instruction: **English**
Duration of basic medical degree course, including practical training: **5 years**
Entrance examination: **No**
Foreign students eligible: **Yes**

MEDICAL SCHOOL
UNIVERSITY OF EDINBURGH
TEVIOT PLACE
EDINBURGH EH8 9AG
Year instruction started: **1728**
Language of instruction: **English**
Duration of basic medical degree course, including practical training: **5 years**
Entrance examination: **No**
Foreign students eligible: **Yes**

·FACULTY OF MEDICINE
UNIVERSITY OF GLASGOW
GLASGOW G12 8QQ
Tel.: +44 (141) 330 4424
Fax: +44 (141) 330 5440
Year instruction started: **1637**
Language of instruction: **English**
Duration of basic medical degree course, including practical training: **5 years**
Entrance examination: **No**
Foreign students eligible: **Yes**

MEDICAL SCHOOL[1]
UNIVERSITY OF ST ANDREWS
OLD UNION BUILDING
ST ANDREWS KY16 9AJ
Tel.: +44 (1334) 476 161
Fax: +44 (1334) 462 144
Year instruction started: **1886**
Language of instruction: **English**
Duration of basic medical degree course, including practical training: **6 or 7 years**
Entrance examination: **No**
Foreign students eligible: **Yes**

■ **WALES**
COLLEGE OF MEDICINE
UNIVERSITY OF WALES
HEATH PARK
CARDIFF CF4 4XN
Tel.: +44 (1222) 742 028
Fax: +44 (1222) 742 914
Year instruction started: **1931**
Language of instruction: **English**
Duration of basic medical degree course, including practical training: **5 years**
Entrance examination: **No**
Foreign students eligible: **Yes**

UNITED REPUBLIC OF TANZANIA

Total population in 1995: **30 799 000**
Number of physicians per 100 000 population (1993): **4**
Number of medical schools: **2**
Duration of basic medical degree course, including practical training: **5 years**
Title of degree awarded: **Doctor of Medicine**
Medical registration/licence to practise: —
Work in government service after graduation: —
Agreements with other countries: —

---

[1] Students study for 3 or 4 years at St Andrews to obtain a Bachelor of Science degree and then continue at Manchester University for 3 years of clinical training.

COLLEGE OF HEALTH SCIENCES
INSTITUTE OF PUBLIC HEALTH
UNIVERSITY OF DAR ES SALAAM
UNITED NATIONS ROAD
PO BOX 65015
UPANGA
DAR ES SALAAM
Year instruction started: **1963**

KILIMANJARO CHRISTIAN MEDICAL COLLEGE
TUMAINI UNIVERSITY
PO BOX 3010
MOSHI
Tel.: +255 (55) 543 77/543 78/543 79
Fax: +255 (55) 543 81
E-mail: jhunter@maf.org
Year instruction started: **1997**

UNITED STATES OF AMERICA

Total population in 1995: **269 444 000**
Number of physicians per 100 000 population (1993): **245**
Number of medical schools: **141 (includes schools of osteopathic medicine)**
Duration of basic medical degree course, including practical training: **4–8 years**
Title of degree awarded: **Doctor of Medicine (MD) or Doctor of Osteopathy (DO)**
Medical registration/licence to practise: **The licence to practise medicine is granted by the individual states. Completion of an acceptable programme of medical education followed by 1–3 years of accredited residency training and an examination acceptable to the licensing board is required. Some states have separate licensing boards for osteopathic medicine. Information concerning special requirements for osteopaths can be obtained from the Federation of State Medical Boards, 400 Fuller Wiser Road, Suite 300, Euless, TX 76039-3855.**

Graduates of foreign medical schools must be certified by the Educational Commission for Foreign Medical Graduates (ECFMG^SM), 3624 Market Street, Philadelphia, PA 19104-2685, to be eligible to enter accredited programmes of graduate medical education (GME). ECFMG certification is also a prerequisite for licensure to practise medicine in most states and is one of the eligibility requirements to taking Step 3 of the United States Medical Licensing Examination™ (USMLE™). Students and graduates of foreign medical schools should refer to the current edition of the ECFMG information booklet for detailed information on eligibility and requirements for ECFMG certification. Graduates of foreign medical schools who are not

citizens or permanent residents of the USA must have been legally admitted to the country before beginning graduate medical education.

Work in government service after graduation: **Not obligatory**

Agreements with other countries: **The North American Free Trade Agreement has provisions concerning the recognition of professional degrees in Canada, Mexico and the USA.**

■ ALABAMA

UNIVERSITY OF ALABAMA SCHOOL OF MEDICINE
1670 UNIVERSITY BOULEVARD
BIRMINGHAM 35294-0019
Tel.: +1 (205) 934 1111
Fax: +1 (205) 934 0333
E-mail: dboulware@uasom.meis.uab.edu
Year instruction started: **1945**
Language of instruction: **English**
Entrance examination: **Yes**
Foreign students eligible: **Yes**

UNIVERSITY OF SOUTH ALABAMA COLLEGE OF MEDICINE
1005 MEDICAL SCIENCES BUILDING
307 UNIVERSITY BOULEVARD
MOBILE 36688
Tel.: +1 (334) 460 7174
Fax: +1 (334) 460 6761
E-mail: schoultz@jaguar1.usouthal.edu
Year instruction started: **1973**
Language of instruction: **English**
Duration of basic medical degree course, including practical training: **4 years**
Entrance examination: **Yes**
Foreign students eligible: **No**

■ ARIZONA

UNIVERSITY OF ARIZONA COLLEGE OF MEDICINE
1501 N. CAMPBELL AVENUE
PO BOX 245017
TUCSON 87524
Tel.: +1 (520) 626 4555
Fax: +1 (520) 626 4884
Year instruction started: **1967**
Language of instruction: **English**
Duration of basic medical degree course, including practical training: **4 years**
Entrance examination: **Yes**
Foreign students eligible: **No**

■ ARKANSAS
COLLEGE OF MEDICINE
UNIVERSITY OF ARKANSAS FOR MEDICAL SCIENCES
4301 WEST MARKHAM
LITTLE ROCK 72205
Year instruction started: **1879**

■ CALIFORNIA
DAVIS SCHOOL OF MEDICINE
UNIVERSITY OF CALIFORNIA
DAVIS 95616
Year instruction started: **1968**

IRVINE COLLEGE OF MEDICINE
UNIVERSITY OF CALIFORNIA
IRVINE 92717
Year instruction started: **1963**[1]

SCHOOL OF MEDICINE
UNIVERSITY OF CALIFORNIA AT SAN DIEGO
PO BOX 109
LA JOLLA 92093
Year instruction started: **1968**

LOMA LINDA UNIVERSITY SCHOOL OF MEDICINE
LOMA LINDA 92354
Year instruction started: **1909**

LOS ANGELES SCHOOL OF MEDICINE
UNIVERSITY OF CALIFORNIA
10833 LE CONTE AVENUE
PO BOX 951722
LOS ANGELES 90095
Year instruction started: **1951**
Language of instruction: **English**
Duration of basic medical degree course, including practical training: **4 years**
Entrance examination: **Yes**

UNIVERSITY OF SOUTHERN CALIFORNIA SCHOOL OF MEDICINE
2025 ZONAL AVENUE
LOS ANGELES 90033
Year instruction started: **1885**

---

[1] As a school of allopathic medicine; since 1896 as a college of osteopathic medicine.

COLLEGE OF OSTEOPATHIC MEDICINE OF THE PACIFIC
WESTERN UNIVERSITY OF HEALTH SCIENCES
COLLEGE PLAZA
309 EAST SECOND STREET
POMONA 91766-1889
Tel.: +1 (909) 469 5414
Fax: +1 (909) 469 5535
Year instruction started: **1978**
Language of instruction: **English**
Duration of basic medical degree course, including practical training: **4 years**
Entrance examination: **Yes**
Foreign students eligible: **Yes**

SAN FRANCISCO SCHOOL OF MEDICINE
UNIVERSITY OF CALIFORNIA
THIRD STREET AND PARNASSUS AVENUE
SAN FRANCISCO 94143-0410
Year instruction started: **1864**
Language of instruction: **English**
Duration of basic medical degree course, including practical training: **4 years**
Entrance examination: **Yes**
Foreign students eligible: **Yes**

STANFORD UNIVERSITY SCHOOL OF MEDICINE
300 PASTEUR DRIVE
STANFORD 94305-5302
Tel.: +1 (415) 723 6436
Fax: +1 (415) 725 7368
Year instruction started: **1908**[1]
Language of instruction: **English**
Duration of basic medical degree course, including practical training: **4 years**
Entrance examination: **Yes**
Foreign students eligible: **Yes**

■ **COLORADO**
SCHOOL OF MEDICINE
UNIVERSITY OF COLORADO
4200 EAST 9TH AVENUE C290
DENVER 80262
Tel.: +1 (303) 315 7565
Fax: +1 (303) 315 8494

---

[1] From 1859 to 1908 as Cooper Medical College.

Year instruction started: **1883**
Language of instruction: **English**
Entrance examination: **Yes**
Foreign students eligible: **Yes**

■ CONNECTICUT

UNIVERSITY OF CONNECTICUT SCHOOL OF MEDICINE
263 FARMINGTON AVENUE
FARMINGTON 06030-1915
Tel.: +1 (860) 679 2385
Fax: +1 (860) 679 1282
Year instruction started: **1968**
Language of instruction: **English**
Duration of basic medical degree course, including practical training: **4 years**
Entrance examination: **Yes**
Foreign students eligible: **Yes**

YALE UNIVERSITY MEDICAL SCHOOL
333 CEDAR STREET
PO BOX 208055
NEW HAVEN 06520-8055
Tel.: +1 (203) 785 4672
Fax: +1 (203) 785 7437
Year instruction started: **1813**
Language of instruction: **English**
Duration of basic medical degree course, including practical training: **4 years**
Entrance examination: **Yes**
Foreign students eligible: **Yes**

■ DISTRICT OF COLUMBIA

GEORGETOWN UNIVERSITY SCHOOL OF MEDICINE
3900 RESERVOIR ROAD NW
WASHINGTON 20007
Year instruction started: **1851**

GEORGE WASHINGTON UNIVERSITY SCHOOL OF MEDICINE AND HEALTH
    SCIENCES
2300 EYE STREET NW
WASHINGTON 20037
Tel.: +1 (202) 994 3506
Fax: +1 (202) 994 1753

Year instruction started: **1825**
Language of instruction: **English**
Duration of basic medical degree course, including practical training: **4 years**
Entrance examination: **Yes**
Foreign students eligible: **Yes**

HOWARD UNIVERSITY COLLEGE OF MEDICINE
520 WEST STREET NW
WASHINGTON 20059
Year instruction started: **1868**

■ **FLORIDA**
UNIVERSITY OF FLORIDA COLLEGE OF MEDICINE
1600 ARCHER ROAD
PO BOX 100215
GAINESVILLE 32610
Tel.: +1 (904) 392 0034
Fax: +1 (904) 392 6482
E-mail: robert_watson@qm.server.ufl.edu
Year instruction started: **1956**
Language of instruction: **English**
Duration of basic medical degree course, including practical training: **4 years**
Entrance examination: **Yes**
Foreign students eligible: **Yes**

UNIVERSITY OF MIAMI SCHOOL OF MEDICINE
1600 NW 10TH AVENUE
PO BOX 016159
MIAMI 33101
Tel.: +1 (305) 213 6545
Fax: +1 (305) 243 6548
Year instruction started: **1952**
Language of instruction: **English**
Duration of basic medical degree course, including practical training: **4 years**
Entrance examination: **Yes**
Foreign students eligible: **No**

NOVA SOUTHEASTERN UNIVERSITY COLLEGE OF OSTEOPATHIC MEDICINE
1750 NE 167TH STREET
NORTH MIAMI BEACH 33162-3017
Tel.: +1 (305) 949 4000
Fax: +1 (305) 945 9674

Year instruction started: **1981**
Language of instruction: **English**
Duration of basic medical degree course, including practical training: **4 years**
Entrance examination: **Yes**
Foreign students eligible: **Yes**

UNIVERSITY OF SOUTH FLORIDA COLLEGE OF MEDICINE
12901 BRUCE B. DOWNS BOULEVARD
PO BOX 53
TAMPA 33612-4799
Tel.: +1 (813) 974 4950
Fax: +1 (813) 974 5556
E-mail: jcurran@com1.med.usf.edu
Year instruction started: **1970**
Language of instruction: **English**
Duration of basic medical degree course, including practical training: **4 years**
Entrance examination: **Yes**
Foreign students eligible: **No**

■ GEORGIA
EMORY UNIVERSITY SCHOOL OF MEDICINE
1440 CLIFTON ROAD NE
ATLANTA 30322-4510
Tel.: +1 (404) 727 5640
Fax: +1 (404) 727 0473
Year instruction started: **1915**
Language of instruction: **English**
Duration of basic medical degree course, including practical training: **4 years**
Entrance examination: **Yes**
Foreign students eligible: **Yes**

MOREHOUSE SCHOOL OF MEDICINE
720 WESTVIEW DRIVE SW
ATLANTA 30310-1495
Tel.: +1 (404) 752 1650
Fax: +1 (404) 752 1512
Year instruction started: **1978**
Language of instruction: **English**
Duration of basic medical degree course, including practical training: **4 years**
Entrance examination: **Yes**
Foreign students eligible: **Yes**

MEDICAL COLLEGE OF GEORGIA
1126 15TH STREET
AUGUSTA 30912-4765
Tel.: +1 (706) 721 3217
Year instruction started: **1828**
Language of instruction: **English**
Duration of basic medical degree course, including practical training: **4 years**
Entrance examination: **Yes**
Foreign students eligible: **No**

MERCER UNIVERSITY SCHOOL OF MEDICINE
1550 COLLEGE STREET
MACON 31207
Year instruction started: **1982**

■ **HAWAII**
JOHN A. BURNS SCHOOL OF MEDICINE
UNIVERSITY OF HAWAII
1960 EAST–WEST ROAD
HONOLULU 96822
Year instruction started: **1967**

■ **ILLINOIS**
NORTHWESTERN UNIVERSITY MEDICAL SCHOOL
303 EAST CHICAGO AVENUE
PO BOX W125
CHICAGO 60611-3008
Tel.: +1 (312) 503 9443
Fax: +1 (312) 908 5502
Year instruction started: **1859**
Language of instruction: **English**
Duration of basic medical degree course, including practical training: **4 years**
Entrance examination: **Yes**
Foreign students eligible: **Yes**

RUSH MEDICAL COLLEGE
RUSH UNIVERSITY
600 SOUTH PAULINE STREET
CHICAGO 60611
Year instruction started: **1971**

PRITZKER SCHOOL OF MEDICINE
UNIVERSITY OF CHICAGO
BIOLOGICAL SCIENCES LEARNING CENTER
924 EAST 57TH STREET
CHICAGO 60637-5416
Tel.: +1 (773) 702 1939
Fax: +1 (773) 702 2598
E-mail: heather@prufrock.bsd.uchicago.edu
Year instruction started: **1927**
Language of instruction: **English**
Duration of basic medical degree course, including practical training: **4 years**
Entrance examination: **Yes**
Foreign students eligible: **Yes**

UNIVERSITY OF ILLINOIS COLLEGE OF MEDICINE AT CHICAGO
1819 WEST POLK STREET
CHICAGO 60612-7332
Tel.: +1 (312) 996 3500
Fax: +1 (312) 996 9006
E-mail: comd@uic.edu
Year instruction started: **1881**
Language of instruction: **English**
Duration of basic medical degree course, including practical training: **4 years**
Entrance examination: **Yes**
Foreign students eligible: **No**

CHICAGO COLLEGE OF OSTEOPATHIC MEDICINE
MIDWESTERN UNIVERSITY
555 31ST STREET
DOWNERS GROVE 60515
Tel.: +1 (708) 515 6059
Year instruction started: **1900**
Language of instruction: **English**
Duration of basic medical degree course, including practical training: **4 years**
Entrance examination: **Yes**
Foreign students eligible: **Yes**

STRITCH SCHOOL OF MEDICINE
LOYOLA UNIVERSITY OF CHICAGO
2160 SOUTH FIRST AVENUE
MAYWOOD 60153
Year instruction started: **1909**

THE CHICAGO MEDICAL SCHOOL
FINCH UNIVERSITY OF HEALTH SCIENCES
3333 GREEN BAY ROAD
NORTH CHICAGO 60064-3095
Tel.: +1 (847) 578 3000
Fax: +1 (847) 578 3401
Year instruction started: **1912**
Language of instruction: **English**
Duration of basic medical degree course, including practical training: **4 years**
Entrance examination: **Yes**
Foreign students eligible: **Yes**

UNIVERSITY OF ILLINOIS COLLEGE OF MEDICINE AT PEORIA
1 ILLINI DRIVE
PO BOX 1649
PEORIA 61605
Tel.: +1 (309) 671 8407
Fax: +1 (309) 671 8452
E-mail: ajp@uic.edu
Year instruction started: **1970**
Language of instruction: **English**
Duration of basic medical degree course, including practical training: **4 years**
Entrance examination: **Yes**
Foreign students eligible: **No**

UNIVERSITY OF ILLINOIS COLLEGE OF MEDICINE AT ROCKFORD
1601 PARKVIEW AVENUE
ROCKFORD 61107
Tel.: +1 (815) 395 5600
Fax: +1 (815) 395 5887
E-mail: buzs@uic.edu
Year instruction started: **1971**
Language of instruction: **English**
Duration of basic medical degree course, including practical training: **4 years**
Entrance examination: **Yes**
Foreign students eligible: **Yes**

SOUTHERN ILLINOIS UNIVERSITY SCHOOL OF MEDICINE
801 NORTH RUTLEDGE STREET
PO BOX 19230
SPRINGFIELD 62794-1215
Tel.: +1 (217) 782 3318
Fax: +1 (217) 524 0786

Year instruction started: **1970**
Language of instruction: **English**
Duration of basic medical degree course, including practical training: **4 years**
Entrance examination: **Yes**
Foreign students eligible: **No**

UNIVERSITY OF ILLINOIS COLLEGE OF MEDICINE AT URBANA-CHAMPAIGN
MEDICAL SCIENCES BUILDING 190
506 SOUTH MATHEWS STREET
URBANA 61801
Tel.: +1 (217) 333 5469
Fax: +1 (217) 333 8868
E-mail: w-sorlie@staff.uiuc.edu
Year instruction started: **1971**
Language of instruction: **English**
Duration of basic medical degree course, including practical training: **4 years**
Entrance examination: **Yes**
Foreign students eligible: **Yes**

■ **INDIANA**
INDIANA UNIVERSITY SCHOOL OF MEDICINE
635 BARNHILL DRIVE
INDIANAPOLIS 46254
Tel.: +1 (317) 274 7175
Fax: +1 (317) 274 4309
Year instruction started: **1903**
Language of instruction: **English**
Duration of basic medical degree course, including practical training: **4 years**
Entrance examination: **Yes**
Foreign students eligible: **No**

■ **IOWA**
COLLEGE OF OSTEOPATHIC MEDICINE AND HEALTH SCIENCES
3200 GRAND AVENUE
DES MOINES 50312
Tel.: +1 (515) 271 1515
Year instruction started: **1898**
Language of instruction: **English**
Duration of basic medical degree course, including practical training: **4 years**
Entrance examination: **No**
Foreign students eligible: **Yes**

UNIVERSITY OF IOWA COLLEGE OF MEDICINE
100 CMAB
IOWA CITY 52242
Year instruction started: **1870**

■ **KANSAS**
SCHOOL OF MEDICINE
UNIVERSITY OF KANSAS COLLEGE OF HEALTH SCIENCES
3901 RAINBOW BOULEVARD
KANSAS CITY 66160-7116
Tel.: +1 (913) 588 5287
Fax: +1 (913) 588 5259
Year instruction started: **1889**
Language of instruction: **English**
Duration of basic medical degree course, including practical training: **4 years**
Entrance examination: **Yes**
Foreign students eligible: **Yes**

■ **KENTUCKY**
UNIVERSITY OF KENTUCKY COLLEGE OF MEDICINE
800 ROSE STREET
LEXINGTON 40536-0084
Tel.: +1 (606) 323 6582
Fax: +1 (606) 323 2039
Year instruction started: **1960**
Language of instruction: **English**
Duration of basic medical degree course, including practical training: **4 years**
Entrance examination: **Yes**
Foreign students eligible: **Yes**

UNIVERSITY OF LOUISVILLE SCHOOL OF MEDICINE
HEALTH SCIENCES CENTER
LOUISVILLE 40292
Year instruction started: **1837**

■ **LOUISIANA**
LOUISIANA STATE UNIVERSITY SCHOOL OF MEDICINE IN NEW ORLEANS
1542 TULANE AVENUE
NEW ORLEANS 70112
Tel.: +1 (504) 568 4006
Fax: +1 (504) 568 4008

E-mail: wplauc@nomvs.lsumc.edu
Year instruction started: **1931**
Language of instruction: **English**
Duration of basic medical degree course, including practical training: **4 years**
Entrance examination: **No**
Foreign students eligible: **No**

TULANE UNIVERSITY SCHOOL OF MEDICINE
1430 TULANE AVENUE
NEW ORLEANS 70112
Year instruction started: **1834**

LOUISIANA STATE UNIVERSITY SCHOOL OF MEDICINE IN SHREVEPORT
PO BOX 33932
SHREVEPORT 71130
Year instruction started: **1969**

■ **MAINE**
UNIVERSITY OF NEW ENGLAND COLLEGE OF OSTEOPATHIC MEDICINE
ELEVEN HILLS BEACH ROAD
BIDDEFORD 04005
Year instruction started: **1977**

■ **MARYLAND**
THE JOHNS HOPKINS UNIVERSITY SCHOOL OF MEDICINE
720 RUTLAND AVENUE
BALTIMORE 21205-2196
Tel.: +1 (410) 955 8401
Fax: +1 (410) 955 2522
E-mail: cdeangel@welchgate.welch.jhu.edu
Year instruction started: **1893**
Language of instruction: **English**
Duration of basic medical degree course, including practical training: **4 years**
Entrance examination: **Yes**
Foreign students eligible: **Yes**

UNIVERSITY OF MARYLAND SCHOOL OF MEDICINE
655 WEST BALTIMORE STREET
BALTIMORE 21201
Year instruction started: **1807**

F. EDWARD HEBERT SCHOOL OF MEDICINE
UNIFORMED SERVICES UNIVERSITY OF THE HEALTH SCIENCES
4301 JONES BRIDGE ROAD
BETHESDA 20814
Year instruction started: **1976**

■ **MASSACHUSETTS**
BOSTON UNIVERSITY SCHOOL OF MEDICINE
80 EAST CONCORD STREET
BOSTON 02118
Tel.: +1 (617) 638 5300
Fax: +1 (617) 638 5258
Year instruction started: **1873**
Language of instruction: **English**
Duration of basic medical degree course, including practical training: **4 years**
Entrance examination: **No**
Foreign students eligible: **Yes**

HARVARD MEDICAL SCHOOL
25 SHATTUCK STREET
BOSTON 02115
Tel.: +1 (617) 432 0442
Fax: +1 (617) 432 0446
Year instruction started: **1782**
Language of instruction: **English**
Duration of basic medical degree course, including practical training: **4 years**
Entrance examination: **Yes**

TUFTS UNIVERSITY SCHOOL OF MEDICINE
136 HARRISON AVENUE
BOSTON 02111
Tel.: +1 (617) 636 6565
Fax: +1 (617) 636 0375
E-mail: medadmissions@infonet.tufts.edu
Year instruction started: **1893**
Language of instruction: **English**
Duration of basic medical degree course, including practical training: **4 years**
Entrance examination: **Yes**
Foreign students eligible: **Yes**

UNIVERSITY OF MASSACHUSETTS MEDICAL SCHOOL
55 LAKE AVENUE NORTH
WORCESTER 01655
Tel.: +1 (508) 856 4265
Fax: +1 (508) 856 5536
Year instruction started: **1970**
Language of instruction: **English**
Duration of basic medical degree course, including practical training: **4 years**
Entrance examination: **No**
Foreign students eligible: **No**

■ MICHIGAN
UNIVERSITY OF MICHIGAN MEDICAL SCHOOL
1335 CATHERINE STREET
ANN ARBOR 48109
Year instruction started: **1850**

WAYNE STATE UNIVERSITY SCHOOL OF MEDICINE
540 EAST CANFIELD
DETROIT 48201
Year instruction started: **1868**[1]

MICHIGAN STATE UNIVERSITY COLLEGE OF HUMAN MEDICINE
A-239 LIFE SCIENCES BUILDING
EAST LANSING 48824-1317
Tel.: +1 (517) 353 9620
Fax: +1 (517) 432 0021
Year instruction started: **1966**

MICHIGAN STATE UNIVERSITY COLLEGE OF OSTEOPATHIC MEDICINE
A308 EAST FEE HALL
EAST LANSING 48824-1316
Tel.: +1 (517) 355 9616
Fax: +1 (517) 355 9862
Year instruction started: **1970**
Language of instruction: **English**
Duration of basic medical degree course, including practical training: **4 years**
Entrance examination: **Yes**
Foreign students eligible: **Yes**

---

[1] As Detroit Medical College.

■ MINNESOTA

SCHOOL OF MEDICINE
UNIVERSITY OF MINNESOTA AT DULUTH
10 UNIVERSITY DRIVE
DULUTH 55812
Tel.: +1 (218) 726 7571
Fax: +1 (218) 726 6235
Year instruction started: **1972**
Language of instruction: **English**
Duration of basic medical degree course, including practical training: **4 years**
Entrance examination: **Yes**
Foreign students eligible: **No**

UNIVERSITY OF MINNESOTA MEDICAL SCHOOL, MINNEAPOLIS
420 DELAWARE STREET SE
PO BOX 293 UMHC
MINNEAPOLIS 55455
Tel.: +1 (612) 626 4949
Fax: +1 (612) 626 4911
E-mail: cerra001@maroon.tc.umn.edu
Year instruction started: **1888**
Language of instruction: **English**
Duration of basic medical degree course, including practical training: **4 years**
Entrance examination: **Yes**
Foreign students eligible: **No**

MAYO MEDICAL SCHOOL
200 FIRST STREET SW
ROCHESTER 55905
Tel.: +1 (507) 284 8219
Fax: +1 (507) 284 2634
E-mail: mcarey@mayo.edu
Year instruction started: **1972**
Language of instruction: **English**
Duration of basic medical degree course, including practical training: **4 years**
Entrance examination: **Yes**
Foreign students eligible: **No**

■ MISSISSIPPI

UNIVERSITY OF MISSISSIPPI SCHOOL OF MEDICINE
2500 NORTH STATE STREET
JACKSON 39216
Tel.: +1 (601) 984 1010
Fax: +1 (601) 984 1013

Year instruction started: **1903**
Language of instruction: **English**
Duration of basic medical degree course, including practical training: **4 years**
Entrance examination: **Yes**
Foreign students eligible: **No**

■ MISSOURI
COLUMBIA SCHOOL OF MEDICINE
UNIVERSITY OF MISSOURI
1 HOSPITAL DRIVE
COLUMBIA 65212
Tel.: +1 (573) 882 2923
Fax: +1 (573) 884 4808
Year instruction started: **1873**
Language of instruction: **English**
Duration of basic medical degree course, including practical training: **4 years**
Entrance examination: **Yes**
Foreign students eligible: **No**

UNIVERSITY OF HEALTH SCIENCES COLLEGE OF OSTEOPATHIC MEDICINE
2105 INDEPENDENCE BOULEVARD
KANSAS CITY 64124
Tel.: +1 (816) 283 2000
Fax: +1 (816) 283 2349
Year instruction started: **1916**
Language of instruction: **English**
Duration of basic medical degree course, including practical training: **4 years**
Entrance examination: **Yes**
Foreign students eligible: **Yes**

KANSAS CITY SCHOOL OF MEDICINE
UNIVERSITY OF MISSOURI
2411 HOLMES STREET
KANSAS CITY 64108
Year instruction started: **1971**

KIRKSVILLE COLLEGE OF OSTEOPATHIC MEDICINE
800 WEST JEFFERSON STREET
KIRKSVILLE 63501
Tel.: +1 (816) 626 2354
Fax: +1 (816) 626 2080

Year instruction started: **1892**
Language of instruction: **English**
Duration of basic medical degree course, including practical training: **4 years**
Entrance examination: **Yes**
Foreign students eligible: **No**

ST LOUIS UNIVERSITY SCHOOL OF MEDICINE
1402 SOUTH GRAND BOULEVARD
ST LOUIS 63104
Tel.: +1 (314) 577 8622
Fax: +1 (314) 771 9316
E-mail: galofrea@sluvca.slu.edu
Year instruction started: **1903**
Language of instruction: **English**
Duration of basic medical degree course, including practical training: **4 years**
Entrance examination: **Yes**
Foreign students eligible: **Yes**

WASHINGTON UNIVERSITY SCHOOL OF MEDICINE
660 SOUTH EUCLID AVENUE
ST LOUIS 63110-1093
Tel.: +1 (314) 362 6844
Fax: +1 (314) 362 4658
E-mail: wumscoa@wustl.edu
Year instruction started: **1891**
Language of instruction: **English**
Duration of basic medical degree course, including practical training: **4 years**
Entrance examination: **Yes**
Foreign students eligible: **Yes**

■ **NEBRASKA**
CREIGHTON UNIVERSITY SCHOOL OF MEDICINE
2500 CALIFORNIA PLAZA
OMAHA 68178
Tel.: +1 (402) 280 2900
Fax: +1 (402) 280 2599
E-mail: medical@creighton.edu
Year instruction started: **1892**
Language of instruction: **English**
Duration of basic medical degree course, including practical training: **4 years**
Entrance examination: **Yes**
Foreign students eligible: **Yes**

UNIVERSITY OF NEBRASKA COLLEGE OF MEDICINE
600 SOUTH 42ND STREET
PO BOX 986545
OMAHA 68198-1220
Tel.: +1 (402) 559 4204
Fax: +1 (402) 559 4148
Year instruction started: **1918**
Language of instruction: **English**
Duration of basic medical degree course, including practical training: **4 years**
Entrance examination: **Yes**
Foreign students eligible: **No**

■ **NEVADA**
UNIVERSITY OF NEVADA SCHOOL OF MEDICAL SCIENCES
MANVILLE MEDICAL SCIENCE BUILDING
RENO 89557-0046
Year instruction started: **1971**

■ **NEW HAMPSHIRE**
DARTMOUTH MEDICAL SCHOOL
DARTMOUTH–HITCHCOCK MEDICAL CENTER
HANOVER 03755-3833
Tel.: +1 (603) 650 1481
Fax: +1 (603) 650 1614
Year instruction started: **1797**

■ **NEW JERSEY**
NEW JERSEY MEDICAL SCHOOL
UNIVERSITY OF MEDICINE AND DENTISTRY OF NEW JERSEY AT NEWARK
185 SOUTH ORANGE AVENUE
UNIVERSITY HEIGHTS
NEWARK 07103-2714
Tel.: +1 (973) 972 4538
Fax: +1 (973) 972 7104
Year instruction started: **1956**
Language of instruction: **English**
Duration of basic medical degree course, including practical training: **4 years**
Entrance examination: **Yes**
Foreign students eligible: **No**

ROBERT WOOD JOHNSON MEDICAL SCHOOL
UNIVERSITY OF MEDICINE AND DENTISTRY OF NEW JERSEY
675 HOES LANE
PISCATAWAY 08854
Year instruction started: **1966**

SCHOOL OF OSTEOPATHIC MEDICINE
UNIVERSITY OF MEDICINE AND DENTISTRY OF NEW JERSEY
1 MEDICAL CENTER DRIVE
STRATFORD 08084-1501
Tel.: +1 (609) 566 6010
Fax: +1 (609) 566 6895
Year instruction started: **1976**
Language of instruction: **English**
Duration of basic medical degree course, including practical training: **4 years**
Entrance examination: **Yes**
Foreign students eligible: **No**

■ **NEW MEXICO**
UNIVERSITY OF NEW MEXICO SCHOOL OF MEDICINE
HEALTH SCIENCE CENTER
BSMB 177
ALBUQUERQUE 87131-5116
Tel.: +1 (505) 277 2321
Fax: +1 (505) 277 6581
E-mail: pburge@medusa.unm.edu
Year instruction started: **1964**
Language of instruction: **English**
Duration of basic medical degree course, including practical training: **4 years**
Entrance examination: **Yes**
Foreign students eligible: **No**

■ **NEW YORK**
ALBANY MEDICAL COLLEGE OF UNION UNIVERSITY
47 NEW SCOTLAND AVENUE
ALBANY 12208
Tel.: +1 (518) 262 5548
Fax: +1 (518) 262 5029
E-mail: redmonds@ccgateway.amc.edu
Year instruction started: **1839**
Language of instruction: **English**
Duration of basic medical degree course, including practical training: **4 years**
Entrance examination: **Yes**
Foreign students eligible: **Yes**

ALBERT EINSTEIN COLLEGE OF MEDICINE OF YESHIVA UNIVERSITY
1300 MORRIS PARK AVENUE
BRONX 10461
Tel.: +1 (718) 430 2106
Fax: +1 (718) 430 8825
E-mail: admissions@aecom.yu.edu
Year instruction started: **1955**
Language of instruction: **English**
Duration of basic medical degree course, including practical training: **4 years**
Entrance examination: **Yes**
Foreign students eligible: **Yes**

STATE UNIVERSITY OF NEW YORK HEALTH SCIENCE CENTER AT BROOKLYN
450 CLARKSON AVENUE
PO BOX 97
BROOKLYN 11203
Year instruction started: **1860**

SCHOOL OF MEDICINE AND BIOMEDICAL SCIENCES
STATE UNIVERSITY OF NEW YORK AT BUFFALO
40 BIOMEDICAL EDUCATION BUILDING
BUFFALO 14214
Tel.: +1 (716) 829 3467
Fax: +1 (716) 829 2798
Year instruction started: **1846**
Language of instruction: **English**
Duration of basic medical degree course, including practical training: **4 years**
Entrance examination: **Yes**
Foreign students eligible: **No**

COLUMBIA UNIVERSITY COLLEGE OF PHYSICIANS AND SURGEONS
630 WEST 168TH STREET
NEW YORK 10032
Tel.: +1 (212) 305 3595
Fax: +1 (212) 305 3545
E-mail: pt8@columbia.edu
Year instruction started: **1767**
Language of instruction: **English**
Entrance examination: **Yes**
Foreign students eligible: **Yes**

CORNELL UNIVERSITY MEDICAL COLLEGE
1300 YORK AVENUE
NEW YORK 10021
Tel.: +1 (212) 746 5454
Fax: +1 (212) 746 8745
Year instruction started: **1898**
Language of instruction: **English**
Duration of basic medical degree course, including practical training: **4 years**
Entrance examination: **Yes**
Foreign students eligible: **Yes**

MOUNT SINAI SCHOOL OF MEDICINE OF THE CITY UNIVERSITY OF NEW
    YORK
1 GUSTAVE L. LEVY PLACE
NEW YORK 10029
Year instruction started: **1968**

NEW YORK UNIVERSITY SCHOOL OF MEDICINE
550 FIRST AVENUE
NEW YORK 10016
Year instruction started: **1842**

NEW YORK COLLEGE OF OSTEOPATHIC MEDICINE
NEW YORK INSTITUTE OF TECHNOLOGY
WHEATLEY ROAD
PO BOX 170
OLD WESTBURY 11568
Year instruction started: **1977**

UNIVERSITY OF ROCHESTER SCHOOL OF MEDICINE AND DENTISTRY
601 ELMWOOD AVENUE
PO BOX 601
ROCHESTER 14642
Tel.: +1 (716) 275 4539
Fax: +1 (716) 273 1016
E-mail: mdadmish@urmc.rochester.edu
Year instruction started: **1925**
Language of instruction: **English**
Duration of basic medical degree course, including practical training: **4 years**
Entrance examination: **No**
Foreign students eligible: **Yes**

STATE UNIVERSITY OF NEW YORK SCHOOL OF MEDICINE AT STONY
 BROOK
HEALTH SCIENCES CENTER
STONY BROOK 11794-8432
Tel.: +1 (516) 444 2080
Fax: +1 (516) 444 2202
Year instruction started: **1971**
Language of instruction: **English**
Duration of basic medical degree course, including practical training: **4 years**
Entrance examination: **Yes**
Foreign students eligible: **Yes**

STATE UNIVERSITY OF NEW YORK COLLEGE OF MEDICINE AT SYRACUSE
HEALTH SCIENCE CENTER
750 EAST ADAMS STREET
SYRACUSE 13210
Tel.: +1 (315) 464 4515
Fax: +1 (315) 464 5565
Year instruction started: **1834**
Language of instruction: **English**
Duration of basic medical degree course, including practical training: **4 years**
Entrance examination: **Yes**
Foreign students eligible: **Yes**

NEW YORK MEDICAL COLLEGE
ADMINISTRATION BUILDING
SUNSHINE COTTAGE
VALHALLA 10595
Tel.: +1 (914) 993 4900
Fax: +1 (914) 993 4145
Year instruction started: **1860**
Language of instruction: **English**
Duration of basic medical degree course, including practical training: **4 years**
Entrance examination: **Yes**
Foreign students eligible: **Yes**

■ **NORTH CAROLINA**
SCHOOL OF MEDICINE
UNIVERSITY OF NORTH CAROLINA AT CHAPEL HILL
121 MACNIDER 202H
CHAPEL HILL 27599
Year instruction started: **1879**

DUKE UNIVERSITY SCHOOL OF MEDICINE
DUKE UNIVERSITY MEDICAL CENTER
PO BOX 3005
DURHAM 27710
Year instruction started: **1930**

EAST CAROLINA UNIVERSITY SCHOOL OF MEDICINE
MOYE BOULEVARD
GREENVILLE 27858-4354
Tel.: +1 (919) 816 2984
Fax: +1 (919) 816 3312
Year instruction started: **1977**
Language of instruction: **English**
Duration of basic medical degree course, including practical training: **4 years**
Entrance examination: **Yes**
Foreign students eligible: **No**

THE BOWMAN GRAY SCHOOL OF MEDICINE OF WAKE FOREST UNIVERSITY
MEDICAL CENTER BOULEVARD
WINSTON-SALEM 27157
Tel.: +1 (910) 716 2011
Fax: +1 (910) 716 4204
Year instruction started: **1941**
Language of instruction: **English**
Duration of basic medical degree course, including practical training: **4 years**
Entrance examination: **Yes**
Foreign students eligible: **Yes**

■ **NORTH DAKOTA**
UNIVERSITY OF NORTH DAKOTA SCHOOL OF MEDICINE
501 COLOMBIA ROAD NORTH
GRAND FORKS 58202

■ **OHIO**
OHIO UNIVERSITY COLLEGE OF OSTEOPATHIC MEDICINE
102 GROSVENOR AND IRVINE HALLS
ATHENS 45701
Tel.: +1 (614) 593 4313
Fax: +1 (614) 593 2256
Year instruction started: **1974**
Language of instruction: **English**
Duration of basic medical degree course, including practical training: **4 years**
Entrance examination: **Yes**
Foreign students eligible: **No**

UNIVERSITY OF CINCINNATI COLLEGE OF MEDICINE
MAIL LOCATION 552
231 BETHESDA AVENUE
CINCINNATI 45267
Year instruction started: **1819**

CASE WESTERN RESERVE UNIVERSITY SCHOOL OF MEDICINE
10900 EUCLID AVENUE
CLEVELAND 44106-4915
Tel.: +1 (216) 368 2825
Fax: +1 (216) 368 3013
Year instruction started: **1843**
Language of instruction: **English**
Duration of basic medical degree course, including practical training: **4 years**
Entrance examination: **Yes**
Foreign students eligible: **Yes**

THE OHIO STATE UNIVERSITY COLLEGE OF MEDICINE
370 WEST 9TH AVENUE
COLUMBUS 43210-1238
Year instruction started: **1833**

WRIGHT STATE UNIVERSITY SCHOOL OF MEDICINE
3640 COLONEL GLENN HIGHWAY
PO BOX 927
DAYTON 45435
Tel.: +1 (513) 873 3010
Fax: +1 (513) 873 3672
E-mail: dean@med.wright.edu
Year instruction started: **1976**
Language of instruction: **English**
Duration of basic medical degree course, including practical training: **4 years**
Entrance examination: **Yes**
Foreign students eligible: **No**

NORTHEASTERN OHIO UNIVERSITIES COLLEGE OF MEDICINE
4209 STATE ROUTE 44
PO BOX 95
ROOTSTOWN 44272-0095
Tel.: +1 (303) 325 2511
Fax: +1 (303) 325 7943

Year instruction started: **1977**
Language of instruction: **English**
Duration of basic medical degree course, including practical training: **4 years**
Entrance examination: **Yes**
Foreign students eligible: **No**

MEDICAL COLLEGE OF OHIO AT TOLEDO
3000 ARLINGTON AVENUE
PO BOX 10008
TOLEDO 43699-0008
Tel.: +1 (419) 381 4172
Year instruction started: **1969**
Language of instruction: **English**
Duration of basic medical degree course, including practical training: **4 years**
Entrance examination: **Yes**
Foreign students eligible: **No**

■ **OKLAHOMA**
UNIVERSITY OF OKLAHOMA SCHOOL OF MEDICINE
800 NORTHEAST 13TH STREET
OKLAHOMA CITY 73190
Year instruction started: **1900**

OKLAHOMA STATE UNIVERSITY COLLEGE OF OSTEOPATHIC MEDICINE
1111 WEST 17TH STREET
TULSA 74107
Tel.: +1 (918) 561 8201
Fax: +1 (918) 561 8413
E-mail: allen@vms.ocom.okstate.edu
Year instruction started: **1974**
Language of instruction: **English**
Duration of basic medical degree course, including practical training: **4 years**
Entrance examination: **Yes**
Foreign students eligible: **Yes**

■ **OREGON**
THE OREGON HEALTH SCIENCES UNIVERSITY SCHOOL OF MEDICINE
3181 S.W. SAM JACKSON
PARK ROAD L102
PORTLAND 97201
Tel.: +1 (503) 494 4329
Fax: +1 (503) 494 3400

Year instruction started: **1887**
Language of instruction: **English**
Duration of basic medical degree course, including practical training: **4 years**
Entrance examination: **Yes**
Foreign students eligible: **No**

■ **PENNSYLVANIA**
LAKE ERIE COLLEGE OF OSTEOPATHIC MEDICINE
1858 WEST GRANDVIEW BOULEVARD
ERIE 16509
Tel.: +1 (814) 866 6641
Fax: +1 (814) 866 8123
Year instruction started: **1993**
Language of instruction: **English**
Duration of basic medical degree course, including practical training: **4 years**
Entrance examination: **Yes**
Foreign students eligible: **Yes**

THE PENNSYLVANIA STATE UNIVERSITY COLLEGE OF MEDICINE
THE MILTON S. HERSHEY MEDICAL CENTER
500 UNIVERSITY DRIVE
PO BOX 850
HERSHEY 17033
Year instruction started: **1967**

MEDICAL COLLEGE OF PENNSYLVANIA AND HAHNEMANN UNIVERSITY
2900 QUEEN LANE
PHILADELPHIA 19129
Tel.:+1 (215) 991 8100
Fax: +1 (215) 843 0214
Year instruction started: **1848**
Language of instruction: **English**
Duration of basic medical degree course, including practical training: **4 years**
Entrance examination: **Yes**
Foreign students eligible: **Yes**

PHILADELPHIA COLLEGE OF OSTEOPATHIC MEDICINE
4150 CITY AVENUE
PHILADELPHIA 19131
Year instruction started: **1899**

TEMPLE UNIVERSITY SCHOOL OF MEDICINE
3400 NORTH BROAD STREET
PHILADELPHIA 19140
Tel.: +1 (215) 707 4613
Fax: +1 (215) 707 2940
Year instruction started: **1901**
Language of instruction: **English**
Duration of basic medical degree course, including practical training: **4 years**
Entrance examination: **No**
Foreign students eligible: **Yes**

JEFFERSON MEDICAL COLLEGE
THOMAS JEFFERSON UNIVERSITY
1025 WALNUT STREET
PHILADELPHIA 19107-5083
Tel.: +1 (215) 955 6980
Fax: +1 (215) 923 6939
E-mail: dean.jmc@mail.tju.edu
Year instruction started: **1824**
Language of instruction: **English**
Duration of basic medical degree course, including practical training: **4 years**
Entrance examination: **Yes**
Foreign students eligible: **Yes**

UNIVERSITY OF PENNSYLVANIA SCHOOL OF MEDICINE
3450 HAMILTON WALK
SUITE 100
PHILADELPHIA 19104-6087
Tel.: +1 (215) 898 8034
Fax: +1 (215) 898 0833
Year instruction started: **1765**
Language of instruction: **English**
Duration of basic medical degree course, including practical training: **4 years**
Entrance examination: **No**
Foreign students eligible: **Yes**

UNIVERSITY OF PITTSBURGH SCHOOL OF MEDICINE
3550 TERRACE STREET
M240 SCAIFE HALL
PITTSBURGH 15261
Tel.: +1 (412) 648 8975
Fax: +1 (412) 648 1236

Year instruction started: **1886**
Language of instruction: **English**
Duration of basic medical degree course, including practical training: **4 years**
Entrance examination: **Yes**
Foreign students eligible: **No**

■ **RHODE ISLAND**
BROWN UNIVERSITY SCHOOL OF MEDICINE
97 WATERMAN STREET
PO BOX G
PROVIDENCE 02912
Tel.: +1 (401) 863 2894
Fax: +1 (401) 863 2660
E-mail: stephen_r_smith@brown.edu
Year instruction started: **1963**
Language of instruction: **English**
Duration of basic medical degree course, including practical training: **4–8 years**
Entrance examination: **No**
Foreign students eligible: **Yes**

■ **SOUTH CAROLINA**
COLLEGE OF MEDICINE
MEDICAL UNIVERSITY OF SOUTH CAROLINA
171 ASHLEY AVENUE
CHARLESTON 29425
Year instruction started: **1824**

UNIVERSITY OF SOUTH CAROLINA SCHOOL OF MEDICINE
COLUMBIA 29208
Tel.: +1 (803) 733 3325
Fax: +1 (803) 733 3328
Year instruction started: **1977**

■ **SOUTH DAKOTA**
UNIVERSITY OF SOUTH DAKOTA MEDICAL SCHOOL
2501 WEST 22ND STREET
SIOUX FALLS 57105
Year instruction started: **1907**

■ **TENNESSEE**
JAMES H. QUILLEN COLLEGE OF MEDICINE
EAST TENNESSEE STATE UNIVERSITY
FIFTH STREET
PO BOX 70571
JOHNSON CITY 37601

Tel.: +1 (423) 929 6327
Fax: +1 (423) 975 8340
E-mail: wootend@etsuserv.east-tenn-st.edu
Year instruction started: **1978**
Language of instruction: **English**
Duration of basic medical degree course, including practical training: **4 years**
Entrance examination: **Yes**
Foreign students eligible: **No**

THE UNIVERSITY OF TENNESSEE COLLEGE OF MEDICINE AT MEMPHIS
62 SOUTH DUNLAP
420 HYMAN BOULEVARD
MEMPHIS 38163-2101
Tel.: +1 (901) 448 5506
Fax: +1 (901) 448 7683
Year instruction started: **1911**
Language of instruction: **English**
Duration of basic medical degree course, including practical training: **4 years**
Entrance examination: **Yes**

MEHARRY MEDICAL COLLEGE
105 D.B. TODD JR BOULEVARD
NASHVILLE 37208
Year instruction started: **1875**

VANDERBILT UNIVERSITY SCHOOL OF MEDICINE
21ST AND GARLAND AVENUES
NASHVILLE 37232
Year instruction started: **1875**

■ TEXAS
TEXAS A & M UNIVERSITY COLLEGE OF MEDICINE
147 REYNOLDS MEDICAL BUILDING
COLLEGE STATION 77843-1114
Tel.: +1 (409) 845 7743
Fax: +1 (409) 847 8663
Year instruction started: **1978**
Language of instruction: **English**
Duration of basic medical degree course, including practical training: **4 years**
Entrance examination: **Yes**
Foreign students eligible: **No**

UNIVERSITY OF TEXAS SOUTHWESTERN MEDICAL SCHOOL AT DALLAS
5323 HARRY HINES BOULEVARD
DALLAS 75235-9012
Tel.: +1 (214) 648 3111
Year instruction started: **1943**
Language of instruction: **English**
Duration of basic medical degree course, including practical training: **4 years**
Entrance examination: **Yes**
Foreign students eligible: **No**

TEXAS COLLEGE OF OSTEOPATHIC MEDICINE
UNIVERSITY OF NORTH TEXAS
HEALTH SCIENCE CENTER AT FORT WORTH
3500 CAMP BOWIE BOULEVARD
FORT WORTH 76107-2699
Tel.: +1 (817) 735 2000
Fax: +1 (817) 735 2486
Year instruction started: **1970**
Language of instruction: **English**
Duration of basic medical degree course, including practical training: **4 years**
Entrance examination: **Yes**
Foreign students eligible: **No**

UNIVERSITY OF TEXAS MEDICAL BRANCH AT GALVESTON
301 UNIVERSITY BOULEVARD
GALVESTON 77555-1305
Tel.: +1 (409) 772 1011
Year instruction started: **1891**
Language of instruction: **English**
Entrance examination: **Yes**
Foreign students eligible: **No**

BAYLOR COLLEGE OF MEDICINE
1 BAYLOR PLAZA
HOUSTON 77030
Tel.: +1 (713) 798 4433
Fax: +1 (713) 790 0055
Year instruction started: **1900**
Language of instruction: **English**
Duration of basic medical degree course, including practical training: **4 years**
Entrance examination: **Yes**
Foreign students eligible: **Yes**

UNIVERSITY OF TEXAS MEDICAL SCHOOL AT HOUSTON
PO BOX 20708
HOUSTON 77225
Year instruction started: **1971**

TEXAS TECHNICAL UNIVERSITY SCHOOL OF MEDICINE
HEALTH SCIENCES CENTER
3601 4TH STREET
PO BOX 4569
LUBBOCK 79430
Tel.: +1 (806) 743 3000
Fax: +1 (806) 743 3021
Year instruction started: **1972**
Language of instruction: **English**
Duration of basic medical degree course, including practical training: **4 years**
Entrance examination: **Yes**
Foreign students eligible: **No**

UNIVERSITY OF TEXAS MEDICAL SCHOOL AT SAN ANTONIO
7703 FLOYD CURL DRIVE
SAN ANTONIO 78284-7790
Tel.: +1 (210) 567 4420
Fax: +1 (210) 567 6962
E-mail: youngj@uthscsa.edu
Year instruction started: **1968**
Language of instruction: **English**
Duration of basic medical degree course, including practical training: **4 years**
Entrance examination: **Yes**
Foreign students eligible: **Yes**

■ **UTAH**
UNIVERSITY OF UTAH SCHOOL OF MEDICINE
50 NORTH MEDICAL DRIVE
SALT LAKE CITY 84132
Tel.: +1 (801) 581 7201
Fax: +1 (801) 585 3300
Year instruction started: **1904**
Language of instruction: **English**
Duration of basic medical degree course, including practical training: **4 years**
Entrance examination: **Yes**
Foreign students eligible: **Yes**

■ VERMONT

UNIVERSITY OF VERMONT COLLEGE OF MEDICINE
GIVEN BUILDING
BURLINGTON 05405
Tel.: +1 (802) 656 2156
Fax: +1 (802) 656 8577
Year instruction started: **1822**
Language of instruction: **English**
Duration of basic medical degree course, including practical training: **4 years**
Entrance examination: **Yes**
Foreign students eligible: **Yes**

■ VIRGINIA

UNIVERSITY OF VIRGINIA SCHOOL OF MEDICINE
MCKIM HALL
PO BOX 395
CHARLOTTESVILLE 22908
Tel.: +1 (804) 924 8418
Fax: +1 (804) 982 0874
Year instruction started: **1825**
Language of instruction: **English**
Duration of basic medical degree course, including practical training: **4 years**
Entrance examination: **Yes**
Foreign students eligible: **Yes**

EASTERN VIRGINIA MEDICAL SCHOOL
700 OLNEY ROAD
PO BOX 1980
NORFOLK 23501
Year instruction started: **1973**

MEDICAL COLLEGE OF VIRGINIA
VIRGINIA COMMONWEALTH UNIVERSITY
1101 EAST MARSHALL STREET
PO BOX 980565
RICHMOND 23298
Tel.: +1 (804) 828 9790
Fax: +1 (804) 828 5115
E-mail: jmmessme@gems.vcu.edu
Year instruction started: **1838**
Language of instruction: **English**
Duration of basic medical degree course, including practical training: **4 years**
Entrance examination: **Yes**
Foreign students eligible: **No**

■ WASHINGTON
UNIVERSITY OF WASHINGTON SCHOOL OF MEDICINE
51–64 PACIFIC AVENUE
PO BOX 356340
SEATTLE 98195
Tel.: +1 (206) 543 5560
Fax: +1 (206) 543 3639
E-mail: dhunt@u.washington.edu
Year instruction started: **1947**
Language of instruction: **English**
Duration of basic medical degree course, including practical training: **4 years**
Entrance examination: **Yes**
Foreign students eligible: **No**

■ WEST VIRGINIA
MARSHALL UNIVERSITY SCHOOL OF MEDICINE
1801 SIXTH AVENUE
HUNTINGTON 25755
Tel.: +1 (304) 696 7000
Year instruction started: **1978**
Language of instruction: **English**
Duration of basic medical degree course, including practical training: **4 years**
Entrance examination: **Yes**
Foreign students eligible: **No**

WEST VIRGINIA SCHOOL OF OSTEOPATHIC MEDICINE
400 NORTH LEE STREET
LEWISBURG 24901
Tel.: +1 (304) 645 6270
Fax: +1 (304) 645 4859
Year instruction started: **1972**
Language of instruction: **English**
Duration of basic medical degree course, including practical training: **4 years**
Entrance examination: **Yes**
Foreign students eligible: **No**

WEST VIRGINIA UNIVERSITY SCHOOL OF MEDICINE
ROBERT C. BYRD HEALTH SCIENCES CENTER
PO BOX 9111
MORGANTOWN 26506-9111

Tel.: +1 (304) 293 2408
Fax: +1 (304) 293 7814
Year instruction started: **1910**
Language of instruction: **English**
Duration of basic medical degree course, including practical training: **4 years**
Entrance examination: **Yes**
Foreign students eligible: **Yes**

■ WISCONSIN
UNIVERSITY OF WISCONSIN MEDICAL SCHOOL
1300 UNIVERSITY AVENUE
MADISON 53706
Year instruction started: **1907**

MEDICAL COLLEGE OF WISCONSIN
8701 WATERTOWN PLANK ROAD
PO BOX 25609
MILWAUKEE 53266
Tel.: +1 (414) 456 8296
Year instruction started: **1913**
Language of instruction: **English**
Duration of basic medical degree course, including practical training: **4 years**
Entrance examination: **Yes**
Foreign students eligible: **Yes**

URUGUAY

Total population in 1995: **3 204 000**
Number of physicians per 100 000 population (1993): **309**
Number of medical schools: **1**
Duration of basic medical degree course, including practical training: **8.5 years**
Title of degree awarded: *Doctor en Medicina* (**Doctor of Medicine**)
Medical registration/licence to practise: —
Work in government service after graduation: —
Agreements with other countries: —

FACULTAD DE MEDICINA
UNIVERSIDAD DE LA REPUBLICA DEL URUGUAY
AVENIDA GENERAL FLORES 2125
MONTEVIDEO 11800
Tel.: +598 (2) 943 414
Fax: +598 (2) 943 414

E-mail: postmaster@biname.edu.uy
Year instruction started: **1875**
Language of instruction: **Spanish**
Duration of basic medical degree course, including practical training: **8.5 years**
Entrance examination: **No**
Foreign students eligible: **No**

UZBEKISTAN

Total population in 1995: **23 209 000**
Number of physicians per 100 000 population (1993): **335**
Number of medical schools: **10**
Duration of basic medical degree course, including practical training: **6–7 years (a further year of supervised clinical practice in the area of specialization is required before the degree is awarded)**
Title of degree awarded: **General Practitioner**
Medical registration/licence to practise: **Physicians must register with the local authorities. The licence to practise medicine is granted by the Ministry of Health of the Republic of Uzbekistan, Navoi Street 12, 700011 Tashkent, following an internship of at least 5 years. Foreigners may practise only if they obtain permission from the Ministry of Labour on the basis of a temporary contract with a health organization or institution in Uzbekistan, and hold a degree recognized by the Ministry of Health**
Work in government service after graduation: —
Agreements with other countries: **Agreements are being concluded between countries of the Commonwealth of Independent States.**

ANDIZAN STATE MEDICAL INSTITUTE
PROSPEKT NAVOI 124
ANDIZAN 710015
Year instruction started: **1955**

BUKHARA STATE MEDICAL INSTITUTE
PROSPEKT NAVOI 1
BUKHARA 705018

MEDICAL CENTRE
FERGANA STATE UNIVERSITY
ULICA A. NAVOIJ 13
FERGANA 712000
Tel.: +7 (3722) 248 010

Year instruction started: **1992**
Language of instruction: **Uzbek, Russian**
Duration of basic medical degree course, including practical training: **6 years**
Entrance examination: **Yes**
Foreign students eligible: **No**

FACULTY OF MEDICINE
KARAKALPAK BRANCH OF TASHKENT PAEDIATRIC MEDICAL INSTITUTE
ULICA UNIVERSITETSKAYA 1
NUKUS 742012

SAMARKAND STATE MEDICAL INSTITUTE
ULICA AMIRA-TIMURA 18
SAMARKAND 703000
Year instruction started: **1930**

FIRST TASHKENT STATE MEDICAL INSTITUTE
ULICA KHAMZA 103
TASHKENT 700048
Tel.: +7 (3712) 676 305
Fax: +7 (3712) 336 226
Year instruction started: **1920**
Language of instruction: **Uzbek, Russian**
Duration of basic medical degree course, including practical training: **6–7 years**
Entrance examination: **Yes**
Foreign students eligible: **Yes**

SECOND TASHKENT STATE MEDICAL INSTITUTE
2 FAROBI STREET
TASHKENT 700019
Tel.: +7 (3712) 469 648/468 311/467 239
Fax: +7 (3712) 467 001/442 603/443 183
E-mail: eric@tashmi.silk.glas.apc.org
Year instruction started: **1990**
Language of instruction: **Uzbek, Russian**
Duration of basic medical degree course, including practical training: **7 years**
Entrance examination: **Yes**
Foreign students eligible: **Yes**

TASHKENT PEDIATRIC MEDICAL INSTITUTE
ULICA ABIDOVOJ 123
TASHKENT 700140
Tel.: +7 (3712) 603 249

Year instruction started: **1972**
Language of instruction: **Uzbek, Russian**
Duration of basic medical degree course, including practical training: **6 years**
Entrance examination: **Yes**

TASHKENT PHARMACEUTICAL INSTITUTE
AIBEK STREET 45
TASHKENT 700015

MEDICAL CENTRE
URGENCH BRANCH OF FIRST TASHKENT STATE MEDICAL INSTITUTE
AL KHORAZMI STREET 25
URGENCH 740000
Tel.: +7 (3620) 615 44
Year instruction started: **1992**
Language of instruction: **Uzbek, Russian**
Duration of basic medical degree course, including practical training: **7 years**
Entrance examination: **Yes**

VANUATU

Total population in 1995: **174 000**
Number of physicians per 100 000 population (1993): —
Number of medical schools: **None**
Medical registration/licence to practise: **Registration is obligatory with the Health Practitioners Board of the Ministry of Health (correspondence should be addressed to the Minister of Health, Private Mail Bag 009, Port Vila). The licence to practise medicine is granted to holders of a degree from a recognized medical school provided that their qualifications entitle them to practise in the country in which the degree or diploma was granted. Foreigners may be granted a 2-year licence to practise.**
Work in government service after graduation: **Obligatory**
Agreements with other countries: **None**

VENEZUELA

Total population in 1995: **22 311 000**
Number of physicians per 100 000 population (1993): **194**
Number of medical schools: **9**
Duration of basic medical degree course, including practical training: **6.5–7 years (a period of practice in a rural area is required before the degree is awarded)**
Title of degree awarded: *Médico Cirujano* **(Physician and Surgeon)**

Medical registration/licence to practise: **Registration is obligatory with the**
Ministerio de Sanidad y Asistencia Social, Edificio Sur, Piso 9, Centro Simón
Bolivar, Caracas 1010, **as well as with the** *Colegio de Medicos* **(medical**
board) of the State in which the graduate intends to practise medicine. The
licence to practise is granted by the *Ministerio de Sanidad y Asistencia*
Social **to holders of a degree issued or validated by a a recognized Venezue-**
lan university. Foreigners may practise only if they have permanent resi-
dence status.

Work in government service after graduation: **Obligatory (all physicians must**
work for a time in a rural area)

Agreements with other countries: **Agreements exist with Bolivia, Colombia,**
Ecuador and Peru.

FACULTAD DE CIENCIAS DE LA SALUD
UNIVERSIDAD DE CARABOBA
NUCLEO
ARAGUA
Year instruction started: **1974**

ESCUELA DE MEDICINA "DR PABLO ACOSTA ORTIZ"
UNIVERSIDAD CENTRO-OCCIDENTAL "LISANDRO ALVARADO"
AVENIDA LIBERATOR CON AVENIDA ANDRES
APDO 516
BARQUISIMETO
Tel.: +58 (51) 519 798/519 898
Fax: +58 (51) 519 589
Year instruction started: **1963**
Language of instruction: **Spanish**
Duration of basic medical degree course, including practical training: **6.5 years**
Entrance examination: **Yes**
Foreign students eligible: **Yes**

ESCUELA DE MEDICINA JOSE MARIA VARGAS
UNIVERSIDAD CENTRAL DE VENEZUELA
ESQUINA SAN LORENZO Y SAN JOSE
APDO 6750
CARACAS 1010
Tel.: +58 (2) 562 9509
Fax: +58 (2) 562 9928
Year instruction started: **1989**
Language of instruction: **Spanish**
Duration of basic medical degree course, including practical training: **6.5 years**
Entrance examination: **Yes**
Foreign students eligible: **Yes**

ESCUELA DE MEDICINA "LUIS RAZETTI"
UNIVERSIDAD CENTRAL DE VENEZUELA
CIUDAD UNIVERSITARIA
CARACAS 1050
Tel.: +58 (2) 606 7770
Fax: +58 (2) 605 3522
Year instruction started: **1883**
Language of instruction: **Spanish (knowledge of English required)**
Duration of basic medical degree course, including practical training: **6.5 years**
Entrance examination: **Yes**
Foreign students eligible: **Yes**

ESCUELA DE MEDICINA
UNIVERSIDAD DE ORIENTE
AVENIDA JOSE MENDEZ
APDO 94
CIUDAD BOLIVAR 8001-A
Year instruction started: **1962**

PROGRAMA DE MEDICINA DEL AREA CIENCIAS DE LA SALUD
UNIVERSIDAD NACIONAL EXPERIMENTAL FRANCISCO DE MIRANDA
EDIFICIO SANTA ANA, ENTRE CALLES FALCON Y ZAMORA
CORO 4101
Tel.: +58 (68) 514 882/519 443/517 581
Fax: +58 (68) 514 882
Year instruction started: **1979**
Language of instruction: **Spanish**
Duration of basic medical degree course, including practical training: **6.5 years**
Entrance examination: **Yes**

ESCUELA DE MEDICINA
UNIVERSIDAD DE ZULIA
AVENIDA 20
APDO 15165
MARACAIBO 4003-A
Tel.: +58 (61) 598 396
Fax: +58 (61) 598 361
Year instruction started: **1946**
Language of instruction: **Spanish**
Entrance examination: **Yes**
Foreign students eligible: **Yes**

ESCUELA DE MEDICINA
UNIVERSIDAD DE LOS ANDES
CALLE 35
EDIFICIO DECANATO DE LA FACULTAD DE MEDICINA
APDO 103
MERIDA 5101
Tel.: +58 (74) 403 041/403 042
Fax: +58 (74) 403 045
E-mail: vicunan@ing.ula.ve
Year instruction started: **1854**
Language of instruction: **Spanish**
Duration of basic medical degree course, including practical training: **6.5 years**
Entrance examination: **Yes**
Foreign students eligible: **Yes**

FACULTAD CIENCIAS DE LA SALUD
UNIVERSIDAD EXPERIMENTAL ROMULO GALLEGOS
SAN JUAN DE LOS MORROS

VIET NAM

Total population in 1995: **75 181 000**
Number of physicians per 100 000 population (1993): —
Number of medical schools: **9**
Duration of basic medical degree course, including practical training: **6 years**
Title of degree awarded: **Doctor of Medicine**
Medical registration/licence to practise: **Registration is obligatory with the health service of the province concerned, which grants the licence to practise medicine according to local needs.**
Work in government service after graduation: **Obligatory (5 years)**
Agreements with other countries: —

BAC THAI MEDICAL SCHOOL
BAC THAI
Year instruction started: **1968**

ECOLE DE MEDECINE
TAY NGUYEN UNIVERSITE
KM 4, DUONG 14
BUON ME THUOT
Tel.: +84 (150) 522 92/524 94/555 72

Year instruction started: **1977**
Language of instruction: **Russian, French, English**
Duration of basic medical degree course, including practical training: **6 years**
Entrance examination: **Yes**
Foreign students eligible: **Yes**

MEDICAL FACULTY
CAN THO UNIVERSITY
CAN THO
Year instruction started: **1979**

HAI PHONG MEDICAL SCHOOL
213 TRAN QUOC TOAN (LACH TRAY) STREET
HAI PHONG
Tel.: +84 (31) 847 907/852 225
Fax: +84 (31) 852 224
Year instruction started: **1979**
Language of instruction: **Vietnamese**
Duration of basic medical degree course, including practical training: **6 years**
Entrance examination: **Yes**
Foreign students eligible: **No**

HANOI MEDICAL SCHOOL
13 TON THAT TUNG STREET
DONG DA
HANOI 10000
Tel.: +84 (4) 852 3798
Fax: +84 (4) 852 5115
Year instruction started: **1902**
Language of instruction: **Vietnamese**
Duration of basic medical degree course, including practical training: **6 years**
Entrance examination: **Yes**
Foreign students eligible: **Yes**

CENTRE UNIVERSITAIRE DE FORMATION ET PERFECTIONNEMENT DES
    PROFESSIONELS DE SANTE DE HO CHI MINH VILLE
520 NGYUEN TRI PHUONG Q10
HO CHI MINH
Tel.: +84 (8) 865 0021
Fax: +84 (8) 865 0025

Year instruction started: **1989**
Language of instruction: **Vietnamese**
Duration of basic medical degree course, including practical training: **6 years**
Entrance examination: **Yes**
Foreign students eligible: **No**

FACULTE DE MEDECINE
UNIVERSITE DES SCIENCES MEDICALES DE HO CHI MIN VILLE
217 AN DUONG VUONG, QUN 5
HO CHI MINH 15000
Tel.: +84 (8) 558 411
Fax: +84 (8) 552 304
Year instruction started: **1975**
Language of instruction: **Vietnamese**
Duration of basic medical degree course, including practical training: **6 years**
Entrance examination: **Yes**
Foreign students eligible: **Yes**

HUE MEDICAL SCHOOL
1 NGOGUYEN STREET
HUE 43100
Year instruction started: **1975**

FACULTE DE MEDECINE DE THAI BINH
DUONG LY BON
THAI BINH 33000
Tel.: +84 (3) 683 1940
Fax: +84 (3) 633 290
Year instruction started: **1968**
Language of instruction: **Vietnamese, French, English**
Duration of basic medical degree course, including practical training: **6 years**
Entrance examination: **Yes**
Foreign students eligible: **Yes**

YEMEN

Total population in 1995: **15 678 000**
Number of physicians per 100 000 population (1993): **26**
Number of medical schools: **2**
Duration of basic medical degree course, including practical training: **6 or 6.5
    years**

Title of degree awarded: **Bachelor of Medicine and Surgery (MB, BS); Doctor of Medicine (MD)**
Medical registration/licence to practise: —
Work in government service after graduation: —
Agreements with other countries: —

FACULTY OF MEDICINE AND PHARMACY
UNIVERSITY OF ADEN
KHORMAKSAR
PO BOX 878
ADEN
Tel.: +967 (2) 231 751
Fax: +967 (2) 231 751
Year instruction started: **1975**
Language of instruction: **English**
Duration of basic medical degree course, including practical training: **6 years**
Entrance examination: **Yes**
Foreign students eligible: **Yes**

FACULTY OF MEDICINE AND HEALTH SCIENCES
UNIVERSITY OF SANA'A
WADI DHAHER ROAD
PO BOX 13078
SANA'A
Tel.: +967 (1) 234 440
Fax: +967 (1) 234 440
Year instruction started: **1982**
Language of instruction: **Arabic, English**
Duration of basic medical degree course, including practical training: **6.5 years**
Entrance examination: **Yes**
Foreign students eligible: **Yes**

YUGOSLAVIA[1]

Total population in 1995: —
Number of physicians per 100 000 population (1993): —
Number of medical schools: **4**
Duration of basic medical degree course, including practical training: —

---

[1] In the absence of official information since 1992, schools listed under "Yugoslavia" reflect information available as of the sixth edition of the *World directory of medical schools*. Seven schools previously listed under "Yugoslavia", which have been the object of communications from the governments of other Member States since the sixth edition of the *World directory*, appear in the entries related to those Member States.

Title of degree awarded: —
Medical registration/licence to practise: —
Work in government service after graduation: —
Agreements with other countries: —

MEDICINSKI FAKULTET
UNIVERZITETA U BEOGRADU
DR SUBOTICA 8
PO BOX 497
YU-11000 BEOGRAD
Tel.: +381 (11) 685 158
Fax: +381 (11) 684 053
Year instruction started: **1920**

MEDICINSKI FAKULTET
UNIVERZITETA U NISU
BRACE TASKOVICA 81
YU-18000 NIS
Tel.: +381 (18) 330 174
Fax: +381 (18) 338 770
Year instruction started: **1960**

MEDICINSKI FAKULTET
UNIVERZITETA U NOVOM SADU
HAJDUK VELJKOVA 3
YU-21000 NOVI SAD
Tel.: +381 (21) 624 145
Fax: +381 (21) 624 153
E-mail: mf-pejic@uns.ns.ac.yu
Year instruction started: **1960**

MEDICINSKI FAKULTET
UNIVERZITETA U PRISTINI
MARSALA TITA B.B.
YU-38000 PRISTINA
Year instruction started: **1969**

ZAMBIA

Total population in 1995: **8 275 000**
Number of physicians per 100 000 population (1993): —
Number of medical schools: **1**
Duration of basic medical degree course, including practical training: **7 years**

Title of degree awarded: **Bachelor of Medicine and Bachelor of Surgery (MB, ChB)**

Medical registration/licence to practise: **Registration is obligatory with the Medical Council of Zambia, Dental Training School Premises, PO Box 32554, Thornpark, 10101 Lusaka. A temporary licence to practise medicine is granted to graduates who have completed 1 year as an intern in a designated hospital. Graduates with foreign medical qualifications must have their degree validated.**

Work in government service after graduation: **Obligatory (1 year)**

Agreements with other countries: **Agreements exist with China, Cuba, the Netherlands and the United Kingdom.**

SCHOOL OF MEDICINE
UNIVERSITY OF ZAMBIA
PO BOX 50110
LUSAKA
Tel.: +260 (1) 252 641
Fax: +260 (1) 250 753
Telex: 44370 unza-lu za
Year instruction started: **1966**
Language of instruction: **English**
Duration of basic medical degree course, including practical training: **7 years**
Entrance examination: **Yes**
Foreign students eligible: **Yes**

ZIMBABWE

Total population in 1995: **11 439 000**
Number of physicians per 100 000 population (1993): **14**
Number of medical schools: **1**
Duration of basic medical degree course, including practical training: **5 years**
Title of degree awarded: **Bachelor of Medicine and Bachelor of Surgery (MB, ChB)**
Medical registration/licence to practise: **The licence to practise medicine is granted by the Health Professions Council, PO Box A 480, Avondale, Harare, to graduates of a recognized medical school who have completed 2 years as an intern.**
Work in government service after graduation: **Not obligatory**
Agreements with other countries: **None**

THE GODFREY HUGGINS SCHOOL OF MEDICINE
UNIVERSITY OF ZIMBABWE
AVONDALE
PO BOX A 178
AVONDALE
HARARE
Year instruction started: **1963**

Further reading

Defining and measuring the social accountability of medical schools. Geneva, World Health Organization, 1995 (unpublished document WHO/HRH/95.7; available on request from Department of Organization of Health Services Delivery, World Health Organization, 1211 Geneva 27, Switzerland).

Developing protocols for change in medical education. Report of an informal consultation, Seattle, Washington, USA, 11–14 August 1992. Geneva, World Health Organization, 1995 (unpublished document WHO/HRH/95.5; available on request from Department of Organization of Health Services Delivery, World Health Organization, 1211 Geneva 27, Switzerland).

Doctors for health. A WHO global strategy for changing medical education and medical practice for health for all. Geneva, World Health Organization, 1996 (unpublished document WHO/HRH/96.1; available on request from Department of Organization of Health Services Delivery, World Health Organization, 1211 Geneva 27, Switzerland).

Improving the social responsiveness of medical schools. Proceedings of the 1998 Educational Commission for Foreign Medical Graduates/World Health Organization Invitational Conference. *Academic Medicine*, 1999, 74 (8, Suppl.):Svii–Sviii, S1–S94.

Priorities at the interface of health care, medical practice and medical education: report of the Global Conference on International Collaboration on Medical Education and Practice, 12–15 June 1994, Rockford, Illinois, USA. Geneva, World Health Organization, 1995 (unpublished document WHO/HRH/95.2; available on request from Department of Organization of Health Services Delivery, World Health Organization, 1211 Geneva 27, Switzerland).

Towards a global consensus on quality medical education: serving the needs of populations and individuals. Proceedings of the 1994 World Health Organization/Educational Commission for Foreign Medical Graduates Invitational Consultation, Geneva, 3–6 October 1994. *Academic Medicine*, 1995, 70 (7, Suppl.): S1–S90.

Towards the assessment of quality in medical education. Geneva, World Health Organization, 1992 (unpublished document WHO/HRH/92.7; available on request from Department of Organization of Health Services Delivery, World Health Organization, 1211 Geneva 27, Switzerland).

Tuberculosis control and medical schools: report of a WHO workshop, Rome, Italy, 29–31 October 1997. Geneva, World Health Organization, 1998 (unpublished document WHO/TB/98.236; available on request from Stop TB Initiative, World Health Organization, 1211 Geneva 27, Switzerland).

World Health Organization/International Association of Francophone Medical Colleges (CIDMEF). *La faculté de médecine et le médecin praticien du XXIᵉ siècle. Journées d'études internationales, Bruxelles, 9–12 avril 1996 (Faculties of medicine and practising physicians in the twenty-first century. International study days, Brussels, 9–12 April 1996.)* Brussels, Fondation pour l'Etude et la Prévention des Maladies de Civilisation, 1998.

World Health Organization/World Organization of Family Doctors (WONCA). *Making medical practice and medical education more relevant to people's needs: the contribution of the family doctor. Working paper from the Joint WHO/WONCA Conference in Ontario, Canada, 6–8 November 1994.* Geneva, World Health Organization, 1995 (unpublished document; available on request from Department of Organization of Health Services Delivery, World Health Organization, 1211 Geneva 27, Switzerland).